AI-Enabled Multiple-Criteria Decision-Making Approaches for Healthcare Management

Sandeep Kautish
Lord Buddha Education Foundation, Nepal

Gaurav Dhiman
Government Bikram College of Commerce, India & Lebanese American University, Lebanon

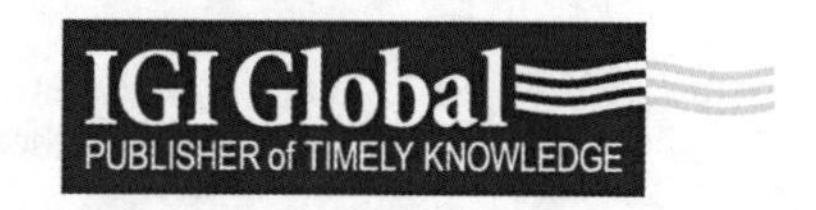

A volume in the Advances in Medical Technologies and Clinical Practice (AMTCP) Book Series

Published in the United States of America by
IGI Global
Medical Information Science Reference (an imprint of IGI Global)
701 E. Chocolate Avenue
Hershey PA, USA 17033
Tel: 717-533-8845
Fax: 717-533-8661
E-mail: cust@igi-global.com
Web site: http://www.igi-global.com

Library of Congress Cataloging-in-Publication Data

Names: Kautish, Sandeep, 1981- editor. | Dhiman, Gaurav, 1993- editor.
Title: AI-enabled multiple criteria decision-making approaches for healthcare management / Sandeep Kautish, and Gaurav Dhiman, editors.
Description: Hershey PA : Engineering Science Reference, [2023] | Includes bibliographical references and index. | Summary: "The success of healthcare decision-making lies in whether healthcare staff, patients, and healthcare organization managers can comprehensively understand the choices and consider future implications to make the best decision possible, so this book investigates practical multiple criteria decision analysis applications and cases for healthcare management"-- Provided by publisher.
Identifiers: LCCN 2022027483 (print) | LCCN 2022027484 (ebook) | ISBN 9781668444054 (hardcover) | ISBN 9781668444061 (paperback) | ISBN 9781668444078 (ebook)
Subjects: LCSH: Medical care--Decision making--Data processing. | Medical informatics. | Multiple criteria decision making. | Artificial intelligence--Medical applications.
Classification: LCC R859.7.D42 A44 2023 (print) | LCC R859.7.D42 (ebook) | DDC 610.285--dc23/eng/20220802
LC record available at https://lccn.loc.gov/2022027483
LC ebook record available at https://lccn.loc.gov/2022027484

This book is published in the IGI Global book series Advances in Medical Technologies and Clinical Practice (AMTCP) (ISSN: 2327-9354; eISSN: 2327-9370)

British Cataloguing in Publication Data
A Cataloguing in Publication record for this book is available from the British Library.

All work contributed to this book is new, previously-unpublished material.
The views expressed in this book are those of the authors, but not necessarily of the publisher.

For electronic access to this publication, please contact: eresources@igi-global.com.

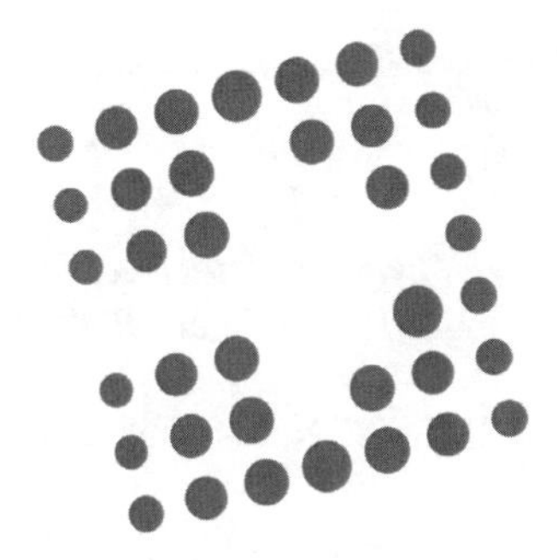

Advances in Medical Technologies and Clinical Practice (AMTCP) Book Series

ISSN:2327-9354
EISSN:2327-9370

MISSION

Medical technological innovation continues to provide avenues of research for faster and safer diagnosis and treatments for patients. Practitioners must stay up to date with these latest advancements to provide the best care for nursing and clinical practices.

The **Advances in Medical Technologies and Clinical Practice (AMTCP) Book Series** brings together the most recent research on the latest technology used in areas of nursing informatics, clinical technology, biomedicine, diagnostic technologies, and more. Researchers, students, and practitioners in this field will benefit from this fundamental coverage on the use of technology in clinical practices.

COVERAGE

- Patient-Centered Care
- Clinical High-Performance Computing
- Diagnostic Technologies
- Medical Imaging
- Nursing Informatics
- Medical Informatics
- Clinical Data Mining
- Nutrition
- Clinical Studies
- Clinical Nutrition

IGI Global is currently accepting manuscripts for publication within this series. To submit a proposal for a volume in this series, please contact our Acquisition Editors at Acquisitions@igi-global.com or visit: http://www.igi-global.com/publish/.

The Advances in Medical Technologies and Clinical Practice (AMTCP) Book Series (ISSN 2327-9354) is published by IGI Global, 701 E. Chocolate Avenue, Hershey, PA 17033-1240, USA, www.igi-global.com. This series is composed of titles available for purchase individually; each title is edited to be contextually exclusive from any other title within the series. For pricing and ordering information please visit http://www.igi-global.com/book-series/advances-medical-technologies-clinical-practice/73682. Postmaster: Send all address changes to above address.

Titles in this Series

For a list of additional titles in this series, please visit:
www.igi-global.com/book-series/advances-medical-technologies-clinical-practice/73682

Exploring the Convergence of Computer and Medical Science Through Cloud Healthcare
Ricardo Queirós (ESMAD, Polytechnic Institute of Porto, Portugal) Bruno Cunha (PORTIC, Portugal) and Xavier Fonseca (PORTIC, Portugal)
Medical Information Science Reference • © 2023 • 300pp • H/C (ISBN: 9781668452608) • US $435.00

The Internet of Medical Things (IoMT) and Telemedicine Frameworks and Applications
Rajiv Pandey (Amity University, India) Amrit Gupta (MRH, SGPGI, Lucknow, India) and Agnivesh Pandey (C.S.J.M. University, India)
Medical Information Science Reference • © 2022 • 325pp • H/C (ISBN: 9781668435335) • US $380.00

Leveraging AI Technologies for Preventing and Detecting Sudden Cardiac Arrest and Death
Pradeep Nijalingappa (Bapuji Institute of Engineering and Technology, Davangere, India) Sandeep Kautish (Lord Buddha Education Foundation, Nepal) Mangesh M. Ghonge (Sandip Institute of Technology and Research Centre, India) and Renjith V. Ravi (MEA Engineering College, India)
Medical Information Science Reference • © 2022 • 263pp • H/C (ISBN: 9781799884439) • US $435.00

Smart Healthcare for Sustainable Urban Development
Rosy Madaan (Manav Rachna International Institute of Research and Studies, India) Komal Kumar Bhatia (J.C. Bose University of Science and Technology, YMCA, India) Supriya P. Panda (Manav Rachna International Institute of Research and Studies, Faridabad, India) Vishal Jain (Sharda University, India) and Payal Gulati (J.C. Bose University of Science and Technology, YMCA, India)
Medical Information Science Reference • © 2022 • 269pp • H/C (ISBN: 9781668425084) • US $325.00

For an entire list of titles in this series, please visit:
www.igi-global.com/book-series/advances-medical-technologies-clinical-practice/73682

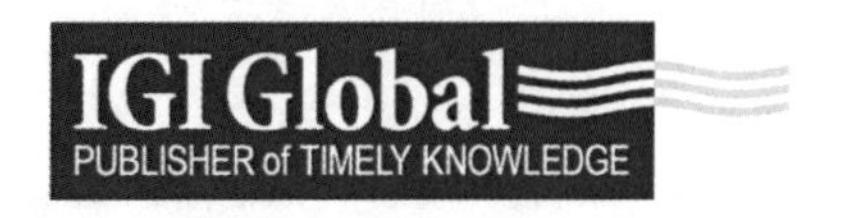

701 East Chocolate Avenue, Hershey, PA 17033, USA
Tel: 717-533-8845 x100 • Fax: 717-533-8661
E-Mail: cust@igi-global.com • www.igi-global.com

Table of Contents

Detailed Table of Contents

Due to the complexity of histopathology tissues, an accurate classification and segmentation of cancer diagnosis is a challenging task in computer vision. The nuclei segmentation of microscopic images is a key prerequisite for cancerous pathological image analysis. However, an accurate nuclei segmentation is a long running major challenge due to the enormous color variability of staining, nuclei shapes, sizes, and clustering of overlapping cells. To address these challenges and early diagnosis as well as reduce the bias decisions of expert lab technician of cancer in clinical practice, the authors study the classification of computer-aided frameworks and automatic nuclei segmentation frameworks based on histopathology images by convolutional deep learning. The authors have used a publicly available PatchCamelyon and 2018 Data Science Bowl histology image dataset for this study. The results are compared and expected to be useful clinically for technician experts in the analysis of cancer diagnosis and the survival chances of patients.

In fields like healthcare, where human intelligence is critical, the introduction of new AI-powered applications is becoming increasingly popular. Technologies have reduced expenses, accelerated drug research, and improved wellness outcomes. AI has become increasingly cognizant of its potential to disrupt the business, as seen by growing funding for the sector in recent years from important stakeholders in both healthcare and risk capital. Traditional approaches include human participation and direct interaction with patients, which are now obsolete due to the advancement of technologies such as messaging bots and intelligent virtual assistants. On the other hand, the internet of things (IoT) is making significant contributions to healthcare, and its gadgets may collect complete health data. Machine intelligence collects and analyses data in established protocols in search of possible health-related predictions. The chapter delves into the aspects of combining AI and IoT to improve efficiency in healthcare systems.

A new paradigm for the solution of problems involving single- and multi-objective fuzzy linear programming is presented in this chapter. As opposed to complex arithmetic and logic for intervals, the method offered uses basic fuzzy mathematical operations for fuzzy integers instead. Using fuzzy numbers to express variables and parameters in a fuzzy linear programming issue (FLPP) is common. However, the authors only talked about FLPP with fuzzy parameters here. Triangular fuzzy numbers are used as fuzzy parameters. Ranking functions are used to convert fuzzy problems into clear ones. Crisp optimization techniques have been used. The proposed solution is tested on a variety of real-world examples that address both of these concerns.

Since 2019, the world has been dealing with an outbreak of the COVID-19 virus. A highly transmissible new coronavirus causes a severe acute respiratory illness. Every country, including India, took steps to battle the virus, such as announcing a phased lockdown. The COVID-19 pandemic has wreaked havoc on India. In reality, the third COVID-19 wave has already begun. The development of COVID-19 vaccinations aided in the healing of the planet. Multiple nations are conducting clinical tests on potential COVID-19 vaccines. India initiated the world's largest vaccination campaign on January 16, 2021. The Indian government has made significant progress in both vaccinating everyone and developing the COVID-19 vaccine. The use of Covaxin and Covishield dosages in different Indian states is investigated in this chapter.

Digital image processing is becoming another ever-growing yet popular field of demands for daily life, ranging from medicine, room evaluation, security, support, and security of the automotive community, among many others. The proposed framework focuses mostly on fuzzy logic structures somewhere in optical image processing. The main goal of most of this work is to demonstrate how fuzzy logic is implemented in image processing with little more than a quick introduction of fuzzy logic and optical image processing. Fuzzy logic, one of those artificial intelligence decision-making approaches, provides even greater room for use. When everything that would also have been allowed access to declarations at all since birth, particularly concerning in popularity in recent years, fuzzy logic as a whole has been proven to be true in virtually all systemic fields. Furthermore, the implications continue to suggest that the previously presented technique is worthy of attention in image processing software systems with the appropriate expansion.

Artificial intelligence (AI)-based image segmentation plays an important role in image processing and computer vision. AI can be used in the medical field (e.g., ophthalmology, disease prediction which involves direct visualization and imaging) as a frequent method for diagnosis. Deep learning comes under machine learning and as a part of AI. Deep learning algorithms have yielded considerable results in the medical field. Diabetic retinopathy is one of the most common causes of blindness, which is diagnosed by examining the appearance of the retina. The diabetic retinopathy stages are determined based on the changes seen in retina or retinal image. This chapter gives a detailed survey on different algorithms used for diagnosing diabetic retinopathy and different deep learning techniques used for medical image segmentation.

Machine learning models are taught how to make a series of decisions depending on a set of inputs in reinforcement learning. The agent learns how to accomplish a goal in an unexpected, maybe complex environment. Reinforcement learning places artificial intelligence in a game-like environment. It solves the problem by trial and error. Artificial intelligence is rewarded or punished based on its actions. Its purpose is to maximize the amount of money paid out in total. In addition to providing the game's rules, the designer does not give any feedback or recommendations on how to win the model. To maximize reward, the model must determine the optimum way to do a job, beginning with purely random trials and progressing to complex techniques and superhuman abilities. Reinforcement learning, with its power of search and diversity of trials, is likely the most effective strategy for hinting at a system's originality. Unlike humans, AI can learn from thousands of concurrent gameplays if a reinforcement learning algorithm is run on sufficiently efficient computer infrastructure.

Internet of nano things (IoNT) is growing at an exponential rate due to a growing population, more communication between devices in networks, sensors, actuators, and so on. This rise shows up in many ways, such as volume, speed, diversity, honesty, and value. Getting important information and insights is hard work and a very important issue. One of the most important ways to solve a problem is to come to a conclusion based on a number of different criteria. This can help you choose the best solution from a number of options. AI-enabled algorithms and decision making that takes into account multiple factors can be useful in big data sets. During the deduction process, AI-enabled algorithms and evaluations based on multiple criteria are used. Because it works well and has a lot of potential, it is used in many different areas, such as computer science and information technology, agriculture, and business.

Preface

Multiple-criteria decision making, including multiple rule-based decision making, multiple-objective decision making, and multiple-attribute decision making, is used by clinical decision makers to analyze healthcare issues from various perspectives. In practical healthcare cases, semi-structured and unstructured decision-making issues involve multiple criteria that may conflict with each other. Thus, the use of multiple-criteria decision making is a promising source of practical solutions for such problems.

AI-Enabled Multiple-Criteria Decision-Making Approaches for Healthcare Management investigates the contributions of practical multiple-criteria decision analysis applications and cases for healthcare management. It also considers the best practices and tactics for utilizing multiple-criteria decision making to ensure the technology is utilized appropriately. Covering key topics such as fuzzy data, augmented reality, blockchain, and data transmission, this reference work is ideal for computer scientists, healthcare professionals, nurses, policymakers, researchers, scholars, academicians, practitioners, educators, and students.

Chapter 1 discusses a very important healthcare topic based on cardiac. It is found that cardiovascular disease is the main cause of mortality globally, killing an estimated 27.9 million people each year and accounting for 31% of all fatalities. Cardiovascular issues are typically the cause of heart failure. It is distinguished by the heart failure to provide adequate blood to the body. When there is insufficient blood flow, all of the body core processes suffer. Heart failure is a disorder or collection of symptoms that cause the heart to weaken. This book chapter will be very beneficial for the researchers doing research in the same field.

Chapter 2 presents the investigation of deep learning architectures for the analysis of cancer diseases using deep neural nets. The investigations are organized into introduction, this section presents the overview of imaging techniques for cancer diagnosis using histopathology images. The next section presents the related works in medical imaging techniques and analysis using deep learning architectures. The architecture of each deep learners are discussed elaborately. Further, the chapter presents the experimental analysis and discussed the outcome of (i) Classification

Performance on PCam Histopathology Patch Dataset, and (ii) Nucleus Segmentation Performance on Data Science Bowl Dataset. The work flows are divided into phases data preparation, training, testing, data augmentation, and evaluation metrics. Finally, the chapter is concluded with a summary on finding and future research.

Chapter 3 discusses industries like healthcare, which have essential human intelligence and the introduction of revolutionary AI powered applications, increasingly in high demand. Technologies have lowered costs, accelerated drug development and increased outcomes for wellness. AI has become increasingly aware of AI potential to revolutionize the industry, with increased funding for the sector in recent years, by key players in both healthcare & risk capital. On the other hand the Internet of Things (IoT) is contributing a lot in healthcare and its devices can collect comprehensive health information. Data collected and analyzed by machine intelligence in standard protocols looking for possible health-related predictions. The proposed chapter gives an insights into the aspects of using AI with IoT with their significance, techniques and applications that could be used in healthcare systems.

Chapter 4 is about wireless body area networks which are a next-generation application that has potential in today's Information Technology and Communication (ITC) system. Doctors may remotely monitor patients using the WBAN programme. WBAN captures medical data and sends it over the internet for processing. There is a requirement to secure the security of such highly sensitive data via the network during remote data access. This has purposefully piqued the academics' attention in providing WBAN security by incorporating blockchain. This chapter explores Internet of Things (IoT) architecture and proposes a lightweight secure access control utilizing blockchain to improve performance. WBAN have reached the revolting future research scope in the health industry.

In Chapter 5, the authors have created a rudimentary AR mobile application that allows you to set 3D virtual items on a tabletop. To create the application, we utilized Android Studio, Java, and Arcore. We also utilized scene form to render the 3D models on an Android mobile device. We also spoke about the principles underlying augmented reality and the applications for which it may be employed. We also highlighted the limitations and challenges that require more study and development in the realm of AR. The placement of 3D animations in the actual environment reflects the unpopular reality of taxpayers. Individual and numerous users can observe and communicate with the things used.

Chapter 6 is a comparative study with linear regression and linear regression with fuzzy data for the same data set. The chapter gave a comparison of LR models and LR models with fuzzy data and actual experimental data using linear regression and linear regression with fuzzy data for the same data set. The introduction portion of the research study on regression analysis provides a general summary of the technique. The approach is represented in the next section. (i) Analysis of linear regression (ii) Fuzzy regression analysis (iii) LR with Fuzzy Data (iv) and an example in terms of numbers from a comparison study utilising experimental data. The computational results that show the best linear models for the data set serve as the chapter's conclusion.

Chapter 7 proposes a new paradigm for the solution of problems involving single- and multi-objective fuzzy linear programming is presented in this paper. As opposed to complex arithmetic and logic for intervals, the method offered uses basic fuzzy mathematical operations for fuzzy integers instead. Using fuzzy numbers to express variables and parameters in a fuzzy linear programming issue (FLPP) is common. However, we have just talked about FLPP with fuzzy parameters here. Triangular fuzzy numbers are used as fuzzy parameters. Ranking functions are used to convert fuzzy problems into clear ones. Crisp optimization techniques have been used to it. The proposed solution is tested on a variety of real-world examples that address both of these concerns.

Chapter 8 discussed the world which has been dealing with an outbreak of the COVID-19 virus. A highly transmissible new coronavirus causes a severe acute respiratory illness. Every country, including India, took steps to battle the virus, such as announcing a phased lockdown. The COVID pandemic has wreaked havoc on India. In reality, the third COVID wave has already begun. The development of COVID vaccinations aided in the healing of the planet. Multiple nations are conducting clinical tests on potential COVID vaccines. India initiated the world's largest vaccination campaign on January 16, 2021. The Indian government has made significant progress in both vaccinating everyone and developing the COVID vaccine. The use of Covaxin and Covishield dosages in different Indian states is investigated in this paper.

Chapter 9 discusses that as of the year 2022, Professor Lotfi Zade's original fuzzy sets have been in existence for over 55 years. Fuzzy sets and their various algorithms have been utilized in a variety of contexts, but their employment in image processing systems has best illustrated their significance as a potent design technique. In this chapter, we have offered a detailed overview of conventional approaches for fuzzy image optimization, including different ways for comparing, contrast adaptation, and occasionally filtering. The majority of this work is devoted to demonstrating how fuzzy logic is applied in image processing, with only a brief introduction to fuzzy logic and optical image processing.

Chapter 10 is about Deep Learning which is a recent fast-growing field in Machine Learning. It leads an important role in many fields, particularly the medical field. One of the important applications of deep learning in the medical field is automated image processing and diagnosing diseases based on the image. There are many automated applications developed using Artificial Intelligence. In the medical field of ophthalmology in which various diagnoses are based on structural changes. Hence in this chapter, the basic features and signs of diabetic retinopathy and the various types of algorithms for image processing in diagnosing and grading diabetic retinopathy are discussed in detail.

Chapter 11 discusses a very important healthcare topic based automatic diseases diagnosing. With its search power and diversity of trials, reinforcement learning is likely the most effective strategy for hinting at a systems originality. If a reinforcement learning algorithm is run on sufficiently efficient computer infrastructure, artificial intelligence, unlike humans, can learn from thousands of concurrent gameplays. This book will go into great detail about reinforcement learning for automated medical diagnosis. This book chapter will be very beneficial for the researchers doing research in the same field.

Chapter 12 discusses an increasing population, more network connections between devices, the Internet of Things, the Internet of Nano Things, sensors, actuators, and other factors all contribute to the exponential growth of the Internet of Nano Things. This might assist you in selecting the best alternative out of several available ones. Big data sets can benefit from AI-enabled algorithms and decision-making that consider a variety of criteria. There is no way around the need to develop more intelligent environments that allow people and robots to work together more successfully and safely. This will be done using a range of artificial intelligence systems and better prediction algorithms.

Sandeep Kautish
Lord Buddha Education Foundation, Nepal

Gaurav Dhiman
Government Bikram College of Commerce, India

Acknowledgment

I am delighted to welcome the readers of my new book, *AI-Enabled Multiple-Criteria Decision-Making Approaches for Healthcare Management*. I congratulate all chapter authors for their valuable submissions and keeping patience during critical review process. I wish to thank all reviewers as well who spared their precious time for the review process.

I am thankful to my wife Yogita and son Devansh and my parents for giving me eternal happiness and support during the entire process.

Last but not the least, I am thankful to almighty god for blessing me with wonderful life and showing me right paths in my all ups and downs during the so far journey of life.

To my loving parents and friends for their divine blessings. ~Gaurav Dhiman

Chapter 1
Real-Time Detection of Cardiac Arrest Using Deep Learning

Pawan Whig
Vivekananda Institute of Professional Studies, India

Ketan Gupta
https://orcid.org/0000-0002-2953-0385
University of the Cumberlands, USA

Nasmin Jiwani
https://orcid.org/0000-0002-7360-0264
University of the Cumberlands, USA

ABSTRACT

The leading cause of death worldwide is cardiac disease, which kills an estimated 27.9 million people each year and is responsible for 31% of all fatalities. Heart failure is frequently brought on by cardiovascular problems. It can be identified by the heart's inability to deliver enough blood to the body. All of the body's fundamental functions are affected when there is insufficient blood flow. Heart failure is a condition or set of symptoms that weakens the heart. Three important aspects form the foundation of the research study's main results. Given that it essentially measures the efficiency of the heart, this is to be expected. The patient's age is the last factor that is most closely associated. The heart's performance progressively deteriorates with age. The data was modeled using machine learning and ANN with an accuracy of about 80%, showing how effective the framework is at detecting cardiac arrest. Deep learning models' accuracy might rise to 90–95%.

DOI: 10.4018/978-1-6684-4405-4.ch001

INTRODUCTION

Every year, about 500,000 Americans die as a result of cardiac arrest, which occurs when the heart abruptly stops beating. People with cardiac arrest become unresponsive and either choke to death or struggle to breathe, a sign known as arrhythmic respiration (Whig et al., 2022). Early CPR can increase a person's chances of life by doubling or tripling them, but it depends on the presence of a volunteer (Anand et al., 2022).

Medical emergencies happen all the time even outside the hospitals, in the privacy of one's home (Alkali et al., 2022; Jiwani et al., 2021). According to new findings, amongst the most common locations for cardiogenic shock is in a people's home, when nobody is expected to be present to react and provide assistance (George et al., 2021).

Research from the University of Iowa has developed a novel tool that may detect heart attack or stroke in patients when they are asleep without wanting to connect with anyone (Parihar & Yadav, n.d.; Sinha & Ranjan, 2015). This new update for a voice assistant, such as Google or Amazon's Alexa, or smartphones recognizes the gasping sound of agonizing respiration and automatically seeks help (Whig & Ahmad, 2019).

The different causes of death are shown in Figure1. The data shows that Sudden Cardiac Arrest is the highest among all other factors, hence it is a very important concern to the discussion in this chapter.

The solid evidence method, which was developed using genuine agonal respiratory instances obtained from Emergency calls, correctly identified arrhythmic respiratory instances 96% at a distance of up to 20 feet (or 6 meters). In July 2019, the results were reported in the journal npj Electronic Health(Rupani & Sujediya, 2016).

"A lot of people have smart speakers in their homes, and these devices have great capabilities that we can make use of," "We imagine a contactless device that monitors the bedroom continually and passively for an agonizing breathing incident and informs anybody nearby to come to perform CPR." If there is no answer, the gadget will immediately dial 911(Channumsin et al., 2015)."

According to 911 call statistics, around 50% of persons who undergo cardiac arrests have agonal breathing, and affected roles who take agonal snorts frequently consume a greater coincidental of survival(Ruchin & Whig, 2015; Shrivastav et al., n.d.). "This type of breathing occurs when a patient has extremely low oxygen levels," explained the University of Washington. "It's a guttural gasping sound, and its peculiarity makes it a useful auditory biomarker to use to determine if someone is having a cardiac arrest(Asopa et al., 2021)."

Figure 1. Data Shows different causes of deaths

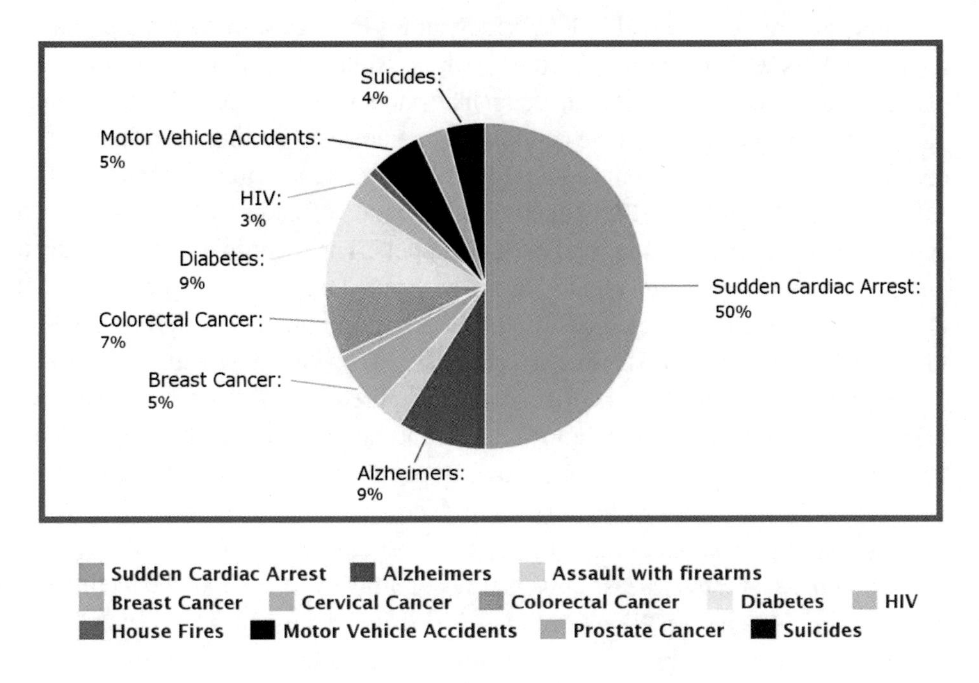

Figure 2. Annual Lives saved after sudden cardiac arrest

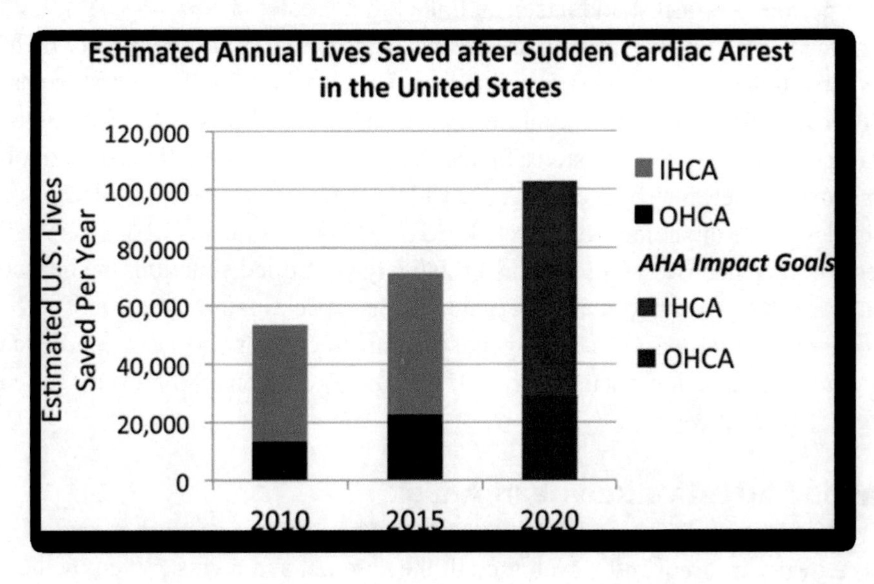

The Estimated Annual Lives saved after sudden cardiac arrest in the United States are shown in Figure 2. Actual 911 calls to Seattle's Emergency Personnel provided the researchers with agonizing breathing noises. Although cardiopulmonary arrest patients are often asleep, by placing their smartphones close to the participant's lips, passersby were able to record the painful gasping noises, enabling the dispatcher to determine whether the patient required rapid CPR. The researchers collected 162 calls between 2009 and 2017, extracting 2.5 seconds of audio at the start of each agonizing breath to compile a total of 236 snippets. The recordings were produced using a variety of connected phones, along with an Alexa Voice, an apple 5s, and a Galaxy Note S3, and the scientists used a variety of ml algorithms to bring a total lot of positive videos to 7,315(Purva Agarwal1, 2016; Rupani & Kumar, 2020).

The scientists used 83 hours of audio data acquired during sleep experiments to create the negative dataset, obtaining 7,305 sound samples(Nadikattu et al., 2020a). These films included common sounds made by people while sleeping. The procedure was then evaluated to ensure that do not mistakenly label another form of breathing, such as snoring, as agonal breathing. Out-of-hospital cardiac arrest (OHCA) is a prominent reason for the disease universal, accounting for about 300,000 fatalities in North America each year(Whig & Ahmad, 2017b). The presence of a certain sort of disorganized breathing, known as agonal breathing, is a relatively underappreciated diagnostic feature of cardiac arrest Agonal breathing is a brainstem reaction that occurs in the presence of acute hypoxia. Agonal breathing implies a relatively short period after arrest and has been linked to a greater chance of survival(Whig & Ahmad, 2017a). The growing use of smartphones and smart speakers (which are predicted to be in 72 percentage points from Us homes by 2020) provides a chance to uncover this audio marker and link cardiac arrest sufferers to EMS or anybody who can offer chest compressions. In this study, we hypothesized that commonplace consumer gadgets may be used to properly identify OHCA-related agonal respiration episodes inside the home (Rupani et al., 2018; Whig & Ahmad, 2016a). As the first piece of evidence, we will focus on a relatively controlled situation: the bedroom, which is where the bulk of OHCA incidents in a special family happen.

Accessing real-world data on agonal breathing occurrences is a major difficulty for algorithm creation for this purpose; because agonal breathing events are very rare, data are scarce.

Cardiac Arrest versus Heart Attack

Those terms are frequently, even though they are not synonyms. When the heart's blood supply is impeded, a heart attack ensues, whereas the heart happens whenever the heart defects and stops beating. The difference between a heart attack and sudden cardiac arrest is that a heart attack is a "circulation" problem, but the heart is an "electrical" problem (Bhatia & Whig, 2013a).

Whenever an artery gets blocked, O_2 blood cannot reach a section of the cardiac, and a stroke occurs. The region of the heart that is normally fed by that artery begins to die if the blocked artery is not quickly reopened. The longer someone goes without treatment, the worse the repercussions grow (Sharma et al., n.d.).

The heart condition can manifest itself in a variety of ways. However, before a heart attack, symptoms usually come gradually and continue for hours, days, or weeks. Its heart generally keeps beating during a heart attack, except in situations of sudden cardiac arrest. The features of this condition in women may vary from those in males(Shridhar & Whig, 2014; Whig & Ahmad, 2014a, 2014b). Heart attack due to blood clots and cholesterol deposition in the artery is shown in Figure 3.

Figure 3. Heart attack due to blood clot and cholesterol deposition

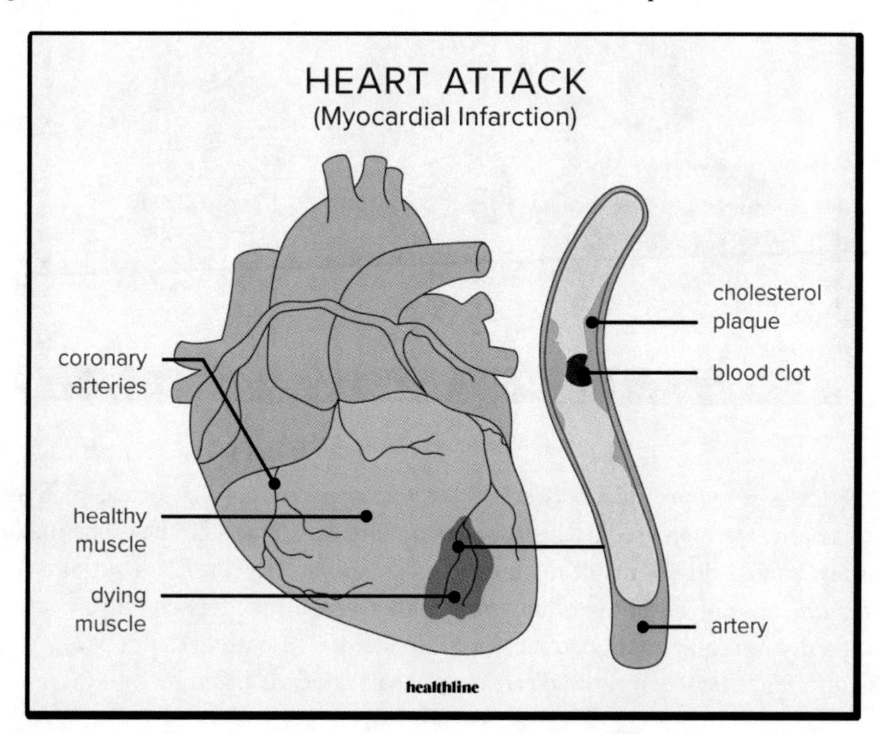

Unexpected cardiac capture happens unexpectedly and without caution. It is caused by an electric fault in the sentiment, which results in an asymmetrical pulse. The sentiment cannot be heart plasma to the intellect, or lungs if its pumping activity is disturbed (Whig & Ahmad, 2011). A person loses consciousness and has no pulse seconds later. If the sufferer does not get care, death happens within minutes(Bhatia & Whig, 2014; Whig & Ahmad, 2014d). The difference between heart attack and Cardiac Arrest is shown in Figure 4.

Figure 4. Difference in heart attack and Cardiac Arrest

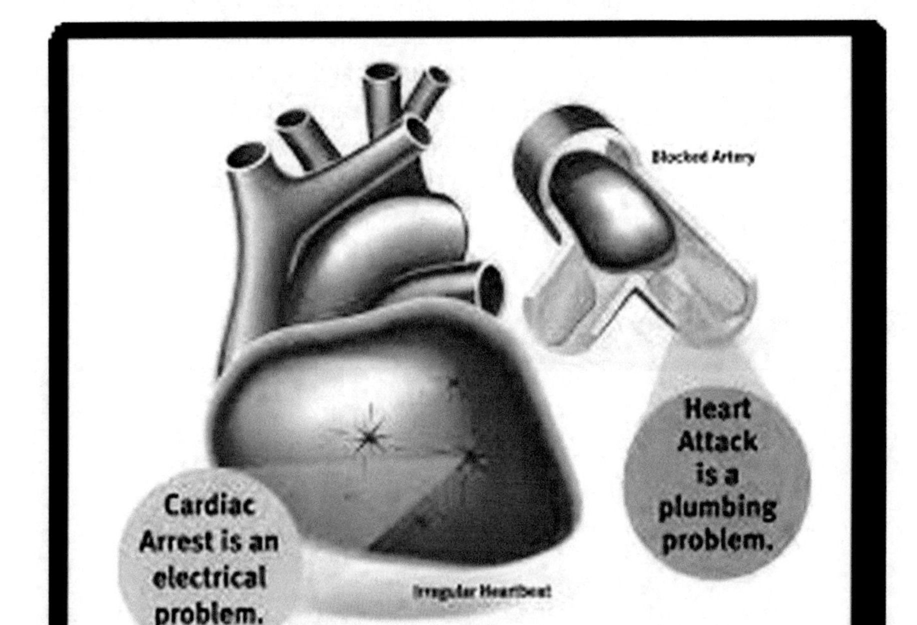

There is a relationship between these two separate cardiac diseases. Sudden cardiac arrest is increased by heart attacks(Whig & Ahmad, 2013b). The majority of heart attacks do not result in abrupt cardiac arrest. However, a heart attack is a common cause of abrupt cardiac arrest. Other heart disorders can also cause the heart's rhythm to be disrupted and result in sudden detention(Khera et al., 2021). The difference between cardiac arrest and heart attack is listed in Table 1.

Table 1. Heart attack vs Cardiac arrest

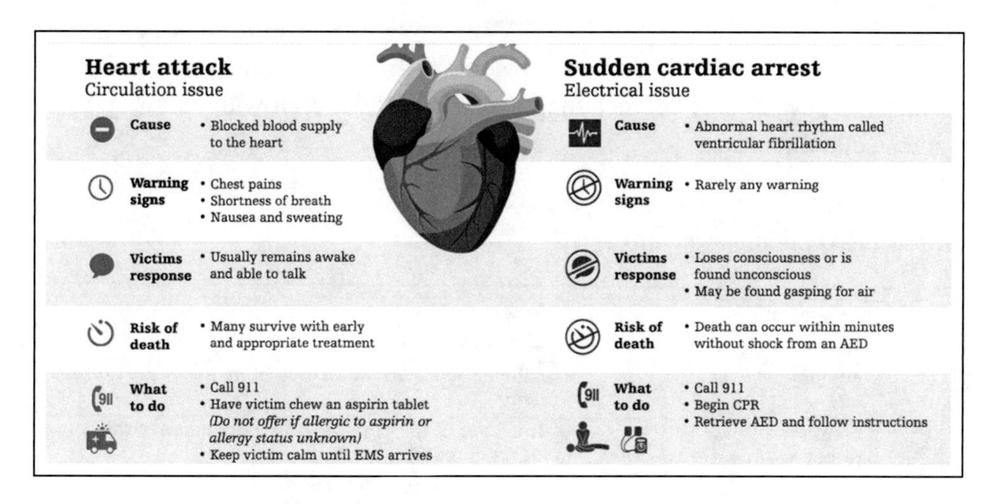

	Heart attack Circulation issue	Sudden cardiac arrest Electrical issue
Cause	• Blocked blood supply to the heart	• Abnormal heart rhythm called ventricular fibrillation
Warning signs	• Chest pains • Shortness of breath • Nausea and sweating	• Rarely any warning
Victims response	• Usually remains awake and able to talk	• Loses consciousness or is found unconscious • May be found gasping for air
Risk of death	• Many survive with early and appropriate treatment	• Death can occur within minutes without shock from an AED
What to do	• Call 911 • Have victim chew an aspirin tablet *(Do not offer if allergic to aspirin or allergy status unknown)* • Keep victim calm until EMS arrives	• Call 911 • Begin CPR • Retrieve AED and follow instructions

MACHINE LEARNING

Machine learning, a type of artificial intelligence, can predict the probability of that heart failure using a combination of temporal and weather information (Khera et al., 2021).

Automation is the research of computational models that are premised on the notion that machines can learn through data and find patterns to guide decisions with minimal intervention. As per the research, the danger of cardiac arrest was greatest on Sunday, Monday, and public holidays, as well as when temperatures dropped substantially within or between days. Such data, per the scientists, might be used as an early warning system for residents, decreasing their danger and enhancing their survival chances, as well as increasing emergency medical care readiness (Nadikattu, 2014).

Cardiac arrest is prevalent throughout the creation; however, it is often linked to dismal survival rates. The risk is influenced by the current meteorological conditions (Bhatia & Whig, 2013b; Nadikattu et al., 2020b).

However, atmospheric information is large and complicated, and ML can identify relationships that standard one-dimensional statistical techniques do not, according to Japanese researchers.

To investigate further, they used everyday climate time data to forecast daily out-of-hospital cardiac arrests. Machine learning was applied to 525,374 of the 1,299,784 incidents that occurred between 2005 and 2013 (Whig & Ahmad, 2013c, 2015).

The findings were then compared against 135,000 instances that occurred in 2015–16 to assess the model's correctness in forecasting the number of daily cases.

Approach Used

The table below displays the data set that was utilized for the analysis and forecast. It includes several criteria, including age and anemia, each with a description as indicated in Table 2.

Table 2. Explanation of Dataset

Parameter	Description
age	Age of the patient
anemia	If the patient had the hemoglobin below the normal range
creatinine phosphokinase	The level of the creatine phosphokinase in the blood in mcg/L
diabetes	If the patient was diabetic
ejection fraction	Ejection fraction is a measurement of how much blood the left ventricle pumps out with each contraction
high_blood_pressure	If the patient had hypertension
platelets	Platelet count of blood in kilo platelets/mL
serum_creatinine	The level of serum creatinine in the blood in mg/dL
serum_sodium	The level of serum sodium in the blood in mEq/L
sex	The Sex of Patient
smoking	If the patient smokes actively or ever did in past
time	It is the time of the patient's follow-up visit for the disease in months
Death_Event	If the patient deceased during the follow-up period

Data Planning and Scrutiny

There are no null values in the dataset. However, numerous outliers must be handled correctly, since the dataset is not adequately distributed. There were two techniques utilized. One without outliers and a feature selection procedure, as well as immediately applying the data to machine learning algorithms, had unimpressive results (Sinha et al., 2015; Whig & Ahmad, 2016b). However, after utilizing the normal distribution of the dataset to overcome the overfitting problem and then employing Isolation Forest to find outliers, the results obtained are extremely encouraging. Various charting approaches were employed to assess the skewness of the data, locate outliers, and examine the data distribution. (Kautish et al. 2022)

Various ML Packages

Machine learning is a field of computer science that deals with how computers can learn from various forms of data. According to Arthur Samuel, the branch of study known as "machine learning" gives computers the capacity to learn without being explicitly instructed(*On the Performance of ISFET-Based Device for Water Quality Monitoring*, n.d.; Whig & Ahmad, 2013a, 2014c). They are frequently used to address a variety of problems in one's life.

In the past, all of the algorithms, mathematical formulae, and statistical calculations were manually coded by individuals doing machine learning tasks (Moorthy et al. 2022). It was a laborious process that took a long time. The various machine learning tools employed in this study are listed in Figure 5 below.

Figure 5. Various Libraries used

```
import NumPy as np
import pandas as pd
import matplotlib.pyplot as plt
from sklearn import preprocessing
from sklearn. Preprocessing import StandardScaler
from sklearn. model_selection import train_test_split
import seaborn as sns
from keras.layers import Dense, BatchNormalization, Dropout, LSTM
from keras.models import Sequential
from tensorflow.keras.utils import to_categorical
from keras import callbacks
from sklearn.metrics import precision_score, recall_score, confusion_matri
x, classification_report, accuracy_score, f1_score
```

Data Evidence

A machine learning function called DataInfo is used to gather the main points of a dataset, including its count and Datatype. the knowledge acquired through data execution. data is displayed in Table 3 below.

Examination of Inequity of Data

An imbalanced dataset has an unequal distribution of classes. On the other hand, a dataset is deemed uneven when the number of samples for a certain issue class varies noticeably, or even drastically (Sharma et al. 2022). The following command is run to verify this, and the outcome is obtained. As can be seen in Fig. 6, the outcome indicates that the data is balanced and prepared for further processing.

Table 3. Data information

```
data info
<class 'pandas. core. frame.DataFrame'>
RangeIndex: 299 entries, 0 to 298
Data columns (total 13 columns):
 #   Column                    Non-Null Count   Dtype
---  ------                    --------------   -----
 0   age                       299 non-null     float64
 1   anaemia                   299 non-null     int64
 2   creatinine phosphokinase  299 non-null     int64
 3   diabetes                  299 non-null     int64
 4   ejection_fraction         299 non-null     int64
 5   high_blood_pressure       299 non-null     int64
 6   platelets                 299 non-null     float64
 7   serum_creatinine          299 non-null     float64
 8   serum_sodium              299 non-null     int64
 9   sex                       299 non-null     int64
 10  smoking                   299 non-null     int64
 11  time                      299 non-null     int64
 12  DEATH_EVENT               299 non-null     int64
dtypes: float64(3), int64(10)
```

Figure 6. Bar graph to show balancing

```
cols= ["#6daa9f","#774571"]
sns. count plot (x= data["DEATH_EVENT"], palette= cols)
```

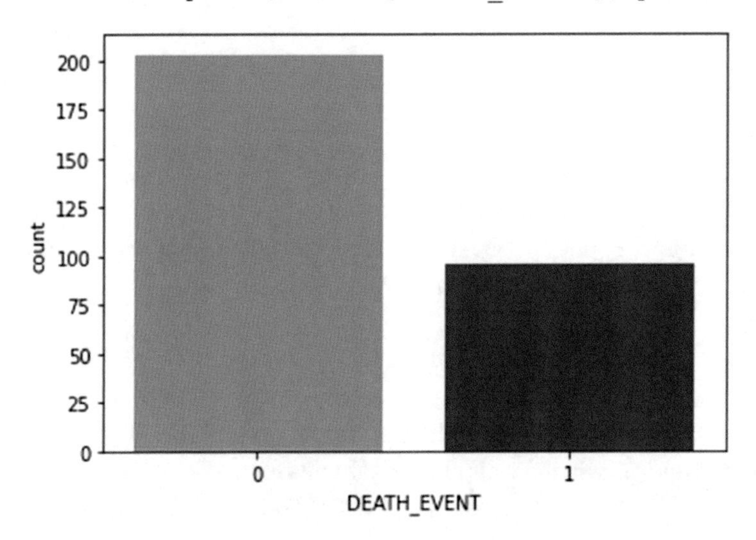

Data Visualization

Using a heat map (or heatmap) to depict the size of a phenomenon in two dimensions as a color map is a data visualization technique. The reader will receive distinct visual cues about how the occurrences are clustered or vary over space as a result of the color shift, which may occur via hue or intensity. Heat map analysis is the process of assessing and analyzing heat map data to learn more about user interaction on a website. Better site designs with lower bounce rates, fewer drop-offs, more pageviews, and greater conversion rates can be produced as a consequence of data research. Figure 7 below displays the heat map between all of the parameters. The heat map's color and value reveal the parameters' relationships with one another, and it is discovered that the majority of the values are positive, fairly correlated, or dependent upon one another. As seen in Figure 7, the two main variables with high dependence to determine whether or not a cardiac arrest is likely are platelets and diabatic (Madhu et al. 2022).

Figure 7. Heat Map using the metadata

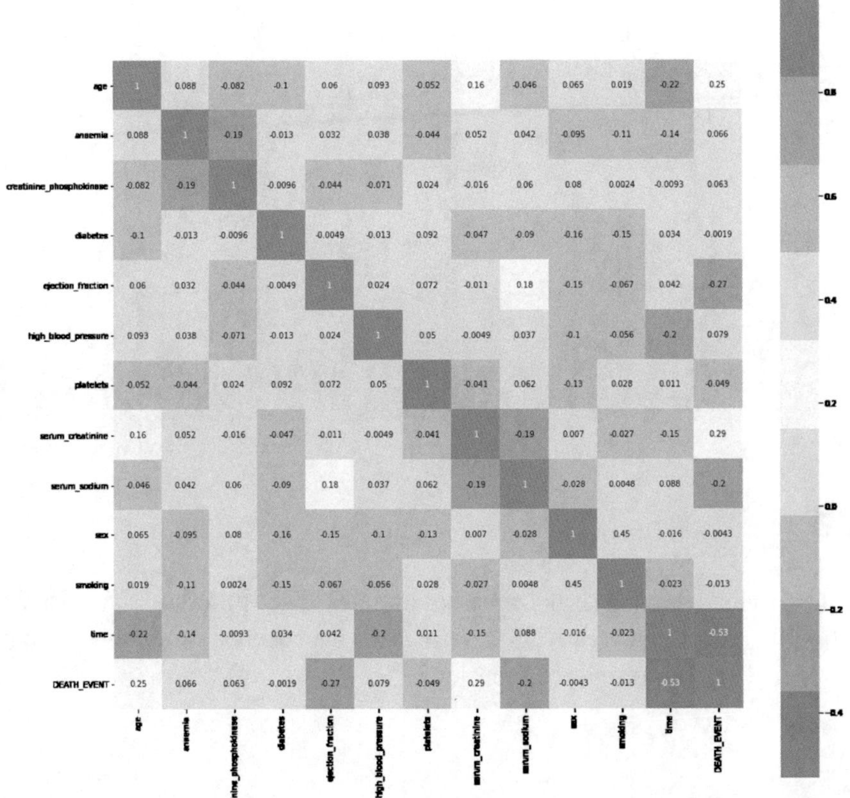

Count Plot

Bar graphs are frequently used seaborn to demonstrate relationships between category data and at least one numerical variable. The independent variable in a count plot is the dependent variable (the number of data points) (the data points). To determine which age group is most impacted by cardiac arrest, the count plot for age and death occurrences is created (Rajawat et al. 2022). According to the graph, cardiac arrest occurs most frequently in people over 60 and much less frequently in children under the age of 10 (Figure 8).

Figure 8 Count Plot for a given dataset

```
#Evauating age distrivution
plt.figure(figsize=(20,12))
#colours =["#774571","#b398af","#f1f1f1" ,"#afcdc7", "#6daa9f"]
Days_of_week=sns.countplot(x=data['age'],data=data, hue ="DEATH_EVENT",pal
ette = cols)
Days_of_week.set_title("Distribution Of Age", color="#774571")
```

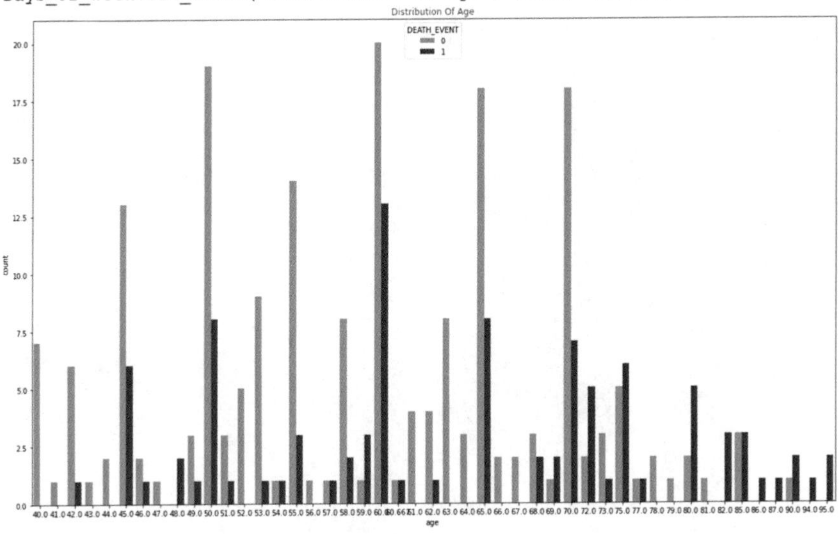

KDE

Similar to a histogram, a kernel density estimate (KDE) plot shows the distribution of observations in a dataset. KDE describes the data using a continuous probability density curve in one or more dimensions.

KDE may produce a less cluttered plot and is easier to comprehend as compared to a histogram, especially when displaying many distributions. However, if the underlying distribution is constrained or irregular, it can result in distortions. Similar to a histogram, the quality of the representation is influenced by the application of the right smoothing parameters.

Using the following command, the Kennel Density Estate graph between age and death event is plotted, and the visualization is shown in Figure 9.

Figure 9 Kernel density estimate Plot

```
sns.kdeplot(x=data["time"], y=data["age"], hue =data["DEATH_EVENT"], palet
te=cols)
```

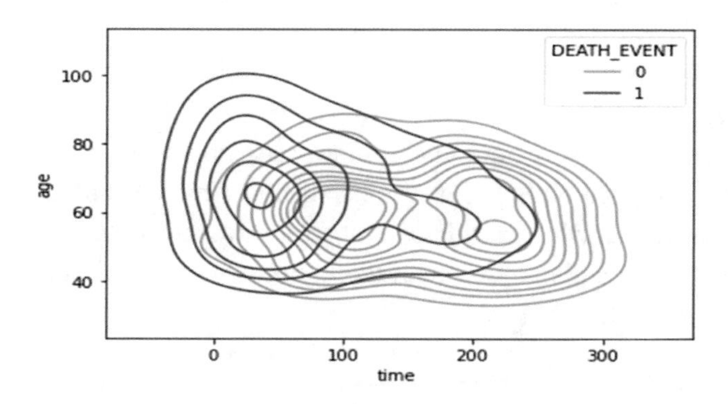

Swarm Box Plot

The only difference between this procedure and strip plot () is that the points are changed to prevent overlap (just along the categorical axis). This shows the value distribution more accurately, but it does not scale well to vast amounts of data. The term “beeswarm” is commonly used to describe this layout style.

When you wish to show all observations as well as a visual representation of the underlying distribution, a swarm plot can be made on its own or in conjunction with a box or violin plot.

Because it shows a large number of quantiles with “letter values,” this sort of graphic was originally called a “letter value” plot. It depicts a nonparametric depiction of distribution with all attributes according to actual data, similar to a box plot. Plotting more quantiles provides more details on the distribution’s shape, especially in the tails. The command used to plot is provided below, and the plots are displayed in Figure 9 underlying distribution. The Swarm and box plot of the

Death event are plotted concerning characteristics like age, cp, ef, platelets, sc, ss, and time.

```
# Boxen and swarm plot of some non binary features.

feature = ["age","creatinine_phosphokinase","ejection_fraction","platelets
","serum_creatinine","serum_sodium", "time"]
for i in feature:
    plt.figure(figsize=(8,8))
    sns.swarmplot(x=data["DEATH_EVENT"], y=data[i], color="black", alpha=0
.5)
    sns.boxenplot(x=data["DEATH_EVENT"], y=data[i], palette=cols)
    plt.show()
```

Describe Command

A Series or DataFrame's numerical values may be utilized to compute statistical statistics like percentile, mean, and standard deviation using the describe () method. It looks at mixed-data-type DataFrame column sets, object series, and numeric column sets. The supplied table lists several statistical findings, and the values of 25% and 75% represent the lower and upper quartiles, respectively, while the value of 50% represents the median along with the minimum and maximum values for each parameter, as seen in Table 4.

Table 4. Statistical investigation

	count	mean	std	min	25%	50%	75%	max
age	299.0	60.833893	11.894809	40.0	51.0	60.0	70.0	95.0
anaemia	299.0	0.431438	0.496107	0.0	0.0	0.0	1.0	1.0
creatinine_phosphokinase	299.0	581.839465	970.287881	23.0	116.5	250.0	582.0	7861.0
diabetes	299.0	0.418060	0.494067	0.0	0.0	0.0	1.0	1.0
ejection_fraction	299.0	38.083612	11.834841	14.0	30.0	38.0	45.0	80.0
high_blood_pressure	299.0	0.351171	0.478136	0.0	0.0	0.0	1.0	1.0
platelets	299.0	263358.029264	97804.236869	25100.0	212500.0	262000.0	303500.0	850000.0
serum_creatinine	299.0	1.393880	1.034510	0.5	0.9	1.1	1.4	9.4
serum_sodium	299.0	136.625418	4.412477	113.0	134.0	137.0	140.0	148.0
sex	299.0	0.648829	0.478136	0.0	0.0	1.0	1.0	1.0
smoking	299.0	0.321070	0.467670	0.0	0.0	0.0	1.0	1.0
time	299.0	130.260870	77.614208	4.0	73.0	115.0	203.0	285.0
DEATH_EVENT	299.0	0.321070	0.467670	0.0	0.0	0.0	1.0	1.0

Figure 10a. Swarm box plot of various parameters with Death event

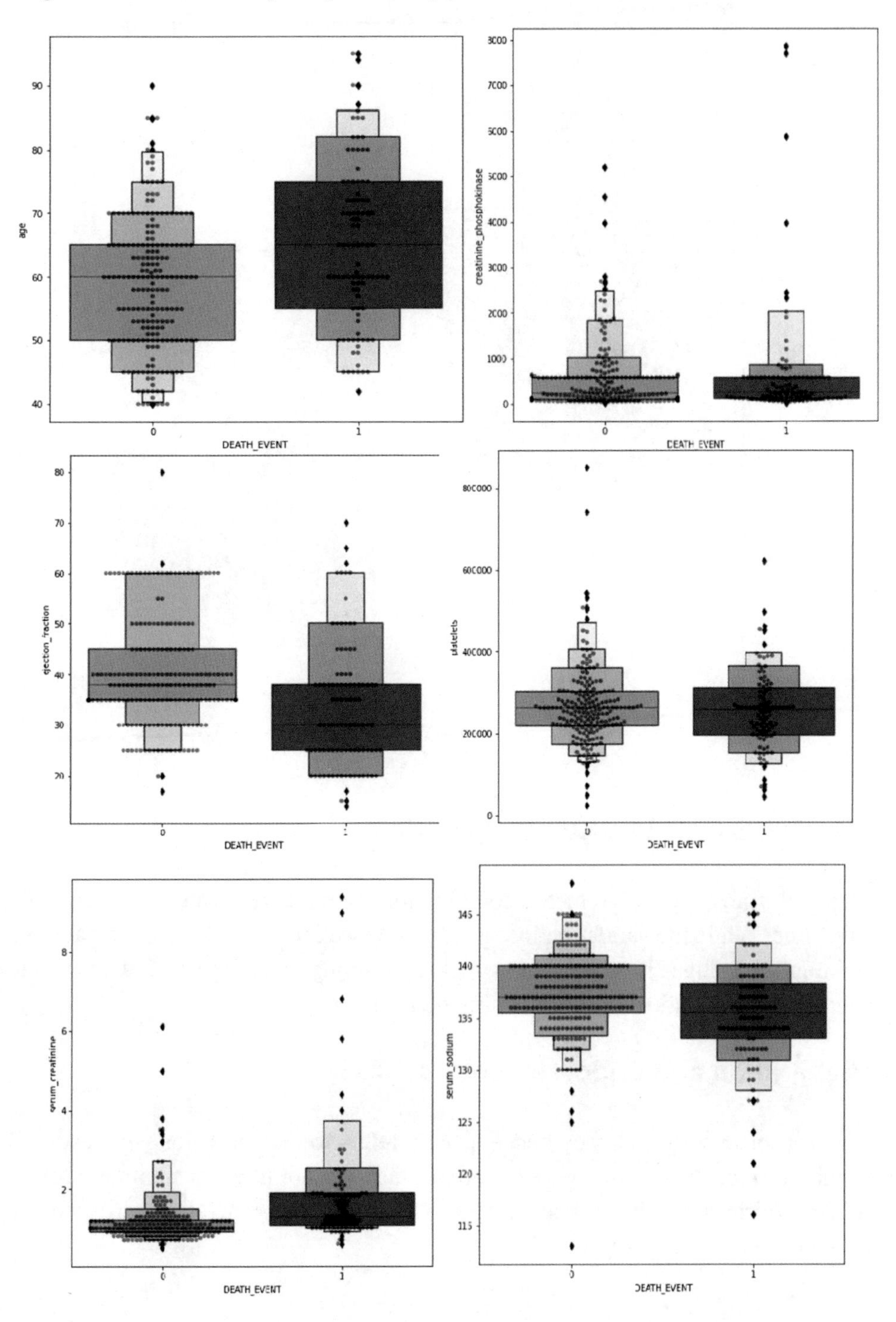

Figure 10b. Swarm box plot of various parameters with Death event

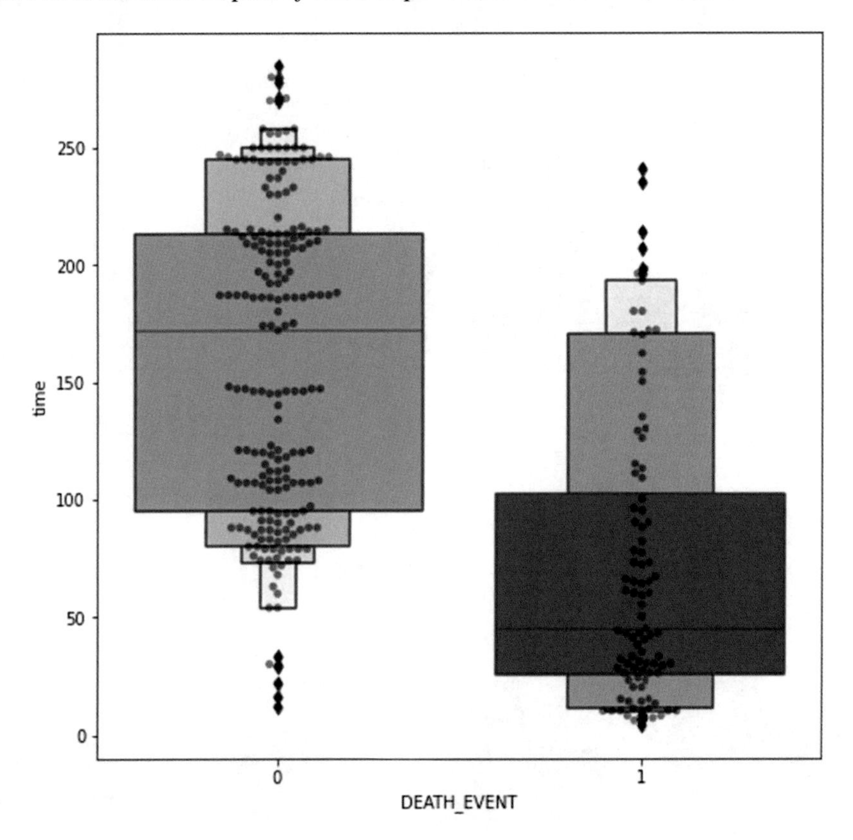

TRAINING AND VALIDATION LOSS

One of the most often used metric combinations is training loss plus validation loss over time. While the validation loss gauges how well the model fits fresh data, the training loss gauges how well the model fits training data. Figure 12 displays the training and validation loss for the provided dataset.

Preparation and Endorsement Accuracy

The test (or testing) accuracy hence usually refers to the validation (or "testing") accuracy, which you compute on a data set that was not used for training but was utilized (during the training process) to verify (or "test") the generalization capability of your model or to "early stop."

Figure 11. Combined Box Plot with parameters

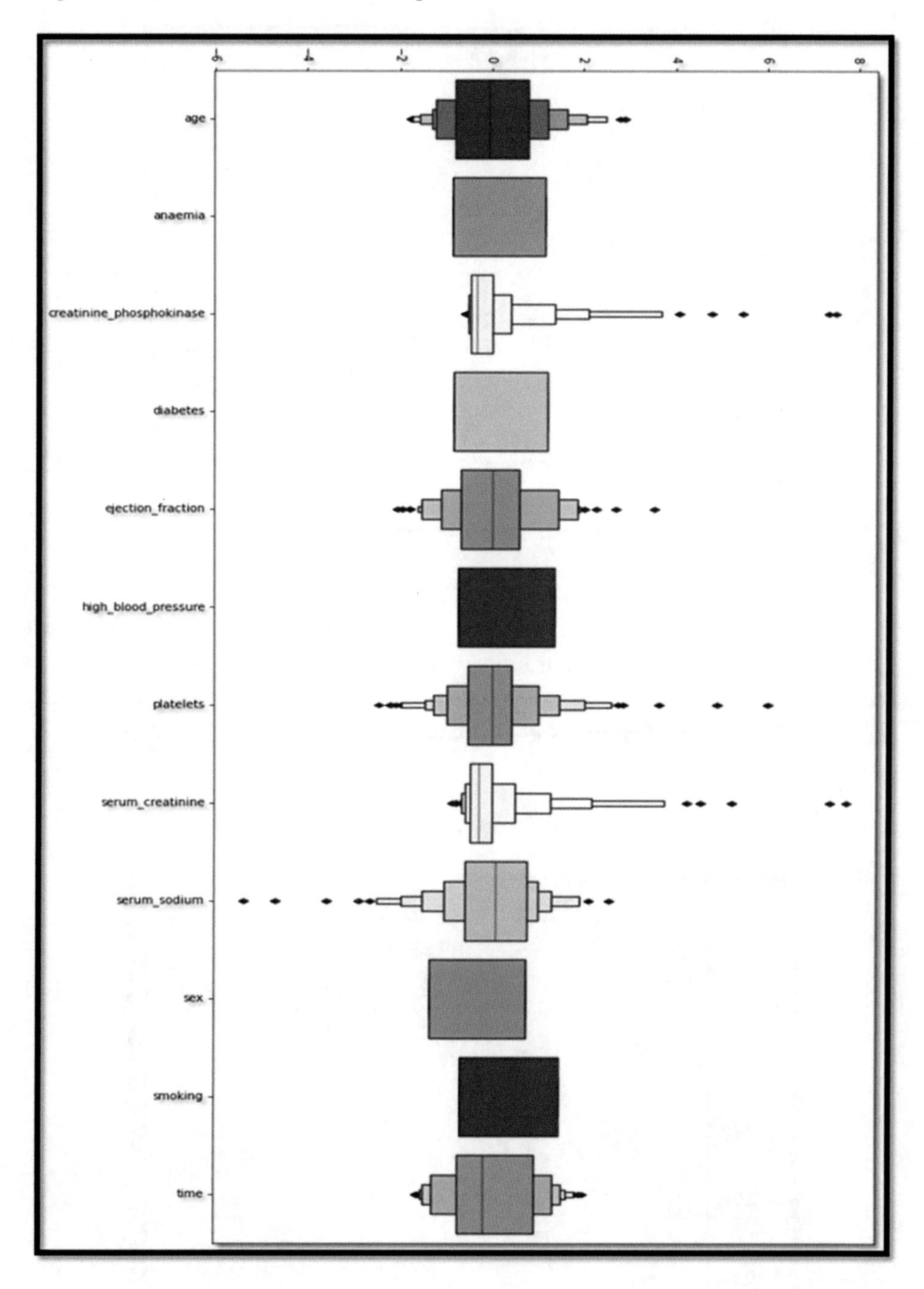

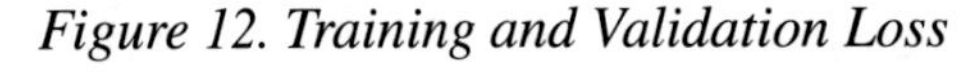

Figure 12. Training and Validation Loss

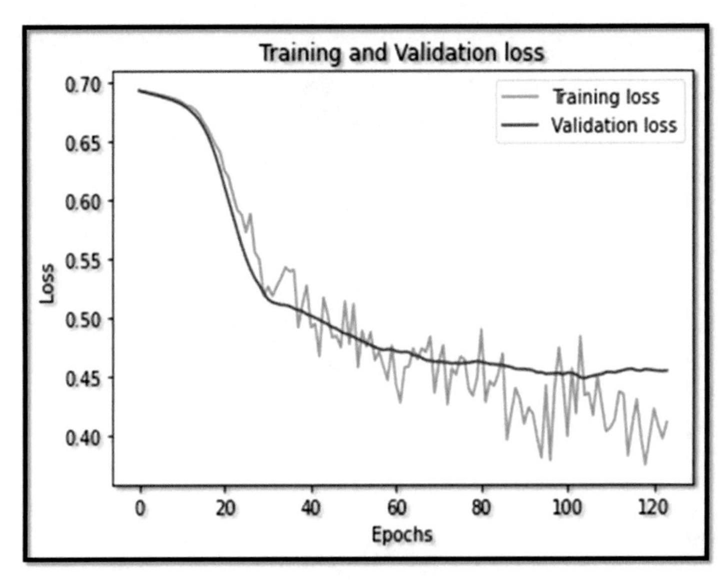

We construct the model with the assistance of the training data, and we assess its performance using both the training and validation sets (evaluation metric is accuracy). The validation's accuracy is just 83 percent, compared to the training's accuracy of 85%. The Training and Validation accuracy is given in Figure 13.

Figure 13 Training and Validation Accuracy

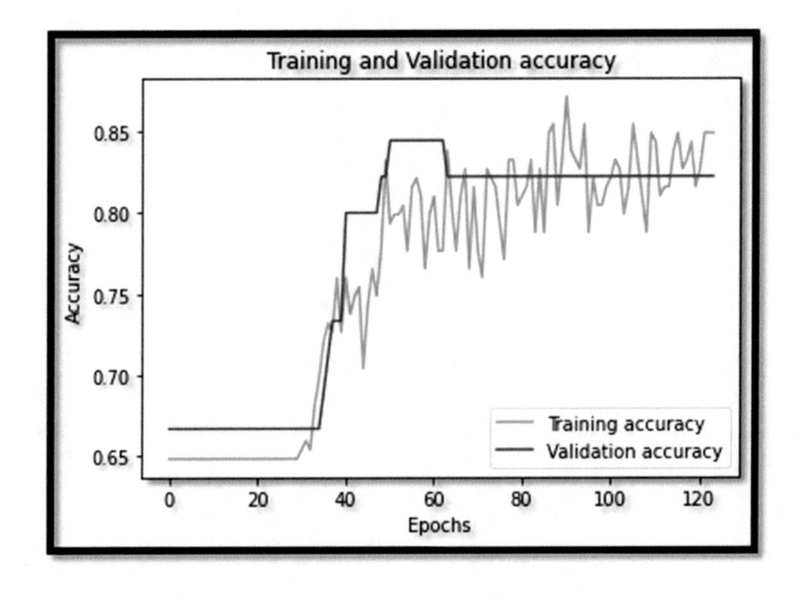

Misperception Matrix

A table displaying how well a classification model—also known as a "classifier"—performs on a set of test data for which the true values are known is called a confusion matrix. In Fig. 12, which represents the confusion matrix for the dataset, the true positive value is 0.65, whereas the false positive value is 0.11, the true negative value is 0.0093, and the false-negative value is 0.11 This score shows that the model fits the data the best. Table 5 displays the accuracy score together with the precision-recall and f1-score.

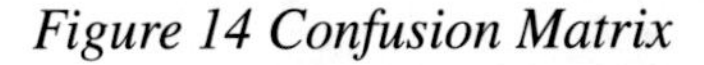

Figure 14 Confusion Matrix

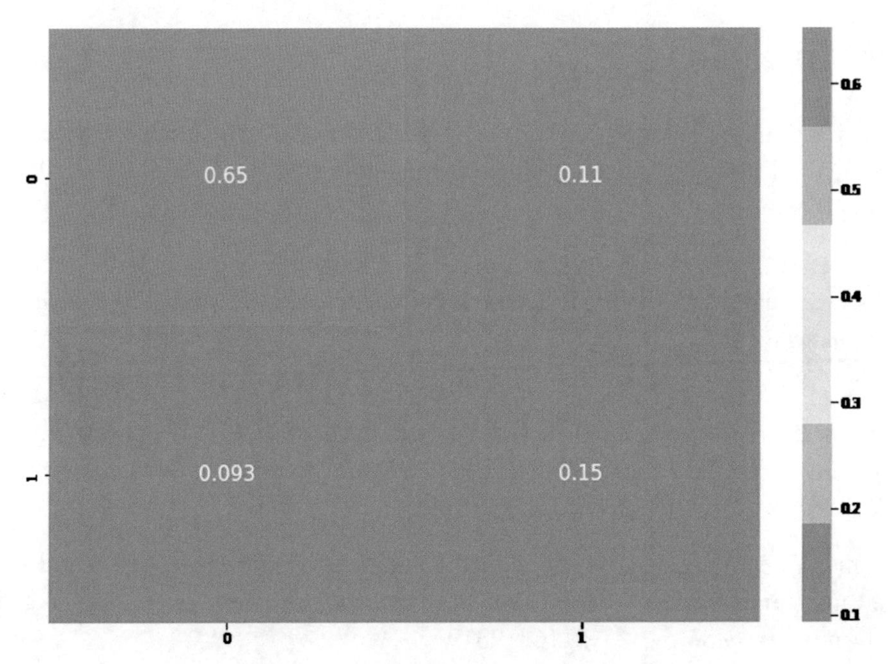

Table 5. Precision-recall and fi-score description

	precision	recall	f1-score	support
0	0.88	0.86	0.87	57
1	0.58	0.61	0.59	18
accuracy			0.80	75
macro avg	0.73	0.74	0.73	75
weighted avg	0.80	0.80	0.80	75

CONCLUSION

In this book chapter, a new framework for real-time cardiac arrest detection using AI and ANN is proposed as a case study. Machine learning is a far more effective method for diagnosing cardiac arrest since it is quick and reliable. Thanks to the usage of ANN, the validation accuracy is 83 percent and the training accuracy is 85 percent, making a respectably significant contribution. Additionally, the accuracy may be increased by enlarging the data and using the deep learning model. ANN is used to build and present the confusion matrix, precision, specificity, sensitivity, and F1 score in tabular form. The findings in the book chapter are plausible, and the researchers will profit from this research study.

REFERENCES

AlkaliY.RoutrayI.WhigP. (2022). Study of various methods for reliable, efficient, and Secured IoT using Artificial Intelligence. *Available at* SSRN 4020364. doi:10.2139/ssrn.4020364

Anand, M., Velu, A., & Whig, P. (2022). Prediction of Loan Behaviour with Machine Learning Models for Secure Banking. *Journal of Computing Science and Engineering: JCSE*, *3*(1), 1–13.

Asopa, P., Purohit, P., Nadikattu, R. R., & Whig, P. (2021). Reducing carbon footprint for sustainable development of smart cities using IoT. *2021 Third International Conference on Intelligent Communication Technologies and Virtual Mobile Networks (ICICV)*, 361–367. 10.1109/ICICV50876.2021.9388466

Bhatia, V., & Whig, P. (2013a). A secured dual-tune multi-frequency-based smart elevator control system. *International Journal of Research in Engineering and Advanced Technology*, *4*(1), 1163–2319.

Bhatia, V., & Whig, P. (2014). Performance analysis of multi-functional bot system design using microcontroller. *International Journal of Intelligent Systems and Applications*, *6*(2), 69–75. doi:10.5815/ijisa.2014.02.09

Channumsin, O., Pimpol, J., Thongsopa, C., & Tangsrirat, W. (2015). VDBA-based floating inductance simulator with a grounded capacitor. *2015 7th International Conference on Information Technology and Electrical Engineering (ICEE)*, 114–117.

George, N., Muiz, K., Whig, P., & Velu, A. (2021, July). The framework of Perceptive Artificial Intelligence using Natural Language Processing (PAIN). *Artificial & Computational Intelligence*.

Jiwani, N., Gupta, K., & Whig, P. (2021). Novel HealthCare Framework for Cardiac Arrest With the Application of AI Using ANN. *2021 5th International Conference on Information Systems and Computer Networks (ISCON)*, 1–5.

Kautish, S., Reyana, A., & Vidyarthi, A. (2022). SDMTA: Attack Detection and Mitigation Mechanism for DDoS Vulnerabilities in Hybrid Cloud Environment. *IEEE Transactions on Industrial Informatics*.

Khera, Y., Whig, P., & Velu, A. (2021). efficient effective and secured electronic billing system using AI. *Vivekananda Journal of Research, 10*, 53–60.

Madhu, G., Govardhan, A., & Ravi, V. (2022). *DSCN-net: a deep Siamese capsule neural network model for automatic diagnosis of malaria parasites detection. Multimed Tools Appl.* doi:10.100711042-022-13008-6

Moorthy, T. V. K., Budati, A. K., Kautish, S., Goyal, S. B., & Prasad, K. L. (2022). Reduction of satellite images size in 5G networks using Machinelearning algorithms. *IET Communications, 16*(5), 584–591. doi:10.1049/cmu2.12354

Nadikattu, R. R., Mohammad, S. M., & Whig, P. (2020a). *Novel economical social distancing smart device for covid-19. International Journal of Electrical Engineering and Technology.*

On the Performance of ISFET-based Device for Water Quality Monitoring. (n.d.). doi:10.4236/ijcns.2011.411087

Parihar, V., & Yadav, S. (2022). *Comparison estimation of effective consumer future preferences with the application of AI.* Academic Press.

Purva Agarwal1, P. W. (2016). A Review-Quaternary Signed Digit Number System by reversible Logic Gate. *International Journal on Recent and Innovation Trends in Computing and Communication, 4*(3).

Rajawat, A. S., Bedi, P., Goyal, S. B., Kautish, S., Xihua, Z., Aljuaid, H., & Mohamed, A. W. (2022). Dark Web Data Classification Using Neural Network. *Computational Intelligence and Neuroscience*.

Ruchin, C. M., & Whig, P. (2015). Design and Simulation of Dynamic UART Using Scan Path Technique (USPT). *International Journal of Electrical, Electronics & Computing in Science & Engineering*.

Rupani, A., & Kumar, D. (2020). *Temperature Effect On Behaviour of Photo Catalytic Sensor (PCS).* Used For Water Quality Monitoring.

Rupani, A., & Sujediya, G. (2016). A Review of FPGA implementation of Internet of Things. *International Journal of Innovative Research in Computer and Communication Engineering*, *4*(9).

Rupani, A., Whig, P., Sujediya, G., & Vyas, P. (2018). Hardware implementation of IoT-based image processing filters. *Proceedings of the Second International Conference on Computational Intelligence and Informatics*, 681–691. 10.1007/978-981-10-8228-3_63

Sharma, C., Sharma, S., Kautish, S., Alsallami, S. A., Khalil, E. M., & Mohamed, A. W. (2022). A new median-average round Robin scheduling algorithm: An optimal approach for reducing turnaround and waiting time. *Alexandria Engineering Journal*, *61*(12), 10527–10538.

Sharma, N. K., Shrivastava, S., & Whig, P. (n.d.). *Optimization of Process Parameters for Developing Stresses in Square Cup by Incremental Sheet Metal (ISM) Technique uses Finite Element Methods*. Academic Press.

Shridhar, J., & Whig, P. (2014). Design and simulation of power-efficient traffic light controller (PTLC). *2014 International Conference on Computing for Sustainable Global Development (INDIACom)*, 348–352. 10.1109/IndiaCom.2014.6828157

Shrivastav, P., Whig, P., & Gupta, K. (n.d.). *Bandwidth Enhancement by Slotted Stacked Arrangement and its Comparative Analysis with Conventional Single and Stacked Patch Antenna*. Academic Press.

Sinha, R., & Ranjan, A. (2015). Effect of Variable Damping Ratio on the design of PID Controller. *2015 4th International Conference on Reliability, Infocom Technologies and Optimization (ICRITO)(Trends and Future Directions)*, 1–4.

Whig, P., & Ahmad, S. N. (2011). Performance analysis and frequency compensation technique for low power water quality monitoring device using ISFET sensor. *International Journal of Mobile and Adhoc Network*, 80–84.

Whig, P., & Ahmad, S. N. (2013a). A novel pseudo NMOS integrated CC -ISFET device for water quality monitoring. *Journal of Integrated Circuits and Systems*. https://www.scopus.com/inward/record.url?eid=2-s2.0-84885357423&partnerID=MN8TOARS

Whig, P., & Ahmad, S. N. (2013b). A novel pseudo-PMOS integrated ISFET device for water quality monitoring. *Active and Passive Electronic Components, 2013*. doi:10.1155/2013/258970

Whig, P., & Ahmad, S. N. (2014a). CMOS integrated VDBA-ISFET device for water quality monitoring. *International Journal of Intelligent Engineering and Systems, 7*(1), 1–7. doi:10.22266/ijies2014.0331.01

Whig, P., & Ahmad, S. N. (2014b). Development of economical ASIC for PCS for water quality monitoring. *Journal of Circuits, Systems, and Computers, 23*(06), 1450079. doi:10.1142/S0218126614500790

Whig, P., & Ahmad, S. N. (2014d). *Simulation of a linear dynamic macro model of the photocatalytic sensor in SPICE. COMPEL The International Journal for Computation and Mathematics in Electrical and Electronic Engineering.*

Whig, P., & Ahmad, S. N. (2015). *Impact of Parameters on Characteristics of Novel PCS.* Academic Press.

Whig, P., & Ahmad, S. N. (2016a). Modeling and simulation of economical water quality monitoring device. *Journal of Aquaculture & Marine Biology, 4*(6), 1–6. doi:10.15406/jamb.2016.04.00103

Whig, P., & Ahmad, S. N. (2016b). *Novel SPICE model for Ultraviolet Photo Catalytic Oxidation (UVPCO).* Sensor for Air and Surface Sanitizers.

Whig, P., & Ahmad, S. N. (2017a). Controlling the Output Error for Photo Catalytic Sensor (PCS) Using Fuzzy Logic. *Journal of Earth Science & Climatic Change, 8*(4), 1–6.

Whig, P., & Ahmad, S. N. (2017b). Fuzzy logic implementation of the photocatalytic sensor. *Int. Robot. Autom. J, 2*(3), 15–19.

Whig, P., & Ahmad, S. N. (2019). Methodology for Calibrating Photocatalytic Sensor Output. *International. Journal of Sustainable Development in Computing Science, 1*(1), 1–10.

Whig, P., Nadikattu, R. R., & Velu, A. (2022). COVID-19 pandemic analysis using the application of AI. *Healthcare Monitoring and Data Analysis Using IoT: Technologies and Applications*, 1.

ADDITIONAL READING

Kouser, S., Velu, A., & Nadikattu, R. R. (2022). Fog-IoT-Assisted-Based Smart Agriculture Application. In *Demystifying Federated Learning for Blockchain and Industrial Internet of Things* (pp. 74–93). IGI Global.

Nadikattu, R. R., & Velu, A. (2022). COVID-19 pandemic analysis using application of AI. *Healthcare Monitoring and Data Analysis Using IoT: Technologies and Applications*, 1.

Sharma, P. (2022). Demystifying Federated Learning for Blockchain: A Case Study. In *Demystifying Federated Learning for Blockchain and Industrial Internet of Things* (pp. 143–165). IGI Global. doi:10.4018/978-1-6684-3733-9.ch006

Velu, A., & Naddikatu, R. R. (2022). The Economic Impact of AI-Enabled Blockchain in 6G-Based Industry. In *AI and Blockchain Technology in 6G Wireless Network* (pp. 205–224). Springer.

Whig, P., Velu, A., & Bhatia, A. B. (2022). Protect Nature and Reduce the Carbon Footprint With an Application of Blockchain for IIoT. In *Demystifying Federated Learning for Blockchain and Industrial Internet of Things* (pp. 123–142). IGI Global. doi:10.4018/978-1-6684-3733-9.ch007

Whig, P., Velu, A., & Nadikattu, R. R. (2022). Blockchain Platform to Resolve Security Issues in IoT and Smart Networks. In *AI-Enabled Agile Internet of Things for Sustainable FinTech Ecosystems* (pp. 46–65). IGI Global. doi:10.4018/978-1-6684-4176-3.ch003

Whig, P., Velu, A., & Ready, R. (2022). Demystifying Federated Learning in Artificial Intelligence With Human-Computer Interaction. In Demystifying Federated Learning for Blockchain and Industrial Internet of Things (pp. 94–122). IGI Global.

KEY TERMS AND DEFINITIONS

ANN: An ANN is based on a collection of connected units or nodes called artificial neurons, which loosely model the neurons in a biological brain.

Cardiac Arrest: The condition usually results from a problem with your heart's electrical system, which disrupts your heart's pumping action and stops blood flow to your body.

CNN: Convolution is a mathematical operation that allows the merging of two sets of information. In the case of CNN, convolution is applied to the input data to filter the information and produce a feature map. This filter is also called a kernel, or feature detector.

Deep Learning: Deep learning is a type of machine learning and artificial intelligence (AI) that imitates the way humans gain certain types of knowledge.

Disorder: A state of confusion.

Healthcare: Health care or healthcare is the improvement of health via the prevention, diagnosis, treatment, amelioration, or cure of disease, illness, injury, and other physical and mental impairments in people. Health care is delivered by health professionals and allied health fields.

Symptoms: A physical or mental problem that a person experiences that may indicate a disease or condition. Symptoms cannot be seen and do not show up on medical tests.

Chapter 2
A Study and Analysis of Deep Neural Networks for Cancer Using Histopathology Images

Anu Singha
Sri Ramachandra Faculty of Engineering and Technology, Sri Ramachandra Institute of Higher Education and Research, Chennai, India

Jayanthi Ganapathy
Sri Ramachandra Faculty of Engineering and Technology, Sri Ramachandra Institute of Higher Education and Research, Chennai, India

ABSTRACT

Due to the complexity of histopathology tissues, an accurate classification and segmentation of cancer diagnosis is a challenging task in computer vision. The nuclei segmentation of microscopic images is a key prerequisite for cancerous pathological image analysis. However, an accurate nuclei segmentation is a long running major challenge due to the enormous color variability of staining, nuclei shapes, sizes, and clustering of overlapping cells. To address these challenges and early diagnosis as well as reduce the bias decisions of expert lab technician of cancer in clinical practice, the authors study the classification of computer-aided frameworks and automatic nuclei segmentation frameworks based on histopathology images by convolutional deep learning. The authors have used a publicly available PatchCamelyon and 2018 Data Science Bowl histology image dataset for this study. The results are compared and expected to be useful clinically for technician experts in the analysis of cancer diagnosis and the survival chances of patients.

DOI: 10.4018/978-1-6684-4405-4.ch002

INTRODUCTION

In health concerns, the cancer diseases become the most common and life-threatening issue. In India, the incidence of any cancer growth rate is increases in young age group at very aggressive Shah, 2020). Cancer starts from a benign state and at the early stages without proper treatment, it becomes malignant when the cells start to grow abnormally. It is started to form a mass or lump via divide infected cells more frequently than normal healthy cells. However, if exposed early, the cancer is a greatly curable disease with 97% chances of survival (Ng, 2009).

The availability of appropriate screening devices is essential for detecting the initial symptoms of cancer. Numerous imaging techniques are used for the screening to detect this disease such as histopathology. To improve the accuracy of the diagnosis for patients, the histopathology images are considered as the gold standard among other imaging techniques (Ng, 2009). Moreover, the histopathological examination can deliver more inclusive and reliable evidence to diagnose cancer and measure its effects on the surrounding tissues (Gurcan et al., 2009; Hipp et al., 2011; Pickles et al., 2015). In this chapter, we have examined these histopathology images.

For analysis of histopathology image, the detection and segmentation of nuclei cells are essential steps. These segmented nuclei are used in the grading diagnosis of many cancers which require comprehensive analysis of the characteristics of the nuclei such as shape, size, gray value, color variation of samples, clusters of nuclei with overlapping, and ratio of nuclei to cytoplasm. It is a major challenge in histopathology images of different patients where the shape and appearance of the different nuclei for disease stages vary greatly. In breast cancer, the identification of the stages of aggressiveness of the disease based upon the Nottingham Histologic Score system which also largely based off the morphologic attributes of the histopathology nuclei (Basavanhally et al., 2011). As a consequence, the accurate segmentation of histopathology image nuclei is a great challenging work in developing automated machine via computer assisted decision support for digital histopathology. Other than these, the segmentation of nuclei of histopathology image is essential to numerous studies, such as feature extraction, cell counts, and classification.

In this chapter, we have examined cancer histopathology images in two ways. First, we examine the patch-based histopathology images for classification either carcinomas metastasis/malignant patch or non-carcinomas/normal patch. Secondly, deep convolutional-de-convolutional segmentation approaches will be analysed to handle accurate segmentation of nuclei.

The contribution of this study will as follow:

1. We have studied the benchmark CNN models for abnormality classification. Unlike the conventional method of using texture feature-based analysis, the

benchmark models make use of the metastatic cancer in small image patches taken from larger digital pathology scans to signify the abnormality.

2. The classification performance of the abnormality classification system has been evaluated with a public PatchCamelyon (PCam) (Bejnordi et al., 2017) histopathologic cancer database by using a series of state-of-the-art classification benchmark systems. The performances will be measured through supervised evaluation metrics like accuracy, recall, precision, F1 score, confusion matrix, and ROC AUC.
3. Encoder-Decoder models has studied to handle nucleus segmentation for breast cancer histopathology images. In Encoder part, it stitches feature maps in the channel dimension to achieve feature fusion and uses a skip structure in Decoder part to combine low- and high-level features to ensure the segmentation effect of the nucleus.
4. The performance of nuclei segmentation has been done with a publicly available dataset i.e. 2018 Data Science Bowl (Kaggle, n.d.).

Literature Review

In this section, we briefly review the development of the early diagnosis of cancer using CAD technologies. The diagnostic accuracy is usually unsatisfactory due to numerous challenges of histology image analysis of the cancer. Therefore, researchers tried to recommend reliable approaches to address these problems to improve the efficacy of early diagnosis of cancer. Now-a-days, deep learning models have shown remarkable performances in several fields of medical imaging that surpassing other conventional techniques (Lee, 2017). The reason behind success of deep learning which performs the nonlinear acts of input data to extract structurally complex features. Along with the help of image processing approaches, it became easier to detect and classify metastasis areas from an infected area (Yasmin et al., 2013). A deep learning-based CAD system were first evaluated by the authors of BreakHis dataset. They entrusted extraction of features and corresponding improve classification results to a deep convolutional neural network AlexNet via transfer learning (Spanhol et al., 2016). (Sun & Binder, 2017) tried to find the best neural network model for classification mission and compared models such as ResNet, GoogleNet, and AlexNet, and finds ResNet as the best model. Authors in (Truong et al., 2020) provides a simple low-cost deep CNN architecture due to the simplicity of architecture. It is for classification of breast cancer histology samples where the model creates patches from sample images to passes them for training. In (Abdel-Zaher & Eldeib, 2016), an unsupervised Deep Belief Network (DBN) is used as first stage for the initialization of the weights and then fed the resultant matrix to the back-propagation neural network as a second stage that utilized supervised manner

(Abdel-Zaher & Eldeib, 2016). Two methods conjugate gradient and Levenberg Marquardt were used in back-propagation. In way of combination of supervised back-propagation and unsupervised DBN shows better results. The multi-classification as benign or malignant and subtypes of breast cancer samples has been carried out by (Gandomkar et al., 2018) using deep residual learning. However, due to the limited training samples and less labeled images available for effective training, these deep learning networks often suffer from overfitting training-validation. Therefore, in recent studies, researchers have united deep learning with traditional machine learning to exploit their individual qualities. For instance, (Araújo et al., 2017) extracted the features by deep CNN (DCNN) and then utilized these features to train a support vector machine (SVM) classifier to label histology sample images of breast. It works on designed patches of 512x512 pixels based on 249 high resolution images and performed four class classification on a dataset released for the bio-imaging breast cancer histology classification challenge 2015 (Pêgo & Aguiar, 2015). (Wang et al., 2016) also used sampling patches to train a convolutional neural network to make patch-level predictions, then created tumor probability heat-maps by aggregated the outcomes of patch-level predictions and made whole slide-level predictions. The network was tested on the Camelyon16 database including 400 Whole Slide Histopathological Images (WSIs) (Bejnordi et al., 2017). (Wang et al., 2020) planned a fused network between machine and deep learning. Where a multi-network feature extraction model to obtain more comprehensive feature representations of breast cancer histological images. As well developed a dual-network orthogonal low-rank learning (DOLL) feature selection method which considers removing the redundant features and obtain complementary features. Another multi-classification study by (Li et al., 2019) proposed an effective scheme to classify the H&E stained of breast histology samples into four classes: normal tissue, benign lesion, in-situ carcinoma and invasive carcinoma. This classification utilized multi-size and discriminative patches of histology images. Recently, (Yari et al., 2020) also applied deep learning for multi-classification of histology diagnosis of breast cancer and achieved good performances.

From above discussion of the surveys, it is noticed that the high-dimensional features will cause the classifier to overfit, high computational costs and affect classification accuracy. The objective of this current research is to present an analysis automated tool for classification of carcinoma metastasis or cancer to lessen human mistakes in the process of diagnosis.

Over the recent times, convolutional neural network-based analysis of several medical image modalities has been demanded highly due to its robust performance. Now, we will present overview of the important recent developments in the medical image segmentation including nuclei of histopathology images. Since most disease analysis highly dependent on cell-level information, the segmentation challenge in computing technology is to investigate all the individual cells to make correct diagnosis.

A fully convolutional network (FCN) (Long et al., 2015) was the initial full convolution neural network which has been introduced for medical image segmentation. To produce fine segmentation, this network defined as a combination of deep semantic information with shallow appearance. (Cui et al., 2019) also introduced an automatic end-to-end fully convolutional neural network nucleus boundary model for segmenting of individual nuclei and their boundaries simultaneously. (Ronneberger et al., 2015) was the first who utilized U-Net as an encoder-decoder model for medical image segmentation tasks. U-Net uses skip connections to integrate low- and high-level information. Later-on, variety of U-Net extensions have been exploited for medical segmentation same purpose. A very popular semantic segmentation model SegNet (Badrinarayanan, 2015) has been utilized by (Lal et al., 2021) and proposed an extension model NucleiSegNet to address the challenges of nuclei segmentation task in histopathology images of liver cancer. The NucleiSegNet architecture consists of three blocks: a robust residual block, a bottleneck block, and an attention decoder block. (Zhao et al., 2017) proposed another semantic segmentation network, namely, PSPNet, inspired by context information of FCN. (Hassan et al., 2021) presented deep semantic nuclei segmentation model based upon PSPSegNet in histopathology images of different organs such as breast, kidney, prostate, and stomach. For histopathology based nuclei segmentation task, (Vu et al., 2019) presented the DRAN model by integrating both nuclei and nuclei contours to achieve accurate nuclei segmentation results. Histopathology nuclei segmentation based on a bending loss regularized network proposed by (Wang et al., 2020). Minimizing bending loss can evade producing contours that comprise multiple nuclei. (Naylor et al., 2019) also presented a model 'DIST' for the segmentation of histopathology image nuclei by employing a regression concept for overlapping nuclei. (Xu et al., 2016) also used stacked sparse autoencoder (SSAE) in breast cancer histopathology images but for detection of nuclei effectively. More survey information about segmentation in histopathology nuclei images can be referred to (Irshad et al., 2013) and (Xing & Yang, 2016).

It is worth noting that color variation in histopathology images, cluster of nuclei with overlapping, shape, and size between different nuclei degrade the performance of the above-mentioned nuclei-segmentation deep CNN models. In this study, we present another analysis of nuclei segmentation models. To demonstrate the effectiveness of the models, we consider histopathology microscopic or fluorescent microscopic images of nuclei cells.

DEEP LEARNING MODELS

A type of deep learning networks, the Convolutional Neural Network (CNN) models, are presented to solve the classification of cancerous histology slide images as well as analysis of nucleus cells. In this section, the models are introduced in two categories as (A) classification deep models, and (B) segmentation deep models.

(A) **Classification based CNN Models:** The trend is observed as the size of the feature maps rises; the resolution of the image decreases in classification CNN models. After the convolutional layers, subsampling is directed using pooling layers such max or average pooling. At last, the fully connected layers along with the SoftMax or Sigmpoid functions are operated to achieve the classifications (Singha et al., 2020). The models which will be discussed are:

(i) *AlexNet:* (Krizhevsky et al., 2017) proposed the AlexNet architecture which was implemented to 227x227 input RGB images. Moreover, this architecture has 8 layers with 5 convolutional layers and 3 of the layers are followed by max-pooling layers while rest of 3 are fully connected layers. The 1000 SoftMax activations were used to classify the outputs. AlexNet has 60M parameters, a significant number of trainable parameters in this architecture may affect the computational actions negatively.

(ii) *VGG 16:* This model was introduced by (Simonyan & Zisserman, 2015), the 16 layers of VGG architecture. It makes the enhancement over AlexNet by substituting large kernel-sized filters of 11 and 5 with multiple 3×3 kernel-sized filters. The final classification consists of 3 fully connected layers. The number of channels increases by a factor of 2 whereas the spatial resolution decreases by half in each stage. Moreover, the simplicity of this network makes it pretty to researchers also due to 138M parameters compared to VGG 19 which has 144M parameters.

(iii) *ResNet 50:* (He et al., 2016) proposed a model called ResNet to have deeper layers with less complexity and shortcut connections which applied reference model VGG-19 and added more layers to ultimately create a plain 50-layer network. The shortcut connections after every two blocks of the convolutional layer aids the network to learn the identity function in a short time with low complexity and to improve it into a deep residual network. The number of the parameters for ResNet-50 is 25.6M.

(iv) *GoogleNet:* This network was proposed by (Zeng et al., 2015) to construct an ideal architecture with more layers (total 22 layers) and fewer parameters to growth the performance. The number of the parameters is 5M only. It is noticeably smaller than that of the ResNet network. Subsequently, the development of a deeper architecture with fewer trainable parameters started from this network.

(v) *DenseNet:* Based upon ResNet identity connections for all the layers, (Huang et al., 2017) presented DenseNet model over 3 sections i.e., dense blocks, transitional layers, and classifier layer. The transitional layer using the 1x1 convolutional layer and pooling layer which reduces the feature maps to a fixed number. As consequence, the number of parameters decreases to a greater extent only 7.98M.

(vi) *MobileNet:* MobileNet is a modernized model that uses depth-wise separable convolutions for embedded vision and mobile applications (Howard et al., 2017). The depth-wise convolution filter executes a single convolution on each input channel, and the point convolution filter combines the output of depth-wise convolution linearly with 1x1 convolutions.

(B) **Segmentation based CNN Models:** Several deep learning-based instance and semantic segmentation methods have been projected in the last decade. In this chapter, we choose three of the most standard networks used for instance segmentation to the nuclei segmentation task. These models are based upon Encoder-Decoder framework. In Encoder part, it stitches feature maps in the channel dimension to achieve feature fusion and uses a skip structure in Decoder part to combine low- and high-level features to ensure the segmentation effect of the nucleus.

(i) *Fully Convolutional Network (FCN):* First (Long et al., 2015) introduced fully convolutional the FCN network that receives an input with arbitrary image size and produces pixel-wise classification as segmentation mask. The main idea behind FCN is to construct a segmentation model by utilizing classification networks such as VGG 16 (Simonyan & Zisserman, 2015) as backbone into fully convolutional networks. The skip connections are used to merge low semantic information over different layers while decoder up-sampling to produce precise segmentation results. The common FCN models are FCN-8 and FCN-16.

(ii) *U-Net:* Inspired by FCN model, (Ronneberger et al., 2015) proposed another well-known encoder-decoder architecture, namely, the U-Net architecture. The encoder path of U-Net follows the typical design of FCN to extract features, and at each step the number of feature channels gets double. The decoder path consists of de-convolution layers where the feature maps from encoder path are concatenated with the corresponding ones to avoid losing spatial information. As a final point, a 1x1 convolution layer is used to produce the segmentation mask.

(iii) *SegNet:* The encoder portion of SegNet (Badrinarayanan, 2015) is analogous to the first 13 convolutional layers of VGG 16, and the decoder portion of SegNet involves a hierarchy of decoders where each max-pooling indices corresponds to an encoder layer during up-sampling. Although U-Net and SegNet have analogous architecture, U-Net does not reuse pooling indices, and it transfers the entire feature map to the corresponding decoder layers and concatenates them with the up-sampled feature maps. This makes U-Net costs more for memory consumptions.

(iv) *Pyramid Scene Parsing Network (PSPNet):* There is a claim that FCN based models do not employ a appropriate tactic to utilize the context of the whole image. Therefore, (Zhao et al., 2017) introduced the PSPNet) which considers the strength of the global context of the image to enhance the local level predictions. They suggested a pyramid pooling module (PPM) to integrate global contextual information. The feature maps from the PPM are pooled at 4 diverse scales corresponding to 4 diverse pyramid levels. Then, the up-sampling and concatenation layers take place to construct the final feature maps, and inputted into a convolution layer to produce the segmentation results.

EXPERIMENT ANALYSIS AND DISCUSSION

This section is divided into two subsections. In subsection (i), we compare and analyse classification network models against PCam histopathology patch dataset (Bejnordi et al., 2017). In subsection (i), we compare and analyse segmentation network models against Data Science Bowl dataset (Kaggle, n.d.).

Classification Performance on PCam Histopathology Patch Dataset

Data Preparation

In this study, a subset of Camelyon16 challenge database is used called PCam dataset. It contains 400 H&E stained whole slide images of sentinel lymph node sections that were acquired and digitized at 2 different centers using a 40x objective. I found that these data were obtained as a result of routine clinical practices and similar to how a trained pathologist would examine similar images for identifying metastases. Moreover, rescaling the whole histology image to the input size for CNN straight will lose huge of detail information. Consequently, we adopts a patch sampling method in order to extract CNN feature information and preserved essential information for classification. In main PCam dataset the duplicate patch images contains due to its probabilistic sampling. However, the version presented on this study does not contain duplicates. Our prepared training data has a class distribution of 60:40 negative and positive samples as shown in Figure 1.

In Figure 2, a positive label indicates that the center 32x32 pixel region of a patch covers at least one pixel of tumor cell. Tumor cell in the outer region of the patch does not impact the label. This outer region of patch is conveyed to enable fully convolutional network that do not use zero-padding.

Figure 1. Prepared data class distribution

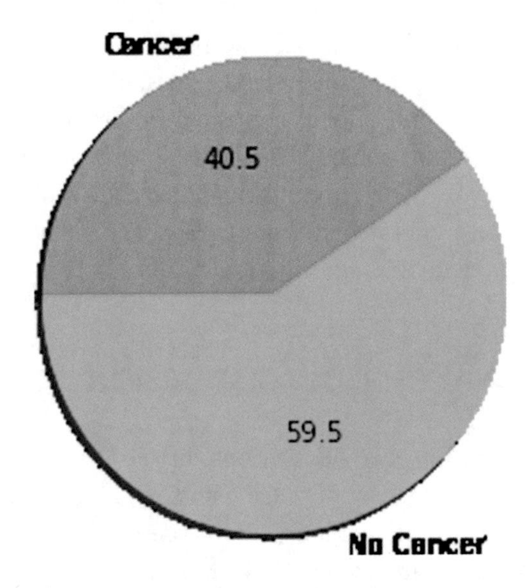

Figure 2. A positive label which at least cover one pixel of tumor tissue at the center 32x32 of a patch of size 96x96

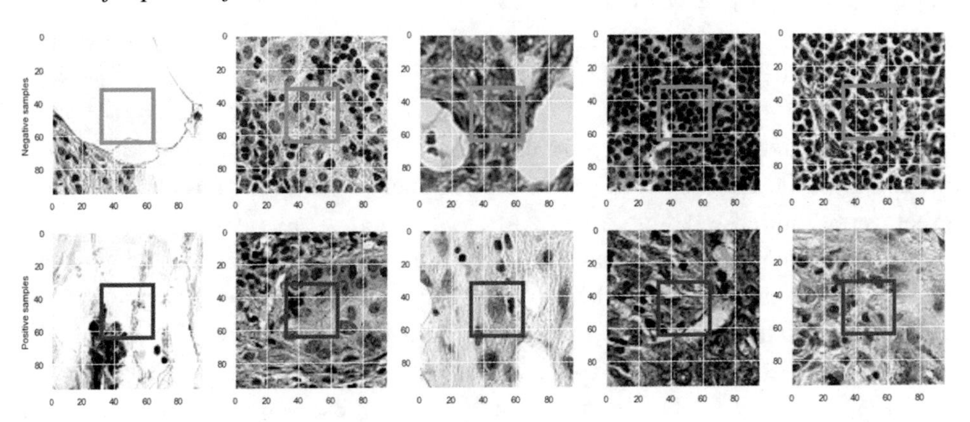

Training and Testing Parameters

We trained the models for about 24 hours for 100 epochs on the training and validation dataset from PCam histology patches. To avoid overfitting issue due to unbalance data sample selection, we have chosen 25000 patches from positive cancer cases and 25000 patches from negative cases of total 50000 samples for training. From this training samples, the splits for training-validation has done at 0.7: 0.3 ratio. Another overfitting avoiding strategy has done through data augmentation. Throughout training, a batch size of 64 used, and the schedule learning rate 0.00015. There a decay learning rate after 5 epochs was set via learning scheduler. If we start at a high learning rate our network model often diverges due to unstable gradients. During testing phase, we collected 2000 patch samples for each positive or negative cases.

Data Augmentation

An augmented patch dataset is created from the normalized patch images in the training set. Patch normalization is performed by subtracting mean values (0.485, 0.456, 0.406) and dividing standard deviation values (0.229, 0.224, 0.225) to the red, green and blue channels separately. For our low GPU memory issues, the finally used dataset has a low number of samples (i.e., cancer: 25000 and no cancer: 25000 and total: 50000). As consequence, the proposed model might be prone to overfit problem. The imbalanced classes can prevent efficient classification performance, however in our case we balanced between selections of class samples. To produce a proficient classification by addressing these two challenges, data augmentation procedures are essential.

Data augmentation through patch rotation by 20-degree, random horizontal flip with probability 0.4, random vertical flip with probability 0.4, pad with reflect mode, and lastly compose all further improves the dataset, and allow to extend the size of the dataset without deteriorating its quality. This is possible because the studied case is orientation invariant, i.e., breast cancer histological images can study by physicians from different directions without altering the diagnosis. Some example patches are shown in Fig. 3.

Evaluation Metric

Specificity (Spec), Precision (Pre), Recall (Rec), F1-score (F1), Matthews Correlation Coefficient MCC, and Accuracy (Acc) are employed as the assessment metric for classification and nuclei segmentation. The calculation formulas are shown in Eqs (1-5). Spec represents the truely negative classification or segmented nuclei rate, Acc represents the ratio of the truely positive classification or segmented nuclei and

Figure 3. Data Augmentation (a) original patch (b) pad with reflect mode (c) horizontal flip with probability 0.4 (d) vertical flip with probability 0.4 (e) rotation with 20 degree (f) compose of all.

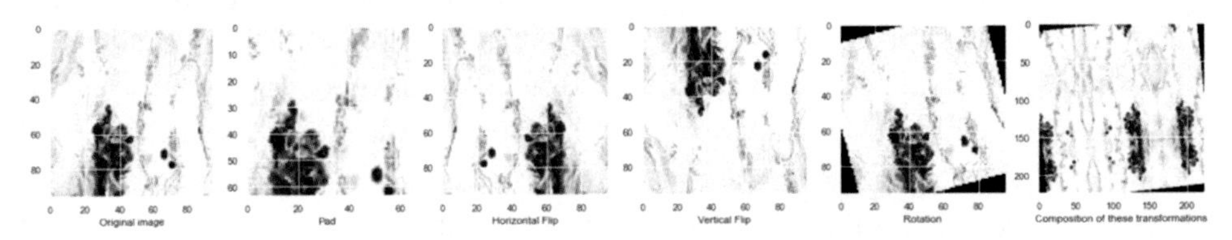

all the background pixels. Among the total amount of classification or segmented nuclei pixels, Precision represents the ratio of truley positive predictive classification or segmented nuclei in label images, and Rec represents the percentage of the total amount of nuclei pixels correctly classified or segmented in label images. F1-score value is used to estimate the harmonic average of the Prec and Rec. F1 could give a biased outcome since it doesn't include TN, and in such cases MCC is a perfect balance metric for evaluating performance. TP, TN, FP, and FN stand for true positive, true negative, false positive, and false negative respectively.

$$Spec = \frac{TN}{TN + FP} \tag{1}$$

$$Rec = \frac{TP}{TP + FN} \tag{2}$$

$$Pre = \frac{TP}{TP + FP} \tag{3}$$

$$F_1 = \frac{2 \times Pre \times Rec}{Pre + Rec} \tag{4}$$

$$MCC = \frac{TP \times TN - FP \times FN}{\sqrt{(TP + FP)(TP + FN)(TN + FP)(TN + FN)}} \tag{5}$$

Comparative Study of via Implementing Above Discussed Classification CNN Models

This section describes the test conducted to evaluate the performance of the comparative analysis over the existing well-known state-of-the-art models such as VGG, ResNet, AlexNet, MobileNet, GoogleNet, and DenseNet. The comparative analysis has done through best performing optimizer such as Adam and SGD in our case. Here we used receiver operating characteristics (ROC) curves that gives the area under the ROC curve (AUC) which is an efficiency measure of the histology patch image features classification.

In Fig. 4 (a), a ROC curve based comparative assessment has shown using Adam optimization strategy. In this case, the ResNet50 and MobileNet models demonstrated the highest accuracy ResNet50 (85%), and MobileNet (83%) models respectively. The AlexNet shows worst performance with covered area of 64% only. In Fig. 4 (b) i.e., based upon SGD+Momentum optimizer, the RestNet50 model also shows the highest performances of 85%, followed by the VGG16 (82%) model. Comparing the performances of Adam and SGD optimizers, it is observed that the performances of the Adagrad and Adadelta approaches gets decreases. Therefore, we haven't presented these two optimizer results.

In a disease diagnosis system, the higher AUC value indicates the better prediction accuracy of the system. Hence, by considering this fact, it can be concluded that the prediction performance of ResNet is better than the other CNN models in the PCam histological dataset.

Figure 4. The ROC curves for comparative evaluation of existing well-known classification state-of-the art models obtained using the PCam dataset. (a) Adam, (b) SGD+Momentum

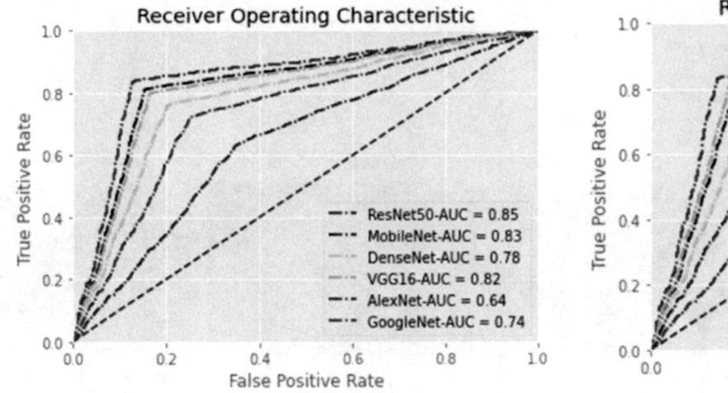

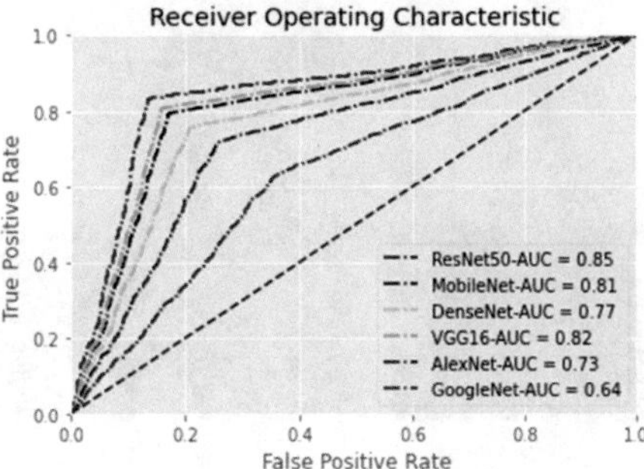

Nucleus Segmentation Performance on Data Science Bowl Dataset

This section is analyzing the performance and compare above discussed segmentation CNN models.

Brief Introduction to Dataset

For experimental evaluation, the 2018 Data Science Bowl (Kaggle, n.d.) has been chosen which consists of 37,333 manually annotated nuclei in 841 2D images from different samples. The nuclei are derived from several organisms including humans, mice, and flies. As well, nuclei have been captured in a variety of conditions such as stains of fluorescent and histology, color of tissues, several magnifications, and illumination effect variations. The training dataset consists of total 670 images along with ground-truth. We have not considered test dataset (total of 68 images) since it doesn't contain of ground-truth. From training dataset, we split 600 for training and rest 70 for testing. The dataset has imbalance distributions of samples of categorical nuclei, as shown in Figure 5.

Figure 5. Dataset sample distributions and variety of sample conditions (Caicedo et al., 2019)

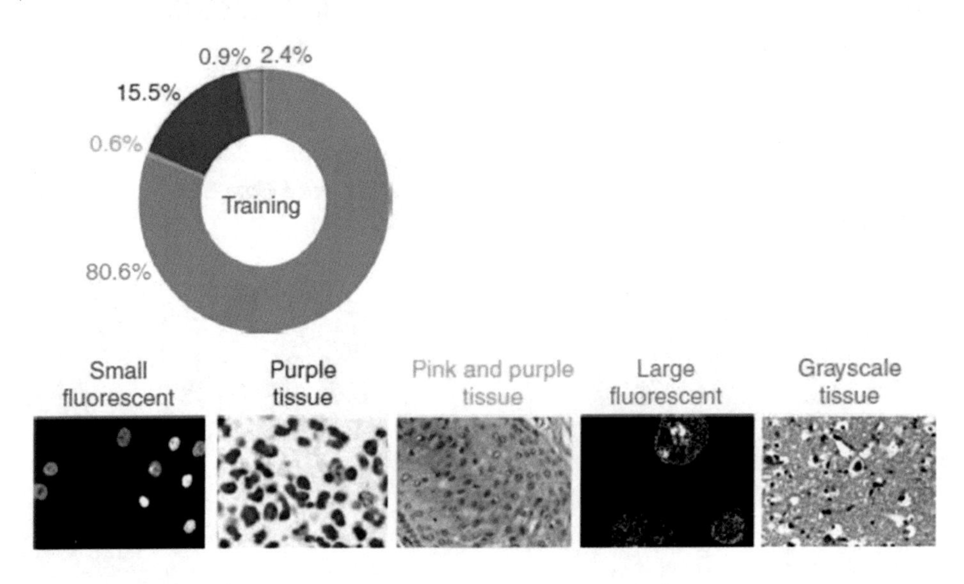

Data Augmentation

Since the used training dataset has a low number of samples, the segmentation CNN models might be prone to over-fit problem. To produce a proficient performance by addressing over-fitting challenge, data augmentation procedures are essential. Data augmentation through sample rotation by 50-degrees, shear with factor 0.5, zoom with factor 0.2, fill mode with reflect, and lastly shift by factor 0.2 both width and height. That allow to extend the size of the dataset without deteriorating its quality.

Training and Testing Parameters

We trained the segmentation-based CNN models for 20 epochs on the training dataset from 2018 Data Science Bowl nuclei images. From this training samples, the splits for training-validation has done at 0.9:0.1 ratio. The overfitting avoiding strategy has done through data augmentation. Throughout training, a batch size of 10 used, and the loss estimating is binary cross entropy. It has been noticed that when the iteration period is about 20, the validation loss/accuracy stops decreasing/increasing which means of leading to the training termination. In fact, the models start to get relatively decent performance when training after the few epochs.

Comparative Study of via Implementing Above Discussed Segmentation CNN Models

In this section, we analyse and compare U-Net (Ronneberger et al., 2015), PSPNet (Zhao et al., 2017), SegNet (Badrinarayanan, 2015), and FCN (Long et al., 2015) versions 8 and 16. All models have their own design of architectures whereas FCNs are used base model VGG for encoder.

Figure 6 shows the boxplots of F1-measure and MCC for all nuclei segmentation models. A boxplot is analysed through a given scores of test images with a specific prototypical five-number of definition summary such as the maximum (max), the minimum (min), the sample median (middle horizontal line), the first quartiles (q1), and third quartiles (q3). As in the figure shows, the FCN 8 and FCN 16 models have not any outliers on F1-score and one outliers on MCC values, however, both the models show lowest performance values of sample median, min, max, q1 and q3. U-Net and SegNet models has the approximately equal median F1-score and MCC, but F1-scores produces the higher number of outliers than MCC evaluation metric values. Whereas PSPNet model promising as a third best model in our comparative evaluation.

Figure 6. Boxplots of F1-score and MCC of the six nuclei segmentation models: (a) F1-score, and (b) MCC

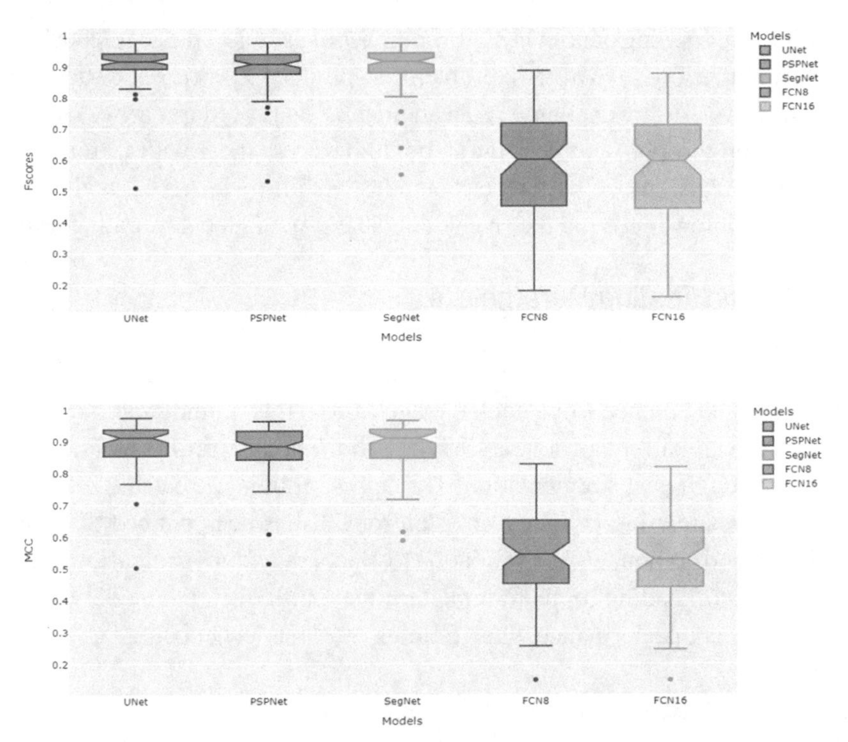

To provide a better visual understanding of the segmentation results, typical segmented outputs of nuclei from different categorical samples are shown in Figure 7 under various state-of-the-art models. In case of grayscale tissue samples, the PSPNet shows most favourable segmented output.

CONCLUSION

In this study, we have studied a Patch-based Histology Classification Networks for automatic classification of PCam breast histology dataset into two class, namely, no cancer and cancer. Finally, the classification models achieve considerable high accuracy and strong robustness. We are expecting these models to be clinically useful for doctors to achieve the early diagnosis of cancer patients. Secondly, this study also analyses deep convolutional encoder-decoder architectures for nuclei segmentation in microscopic pathological images. The 2018 Data Science Bowl dataset has used to demonstrate the segmentation models experimentation. In the process of model training, numerous optimizations have been analysed whereas adamax specified most promising results and improve the segmentation performance. From the comparative studies, it has been observed that grayscale tissue samples segmentation done more accurately by PSPNet.

Figure 7. Typical segmentation results of various nuclei samples from 2018 Data Science Bowl dataset. Column (1) shows original samples, column (2) shows ground-truth binary mask, column (3) shows segmented results under U-Net model, column (4) shows segmented results under PSPNet model, and last column shows segmented results under FCN-8 model.

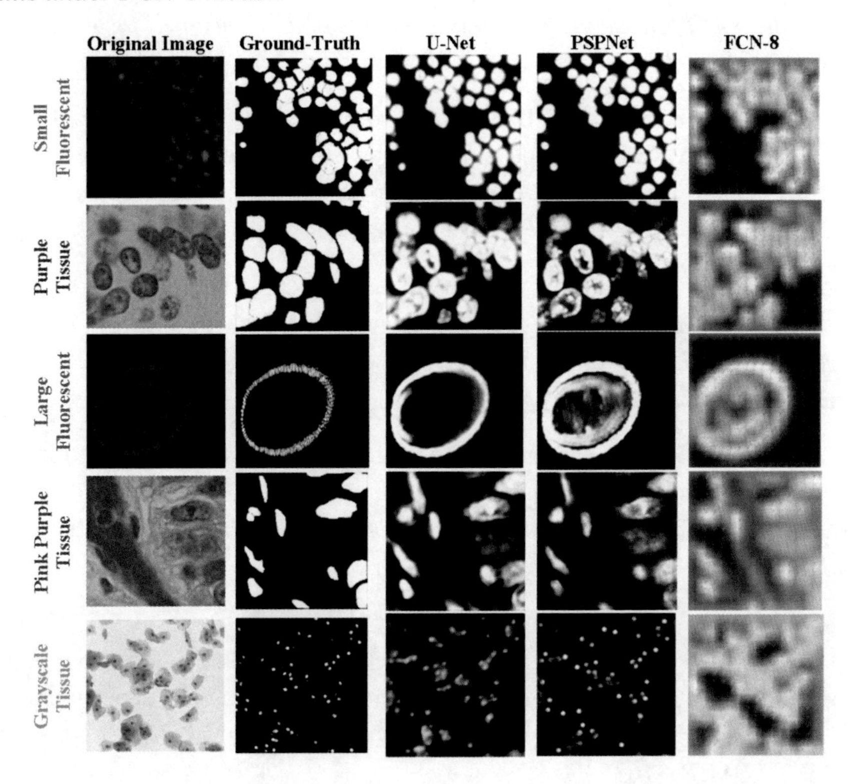

ACKNOWLEDGMENT

The work presented here is being conducted in the Sri Ramachandra Faculty of Engineering and Technology (SRET), Sri Ramachandra Institute of Higher Education and Research, Chennai, India. The authors would also like to thank V. Raju, Provost, SRET for his kind support to carry out this work.

REFERENCES

Abdel-Zaher, A. M., & Eldeib, A. M. (2016). Breast cancer classification using deep belief networks. *Expert Systems with Applications*, *46*, 139–144. doi:10.1016/j.eswa.2015.10.015

Araújo, T., Aresta, G., Castro, E., Rouco, J., Aguiar, P., Eloy, C., Polónia, A., & Campilho, A. (2017). Classification of breast cancer histology images using convolutional neural networks. *PLoS One*, *12*(6), e0177544. doi:10.1371/journal.pone.0177544 PMID:28570557

Badrinarayanan, V., Handa, A., & Cipolla, R. (2015). *SegNet: A deep convolutional encoder-decoder architecture for robust semantic pixel-wise labelling.* https://arxiv.org/abs/1505.07293

Basavanhally, A., Feldman, M. D., Shih, N., Mies, C., Tomaszewski, J.E., Ganesan, S., Madabhushi, A. (2011). Multi-field of view strategy for image-based outcome prediction of multiparametricestrogen receptor-positive breast cancer histopathology: Comparison to oncotype dx. *J Pathol Inform*, *2*(1).

Bejnordi, E. (2017). Diagnostic Assessment of Deep Learning Algorithms for Detection of Lymph Node Metastases in Women With Breast Cancer. *Journal of the American Medical Association*, *318*(22), 2199–2210. doi:10.1001/jama.2017.14585 PMID:29234806

Bejnordi, E., & .... (2017). Diagnostic Assessment of Deep Learning Algorithms for Detection of Lymph Node Metastases in Women With Breast Cancer. *Journal of the American Medical Association*, *318*(22), 2199–2210. doi:10.1001/jama.2017.14585 PMID:29234806

Caicedo, J. C., Goodman, A., Karhohs, K. W., Cimini, B. A., Ackerman, J., Haghighi, M., Heng, C. K., Becker, T., Doan, M., McQuin, C., Rohban, M., Singh, S., & Carpenter, A. E. (2019). Nucleus segmentation across imaging experiments: The 2018 Data Science Bowl. *Nature Methods*, *16*(12), 1247–1253. doi:10.103841592-019-0612-7 PMID:31636459

Cui, Y., Zhang, G., Liu, Z., Xiong, Z., & Hu, J. (2019). A deep learning algorithm for one-step contour aware nuclei segmentation of histopathology images. *Medical & Biological Engineering & Computing*, *57*(9), 2027–2043. doi:10.100711517-019-02008-8 PMID:31346949

Gandomkar, Z., Brennan, P. C., & Mello-Thoms, C. (2018). MuDeRN: Multicategory classification of breast histopathological image using deep residual networks. *Artificial Intelligence in Medicine*, *88*, 14–24. doi:10.1016/j.artmed.2018.04.005 PMID:29705552

Gurcan, M. N., Boucheron, L. E., Can, A., Madabhushi, A., Rajpoot, N. M., & Yener, B. (2009). Histopathological image analysis: A review. *IEEE Reviews in Biomedical Engineering*, *2*, 147–171. doi:10.1109/RBME.2009.2034865 PMID:20671804

Hassan, L., Saleh, A., Abdel-Nasser, M., Omer, O. A., & Puig, D. (2021). Promising Deep Semantic Nuclei Segmentation Models for Multi-Institutional Histopathology Images of Different Organs. *International Journal of Interactive Multimedia and Artificial Intelligence*, *6*(6), 35–45. doi:10.9781/ijimai.2020.10.004

He, K., Zhang, X., Ren, S., & Sun, J. (2016). Deep residual learning for image recognition. *Proc. IEEE Conf. Comput. Vis. Pattern Recognit. (CVPR)*, 770-778.

Hipp, J., Fernandez, A., Compton, C., & Balis, U. (2011). Why a pathology image should not be considered as a radiology image. *Journal of Pathology Informatics*, *2*(1), 26. doi:10.4103/2153-3539.82051 PMID:21773057

Howard, A. G., Zhu, M., & Chen, B. (2017). *Mobilenets: Efficient convolutional neural networks for mobile vision applications*. Academic Press.

Huang, G., Liu, Z., Van Der Maaten, L., & Weinberger, K. Q. (2017). Densely connected convolutional networks. *Proc. IEEE Conf. Comput. Vis. Pattern Recognit. (CVPR)*, 4700-4708.

Irshad, H., Veillard, A., Roux, L., & Racoceanu, D. (2013). Methods for nuclei detection, segmentation, and classication in digital histopathology: A review Current status and future potential. *IEEE Reviews in Biomedical Engineering*, *7*, 97–114. doi:10.1109/RBME.2013.2295804 PMID:24802905

Kaggle. (n.d.). *2018 Data Science Bowl*. https://www.kaggle.com/c/data-science-bowl-2018

Krizhevsky, A., Sutskever, I., & Hinton, G. E. (2017). ImageNet classification with deep convolutional neural networks. *Communications of the ACM*, *60*(6), 84–90. doi:10.1145/3065386

Lal, S., Das, D., Alabhya, K., Kanfade, A., Kumar, A., & Kini, J. (2021). NucleiSegNet: Robust Deep Learning Architecture for the Nuclei Segmentation of Liver Cancer Histopathology Images. *Computers in Biology and Medicine*, *128*, 128. doi:10.1016/j.compbiomed.2020.104075 PMID:33190012

Lee, J. (2017). Lee-deep learning in medical imaging_gen. *Medical, 18*, 570–584. PMID:28670152

Li, Y., Wu, J., & Wu, Q. (2019). Classification of Breast Cancer Histology Images Using Multi-Size and Discriminative Patches Based on Deep Learning. *IEEE Access: Practical Innovations, Open Solutions, 7*, 21400–21408. doi:10.1109/ACCESS.2019.2898044

Long, J., Shelhamer, E., & Darrell, T. (2015). Fully convolutional networks for semantic segmentation. *Proc. IEEE Conf. Comput. Vis. Pattern Recognit. (CVPR)*, 3431-3440.

Naylor, P., Laé, M., Reyal, F., & Walter, T. (2019). Segmentation of nuclei in histopathology images by deep regression of the distance map. *IEEE Transactions on Medical Imaging, 38*(2), 448–559. doi:10.1109/TMI.2018.2865709 PMID:30716022

Ng, E. Y. K. (2009). A review of thermography as promising non-invasive detection modality for breast tumor. *International Journal of Thermal Sciences, 48*(5), 849–859. doi:10.1016/j.ijthermalsci.2008.06.015

Pêgo, A., & Aguiar, P. (2015). Bioimaging. *4th International Symposium in Applied Bioimaging*. http://www.bioimaging2015.ineb.up.pt/dataset.html

Pickles, M. D., Gibbs, P., Hubbard, A., Rahman, A., Wieczorek, J., & Turnbull, L. W. (2015). Comparison of 3.0T magnetic resonance imaging and X-ray mammography in the measurement of ductal carcinoma in situ: A comparison with histopathology. *European Journal of Radiology, 84*(4), 603–610. doi:10.1016/j.ejrad.2014.12.016 PMID:25604907

Ronneberger, O., Fischer, P., & Brox, T. (2015). *U-net: Convolutional networks for biomedical image segmentation*. Available: https://arxiv.org/abs/1505.04597

Shah, S. (2020). Latest Statistics of Breast Cancer in India. *Breast Cancer India*. https://www.breastcancerindia.net/statistics/trends.html

Simonyan, K., & Zisserman, A. (2015). Very deep convolutional networks for large-scale image recognition. *Proc. Int. Conf. Learn. Represent. (ICLR)*, 1-14.

Singha, A., Bhowmik, M. K., & Bhattacherjee, D. (2020). Akin-based Orthogonal Space (AOS): A subspace learning method for face recognition. *Multimedia Tools and Applications, 79*(47-48), 35069–35091. doi:10.100711042-020-08892-9

Spanhol, F. A., Oliveira, L. S., Petitjean, C., & Heutte, L. (2016). Breast cancer histopathological image classification using convolutional neural networks. *Proc. Int. Joint Conf. Neural Netw. (IJCNN)*, 2560-2567. 10.1109/IJCNN.2016.7727519

Sun, J., & Binder, A. (2017). Comparison of deep learning architectures for H&E histopathology images. *Proc. IEEE Conf. Big Data Analytics (ICBDA)*, 43-48. 10.1109/ICBDAA.2017.8284105

Truong, T. D., & Pham, H. T. T. (2020). Breast cancer histopathological image classification utilizing convolutional neural network. *IFMBE Proceedings*, *69*, 531–536. doi:10.1007/978-981-13-5859-3_92

Vu, Q. D., Graham, S., Kurc, T., To, M. N. N., Shaban, M., Qaiser, T., Koohbanani, N. A., Khurram, S. A., Kalpathy-Cramer, J., Zhao, T., Gupta, R., Kwak, J. T., Rajpoot, N., Saltz, J., & Farahani, K. (2019). Methods for segmentation and classification of digital microscopy tissue images. *Frontiers in Bioengineering and Biotechnology*, *7*(53), 1–15. doi:10.3389/fbioe.2019.00053 PMID:31001524

Wang, D., Khosla, A., Gargeya, R., Irshad, H., & Beck, A. H. (2016). *Deep learning for identifying metastatic breast cancer*. Available: https://arxiv.org/abs/1606.05718

Wang, H., Xian, M., & Vakanski, A. (2020). Bending Loss Regularized Network for Nuclei Segmentation in Histopathology Images. *Proc. 2020 IEEE 17th International Symposium on Biomedical Imaging (ISBI)*, 1-5.

Wang, Y., Lei, B., Elazab, A., Tan, E.-L., Wang, W., Huang, F., Gong, X., & Wang, T. (2020). Breast Cancer Image Classification via Multi-Network Features and Dual-Network Orthogonal Low-Rank Learning. *IEEE Access: Practical Innovations, Open Solutions*, *8*, 27779–27792. doi:10.1109/ACCESS.2020.2964276

Xing, F., & Yang, L. (2016). Robust nucleus/cell detection and segmentation in digital pathology and microscopy images: A comprehensive review. *IEEE Reviews in Biomedical Engineering*, *9*, 234–263. doi:10.1109/RBME.2016.2515127 PMID:26742143

Xu, J., Xiang, L., Liu, Q., Gilmore, H., Wu, J., Tang, J., & Madabhushi, A. (2016). Stacked sparse autoencoder (SSAE) for nuclei detection on breast cancer histopathology images. *IEEE Transactions on Medical Imaging*, *35*(1), 119–130. doi:10.1109/TMI.2015.2458702 PMID:26208307

Yari, Y., Nguyen, T. V., & Nguyen, H. T. (2020). Deep Learning Applied for Histological Diagnosis of Breast Cancer. *IEEE Access: Practical Innovations, Open Solutions*, *8*, 162432–162448. doi:10.1109/ACCESS.2020.3021557

Yasmin, M., Sharif, M., & Mohsin, S. (2013). Survey paper on diagnosis of breast cancer using image processing techniques. *Research Journal of Recent Sciences*, *2*, 8898.

Zeng, G., He, Y., Yu, Z., Yang, X., Yang, R., & Zhang, L. (2015). Going deeper with convolutions Christian. *Proc. IEEE Conf. Comput. Vis. Pattern Recognit. (CVPR)*, 1-9.

Zhao, H., Shi, J., Qi, X., Wang, X., & Jia, J. (2017). Pyramid scene parsing network. *Proc. IEEE Conf. Comput. Vis. Pattern Recognit.*, 2881-2890.

ADDITIONAL READING

Ailiang, L., Bingzhi, C., Jiayu, X., Zheng, Z., Guangming, L., & David, Z. (2022). DS-TransUNet: Dual Swin Transformer U-Net for Medical Image Segmentation. *IEEE Transactions on Instrumentation and Measurement*, *71*, 4005615.

Irshad, H., Veillard, A., Roux, L., & Racoceanu, D. (2013). Methods for nuclei detection, segmentation, and classification in digital histopathology: A review Current status and future potential. *IEEE Reviews in Biomedical Engineering*, *7*, 97–114. doi:10.1109/RBME.2013.2295804 PMID:24802905

Kang, Q., Lao, Q., & Fevens, T. (2019). Nuclei segmentation in histopathological images using two-stage learning. In D. Shen (Ed.), *Medical Image Computing and Computer Assisted Intervention* (pp. 703–711). Lecture Notes in Computer Science. Springer. doi:10.1007/978-3-030-32239-7_78

Kong, Y., Genchev, G. Z., Wang, X., Zhao, H., & Lu, H. (2020). Nuclear Segmentation in Histopathological Images Using Two-Stage Stacked U-Nets With Attention Mechanism. *Frontiers in Bioengineering and Biotechnology*, *8*, 573866. doi:10.3389/fbioe.2020.573866 PMID:33195135

Lagree, A., Mohebpour, M., Meti, N., Saednia, K., Lu, F.-I., Slodkowska, E., Gandhi, S., Rakovitch, E., Shenfield, A., Sadeghi-Naini, A., & Tran, W. T. (2021). A review and comparison of breast tumor cell nuclei segmentation performances using deep convolutional neural networks. *Scientific Reports*, *11*(1), 8025. doi:10.103841598-021-87496-1 PMID:33850222

Li, X., Chen, H., Qi, X., Dou, Q., Fu, C.-W., & Heng, P.-A. (2018). H-denseUnet: Hybrid densely connected unet for liver and tumor segmentation from ct volumes. *IEEE Transactions on Medical Imaging*, *37*(12), 2663–2674. doi:10.1109/TMI.2018.2845918 PMID:29994201

Singha, A., & Bhowmik, M. K. (2020). Salient Features for Moving Object Detection in Adverse Weather Conditions during Night Time. *IEEE Transactions on Circuits and Systems for Video Technology*, *30*(10), 3317–3331. doi:10.1109/TCSVT.2019.2926164

Ukwuoma, C. C., Hossain, M. A., Jackson, J. K., Nneji, G. U., Monday, H. N., & Qin, Z. (2022). Multi-Classification of Breast Cancer Lesions in Histopathological Images Using DEEP_Pachi: Multiple Self-Attention Head. *Diagnostics (Basel)*, *12*(5), 1152. doi:10.3390/diagnostics12051152 PMID:35626307

Umer, M. J., Sharif, M., Kadry, S., & Alharbi, A. (2022). Multi-Class Classification of Breast Cancer Using 6B-Net with Deep Feature Fusion and Selection Method. *Journal of Personalized Medicine*, *12*(5), 683. doi:10.3390/jpm12050683 PMID:35629106

Veta, M., Pluim, J. P. W., Diest, P. J. V., & Viergever, M. A. (2014). Breast cancer histopathology image analysis: A review. *IEEE Transactions on Biomedical Engineering*, *61*(5), 1400–1411. doi:10.1109/TBME.2014.2303852 PMID:24759275

KEY TERMS AND DEFINITIONS

Classification CNN Models: Classification CNN models that classify each pixel to identify what is in an image. For example, VGG, ResNet, and AlexNet.

Data Augmentation: These are techniques which is used to increase the amount of image/data by adding slightly transformed/modified copies of already existing images/data or newly created synthetic images/data from existing images/data.

Histopathology: Histopathology is a microscopic examination of a biopsy specimen that is processed onto glass slides. This examination diagnoses the signs of the cancer disease.

Invasive Cancer: The invasive breast cancers may have spread within the breast only, or to nearby lymph nodes. They may have spread to distant body parts.

Metastatic Cancer: The metastatic breast cancers have spread outside of the breast and nearby lymph nodes to distant body parts.

Nuclei: The nuclei of a cancer tissues are larger and darker than that of a normal tissue. Another feature of the nucleus of a cancer tissue is that after being stained with certain dyes, it appears darker when seen under an optical microscope.

Segmentation CNN Models: Segmentation CNN models provide the exact outline of the region of objects, i.e., pixel by pixel details are provided for given objects in an image. For example, U-Net and PSPNet.

Chapter 3
Artificial Intelligence Based on IoT for Healthcare

Supriya M. S.
https://orcid.org/0000-0003-3465-6879
Ramaiah University of Applied Sciences, India

Vismaya K. J.
Ramaiah University of Applied Sciences, India

Ramya B. N.
Ramaiah University of Applied Sciences, India

Nikil Kumar P.
Torry Harris Business Solutions, India

ABSTRACT

In fields like healthcare, where human intelligence is critical, the introduction of new AI-powered applications is becoming increasingly popular. Technologies have reduced expenses, accelerated drug research, and improved wellness outcomes. AI has become increasingly cognizant of its potential to disrupt the business, as seen by growing funding for the sector in recent years from important stakeholders in both healthcare and risk capital. Traditional approaches include human participation and direct interaction with patients, which are now obsolete due to the advancement of technologies such as messaging bots and intelligent virtual assistants. On the other hand, the internet of things (IoT) is making significant contributions to healthcare, and its gadgets may collect complete health data. Machine intelligence collects and analyses data in established protocols in search of possible health-related predictions. The chapter delves into the aspects of combining AI and IoT to improve efficiency in healthcare systems.

DOI: 10.4018/978-1-6684-4405-4.ch003

INTRODUCTION AND BACKGROUND

We refer to ourselves as Humans (Homo sapiens), or "man the wise because intelligence is so vital to us," For thousands of years, scientists have been trying to figure out how we think: how a small amount of stuff can observe, analyse, foresee, and manage a cosmos far larger and more intricate than its own. Artificial Intelligence (AI) enters the picture at this point.

Healthcare, also known as healthcare, is the science of sickness, disease, damage, and other mentally and physically problems in humans by avoiding, detecting, treating, healing from, or curing them. Hospitals, clinics, and community health agencies are all quite different places to work. Healthcare systems are complicated, and we need to understand a variety of topics such as hospital kinds, patient care, insurance, healthcare providers, and legal concerns. This lesson will assist you in learning essential healthcare ideas so that you may succeed at work and comprehend the system.

AI aims to understand as well as construct intelligent beings. AI is a science and engineering field that is still in its infancy. The phrase was coined in 1956, shortly after work began in earnest following World War II. AI is commonly mentioned as the "area I'd most like to be in" by scientists from various areas, in addition to molecular biology. Any physics student would be forgiven for thinking that Galileo, Newton, Einstein, and the others had already figured everything out. However, this AI has positions available for several full-time Einsteins and Edisons. By putting a greater emphasis on digital transformation, more enterprises are being pushed to undertake projects driven by the IoT. These efforts allow businesses to improve consumer experience, generate new business channels, or build new partner ecosystems.

However, acquiring insights might make it difficult to realize these benefits. The sheer volume of data generated by these devices, the diversity of data that comes in, and the speed at which data is collected have posed challenges for businesses in terms of storage, processing power, and analytics.

IoT is growing at a breakneck pace across all industries, but businesses in each confront their own set of obstacles along the way. Enterprises may utilize prescriptive and predictive analytics to make well-informed choices by using all the massive data created by IoT devices and using machine learning models.

SIGNIFICANCE OF ARTIFICIAL INTELLIGENCE AND IOT

In the previous 20 years, artificial intelligence has made significant progress. This AI has established itself as a realistic approach for synthesizing and obtaining cognition. Furthermore, personified AI is now thought to avoid or successfully address many of the basic issues that standard AI faces. Even if there are considerable variations between these criticisms, they all agree on the fact that these systems are simply computational. Without this feature, it is impossible to argue that these systems know what they are doing; they do not examine their criteria. To put it another way, all of this advice is a variant on the challenge of how to build an artificial system in such a way that connected elements of the environment appear as relevant from the viewpoint of the system itself, rather than only from the viewpoint of the human creator or observer.

From periodic to unremitting, from illness to wellbeing and reliability, and from doctor's office to wherever a patient is, clinician-managed to patient-authorized, and restricted data to complete angle, multimodal private public population physical cyber social big data driven, the process has changed dramatically. It is all this healthcare, and this AI has more application in this healthcare (Froese & Ziemke, 2009). Artificial intelligence (AI) has also become entangled with what is termed Tran humanism (TH). AI is conceived and focused upon (with some comment on TH) (Morgan, 2018).

In recent years, data has emerged as a critical source of intelligence, and smart applications are bringing new possibilities to real-world problems including wireless communications, genetics, agriculture, and finance. It is simpler to do the intended task since these applications demand data and offer actionable insights about the user experience. Its operation integrates data, personalizes the customer experience, enhances customer connections, boosts operative effectiveness, and enables new business models (Vashistha et al., 2019).

The range of keen applications that make life simpler, like SG, UAV, and Smart Cities. These applications generate a large quantity of data, which is difficult to store in a database. Furthermore, its transmission creates security problems. To overcome these obstacles, the use of BT, that has a distributed database network, came into play. Satoshi Nakamoto created the term in 2008, and it refers to a moment sequence of vandal documents that are controlled by a group of computers. It is made up of a number of blocks that are linked together using schema in cryptography. Immutability, decentralization, and transparency are the three pillars of BT. these three qualities may be found in a wide range of applications. Consider the presence of digital currency (currency that does not have a physical form) and the study of its appropriateness in smart applications (Vashistha et al., 2019).

IoT has been more industrialized in recent years, and it now has more applications in smart phones and smart cities, making human existence more secure. Sensors will create a huge amount of sensing data as industrialization grows in the IoT.AI plays a critical role in big data analysis as a powerful analytic device that provides scalable and precise data analysis in true. However, AI applied in there are several shortcomings in the development and design of a viable big data analytical tool, including centralized approach, privacy and security, resource limitations, and a lack of training data.

Block chain, on the other hand, as a new technology, supports a decentralized architecture. It encourages the removal of centralized management and can overcome the current AI difficulties by providing a safe distribution of information and services to the network's numerous nodes (Singh et al., 2020).

IoT systems store massive volumes of data collected from sensors all around us. Deep Learning is one of the methods we employ to extract meaningful information from these data. The combination of IoT and deep learning opens many opportunities for exploring the actual world (Zhou et al., 2019).

NEED FOR AI AND IoT IN HEALTHCARE

Not only IoT application in healthcare promises to compute their daily workflow operations but also to improve patients' treatment standard and contentment. To head medical inventory, track patients and assets IoT technologies can be used. The idea of digital medication (pills) is another recent application of IoT in healthcare, applied for oncology and psychiatric treatment. An IoT infrastructure gives connectivity needed to the healthcare system infrastructure. Healthcare stakeholders have smooth connectivity and transmission made by the IoT healthcare ecosystem. IoT devices may aid in the possession, monitoring, tracking, and storage of important medical and health data through this seamless connectivity, allowing doctors to give patients with more accurate diagnoses and high-quality treatment (Zeadallyet & Bello, 2021).

Artificial intelligence (AI) is becoming a norm in healthcare, thanks to the rising adequacy of healthcare data and the fast improvement of analysed tools. Health risk alarm and prediction can be triggered by real-time findings, an artificial intelligence system collects useful data from a large patient population. Many forms of healthcare data, both structured and unstructured, are processed using AI systems. Neural networks, the classic support vector machine, and however, natural language processing is a common AI tool for unstructured data. AI is used in critical illness areas like as cancer, neurology, and cardiology (Jiang et al., 2017).

One of the newest artificial intelligence benefits is machine learning. Because of its successful expansion in biomedical sciences, tools for developing innovative modelling and prediction approaches for clinical application are created (Jiang et al., 2017).

HEALTH CARE SERVICES REALIZED WITH IoT CONCEPT

The present common healthcare services that are recognized with IoT principles include obtaining similar medical data for patients' observation to monitor progress and assisting outpatients in adhering to treatment advice and the usage of suggested drugs. Assistive living, mobile health, and in-home healthcare are further options. The cost of IoT-based healthcare solutions is expected to reach $1 trillion by 2025, according to some forecasts. It is hoped that this method would allow the healthcare business will concentrate its efforts. On other aspects of health that require greater, allowing everyone to receive up-to-date, personalized, accessible, and timely treatment. Healthcare also makes use of a variety of data standards to facilitate communication across processes, employees and equipment. Data document merits, message quality, data excellence, and process value, which might be based on relationships, classifications, purposes, semantics, or syntax, are examples. One such benefit is Health Level 7 (HL7), which is a part of the Information Portability and accountability Act (HIPAA) as well as the Fast Health Interoperability Resource (FHIR) .Finally, there are a variety of country-specific healthcare processes and tactics that must be followed while creating and implementing an IoT-based healthcare system(Zeadallyet & Bello, 2021).The most powerful way to answer present problems is the process of developing biosensors using AI or next- generation biosensors.

Figure 1. AI in Medical Wearable Devices.

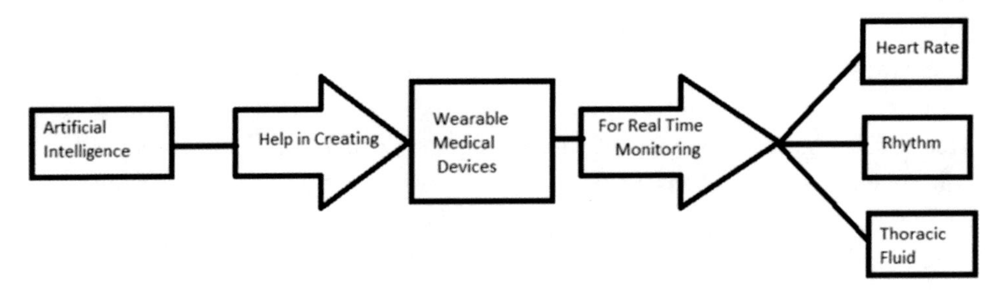

Figure 1 depicts the application of artificial intelligence (AI) to monitor real-time medical issues utilizing wearable medical equipment. Wearable technologies, such as those designed for cardiac disease, big data and the IoT are also on the rise, have the potential to transform healthcare (IoT) (Abie, 2019).

AI-Assisted IoT-Based Healthcare Solutions

A Virtual Assistant for Personal Health An artificial intelligence (AI) system is being used to help and improve assisted living. When patients are outside of the hospital, AI systems act as personal coaches, encouraging them to make specific decisions that are beneficial to their health. To analyse a patient's current mental state, artificial intelligence (AI) systems can issue prescription reminders and use human-like interactions. When clinical healthcare practitioners are absent, monitoring patients' behaviour and issuing proactive warnings to the patients' physicians and clinical professionals is also useful. Other applications of AI include remote surgery, personalized medical therapies for individual patients, and the detection of anomalies in radiographic results (Jiang et al., 2017).

Design Architectures for IoT in Healthcare

It is impossible to overestimate the benefits of investing in various forms of technology to improve healthcare delivery systems. It is critical that all networked systems and devices in the healthcare setting have a robust connection. There have been various recently proposed designs to leverage IoT basic technologies for improved administration and delivery of healthcare services. The architectures of these services differ from one service to the next. This includes defining the aim and targeted healthcare solution for each architecture, in addition to the architectural design components and their operations, together with the service functions that they must support. Information about an alert or warning is sent through notification. Other functional features include Internet connectivity and device identification and connection. When it comes to delivering tailored healthcare solutions and objectives, the IoT architecture relies on several functional services. As a consequence, an IoT-based healthcare system will be developed. There is a significant priority placed on internet connections, device identification and connectivity as well as streaming in real time, analytics and security services. These services may be provided at a cheap cost by leveraging IoT principles and technologies (Zeadallyet & Bello, 2021).

Intelligent Coaching Systems for Healthcare

There has been a fast increase in the number of people, and certain chronic conditions necessitate patients to get continuing medical treatment to aid in their recovery, making home healthcare and rehabilitation IoT architecture increasingly important. Patients with chronic illnesses like dementia and Alzheimer's require care at home. By allowing the creation of coaching systems, the IoT ecosystem has the power to offer high-quality healthcare solutions. Such systems can utilize the information gathered to allocate patients to physically demanding activities in order to keep their health in check. Patients with dementia can benefit from coaching systems since they can maintain and stimulate their mental and physical abilities, as well as sleep better at night. They encourage the patient to remain active and to engage in activities that will help them be energized and active so that they may live as naturally as possible. These mentoring systems that are premised on supercomputing cognitive examples of human memory, help people improve their performance, have the potential to enhance patients' daily life when linked to the Internet of Things idea. Patients with cognitive impairment benefit from the architecture's ability to detect and respond to a wide range of activities, from potentially hazardous situations to abnormal patient behaviour. In addition to memory problems, anxiety and psychotic symptoms, sleep and waking cycle irregularities can also contribute to aberrant behaviour. The components of the cognitive architecture process and interpret data collected from devices. The architecture employs frameworks that replicate the brain's structure and encourage research into how the mind functions. This architecture's healthcare objective is to provide advice and counselling to cognition-impaired individuals. Tutoring patients to avoid taking wrong behaviours is the overall service given. (Zeadallyet & Bello, 2021)

FUTURE IoT HEALTHCARE OPPORTUNITIES

As a result of IoT assistance in healthcare, physicians and health professionals will be able to respond promptly and efficiently to patients' medical requirements, either remotely or face to face, allowing for early treatment and high-quality care.

Public Health

As a result, every government that is in the health care industry considers public health to be a major priority. When used in big data technology in combination and robust predictive analytics algorithms, the Internet of Things can help to enhance public health management by capturing and analysing data.

Remote Surgery

It allows for the delivery of high-quality healthcare to underserved communities where surgical treatment is unavailable. Remote surgery offers the ability to allow healthcare surgical specialists from across the world to cooperate successfully on an operation without having to meet in person. There are several technologies that allow IoT-based remote surgeries to be carried out. Basic remote surgery places the patient and the surgeon in separate locations. The surgical specialist keeps track of every move and action of tele-surgical robot using a dedicated dashboard, allowing him to operate and monitor the surgical robots from afar. It may take some time for remote surgery that combines complex surgical procedures to completely integrate into the healthcare system. A full-fledged IoT ecosystem with comprehensive security services, on the other hand, may assist provide accurate and dependable surgical operations at any time, wherever on the planet.

Patient Participation that Lasts

Patients seldom participate actively in their own treatment plans. Furthermore, people who use wearable devices to monitor their vital signs do not get a unified and integrated view of all the data they collect.IoT technology can push healthcare providers to embrace data standards that allow diverse data sources to be integrated. Implementing the proper data standard is critical to managing chronic illnesses remotely or using predictive analytics. This allows care professionals to easily communicate with patients and urge them to stick to their treatment regimens. Finally, a unified picture of data from several sources would aid in providing high-quality, cost-effective healthcare. (Zeadallyet & Bello, 2021)

Treatments and Services at the Hospital

Patients can benefit from an IoT platform with AI that is well-integrated,that can provide them with efficient and precise health care. Automated prescriptions, drug distribution, and auto diagnostic are examples of these services. Patients may book appointments, get prescriptions, view billing information, and get an automated diagnosis by interacting directly with an always-available system. As a result, healthcare organizations will save money on administrative and operational expenditures. (Zeadallyet & Bello,2021).

Towards an Artificial Intelligence Framework for Data-driven Prediction of Coronavirus Clinical Severity

The virus SARS-CoV, which causes coronavirus illness (COVID-19), has spread to every inhabited continent and has become a pandemic. Given the growing caseload, there is a pressing need to improve clinical abilities in order to distinguish between the numerous moderate cases. This study offers a preliminary assessment of Artificial Intelligence (AI) in relation to COVID-19. (Jiang, Xiangao & Coffee, Megan & Bari, Anasse & Wang, Junzhang & Jiang, Xinyue & Huang, Jianping &

Shi, Jichan & Dai, Jianyi & Cai, Jing & Zhang, Tianxiao & Wu, Zhengxing & He, Guiqing & Huang, Yitong. (2020).)

AI BASED ON IoT TECHNIQUES USED IN HEALTHCARE

The IoT offers a wide range of applications in sectors such as information technology and smart and linked health care, the latter of which is particularly important. The utilization of networked sensors may be employed to bring about a positive transformative shift in the health care background by using our physical and mental health data. This allows monitoring to reach those who otherwise would not have easy access to a reliable health monitoring system. The recorded information or data may then be evaluated using various machine learning algorithms or processes, and then shared with medical experts through wireless connectivity, who can then make appropriate recommendations. These criteria currently exist, but we should aim to enhance them by analysing historical data in order to forecast future difficulties using narrow analytics. This would enable us to shift from a reactive to a proactive strategy by detecting patterns immediately and making recommendations on behalf of the real medical care provider. The technology will be able to provide drive suggestions based on historical and experience data stored in the cloud. The authors developed a methodology for uncovering knowledge in a data base by shedding light on hidden patterns that might aid in making trustworthy judgments. Experiments that are carried out with the help of a few machine learning algorithms or stages (Kaur et al., 2019).

Neural Networks and Deep Learning

The statistical approach of fitting models to data to improve from them is known as machine learning (ML).

It is one of the most common forms of AI; according to a Deloitte study performed in 2018, 1,100 US managers whose company's stayed exploring AI, 63 percent of the companies surveyed were using machine learning in their operations.

Personalized medicine, which forecasts which therapeutic approaches are likely to function well on a patient based on numerous patient characteristics and treatment experiences, is the most prevalent use of classical ML in healthcare. The majority of machine learning and accurate medicine applications need supervised learning, which necessitates the use of a training dataset with a predetermined end variable.

In Figure 2, machine learning methods are employed in medical literature. The information was gathered by searching PubMed for machine learning algorithms in healthcare (Davenport & Kalakota, 2019).

Figure 2. Machine Learning in Literature

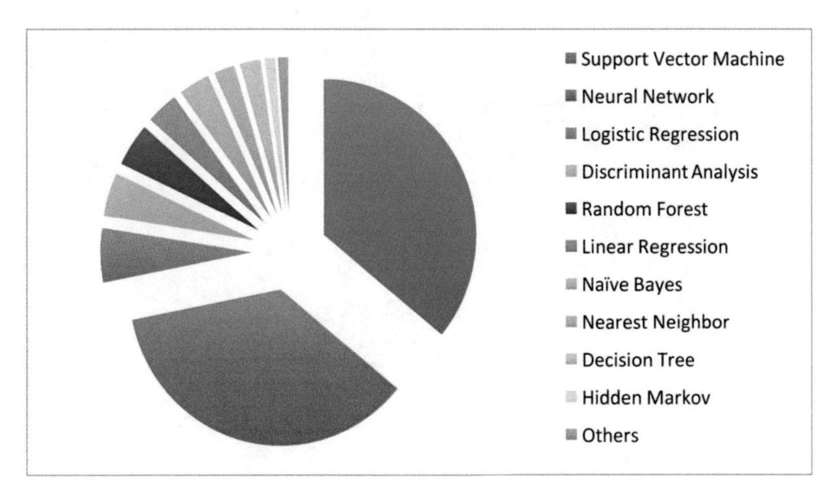

Support Vector Machine

SVM is mostly worn to divide patients into two groups, with Yi as a classifier: Yi = 1 or 1 denotes the ith patient belongs to group 1 or group 2. The main notion is that utilizing a decision boundary, the subjects may be divided into two groups depending on Xij characteristics.

That can be written as:

$$a_i = \sum_{i=1}^{p} w_j X_{ij} + b$$

Equation 1(Davenport & Kalakota, 2019).

Neural networks have been used for categorization applications like predicting whether a patient would acquire a certain ailment since the 1960s. They've also had a lengthy history in medical study, where they've been utilized for things like forecasting whether a patient would acquire a certain ailment. It considers the weights of variables or "features" that connect inputs and outputs, as well as the inputs and outputs themselves. Though the similarity to brain function isn't particularly great, it has been likened to how neurons perceive impulses.

In order to diagnose strokes, Mirtskhulava et colleagues employed a neural network. p=16 shot complaints are the input parameters Xi 1,..., Xip, such as arm or leg par aesthesia, acute disorientation, visual difficulties, mobility problems, and so on. Yi is a binary outcome: Yi =1/0 denotes whether or not the ith patient has

Figure 3. Support Vector Machine Illustration
(Davenport & Kalakota, 2019)

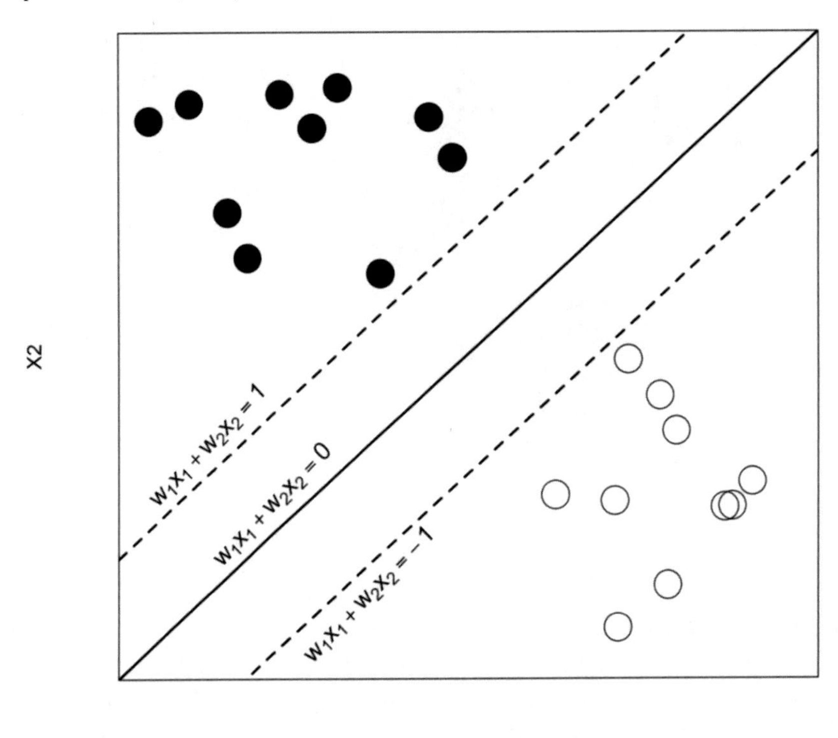

had a stroke. The probability of a stroke, ai, is the output parameter of interest is (Davenport & Kalakota, 2019)

$$a_i = h\left\{\sum_{k=1}^{D} w_{2l} f_k \left(\sum_{l=1}^{p} w_{1l} X_{il} + w_{10}\right) + w_{20}\right\}$$

Equation 2 (Davenport & Kalakota, 2019).

Natural Language Processing

AI experts have been working on understanding human language since the 1950s. Speech recognition, text analysis, translation, and additional language-related goals are among the applications covered by NLP. NLP may be divided into two types: statistical and semantic. Statistical natural language processing is based on ML and

Figure 4. Illustration of Neural Network
(Davenport & Kalakota, 2019).

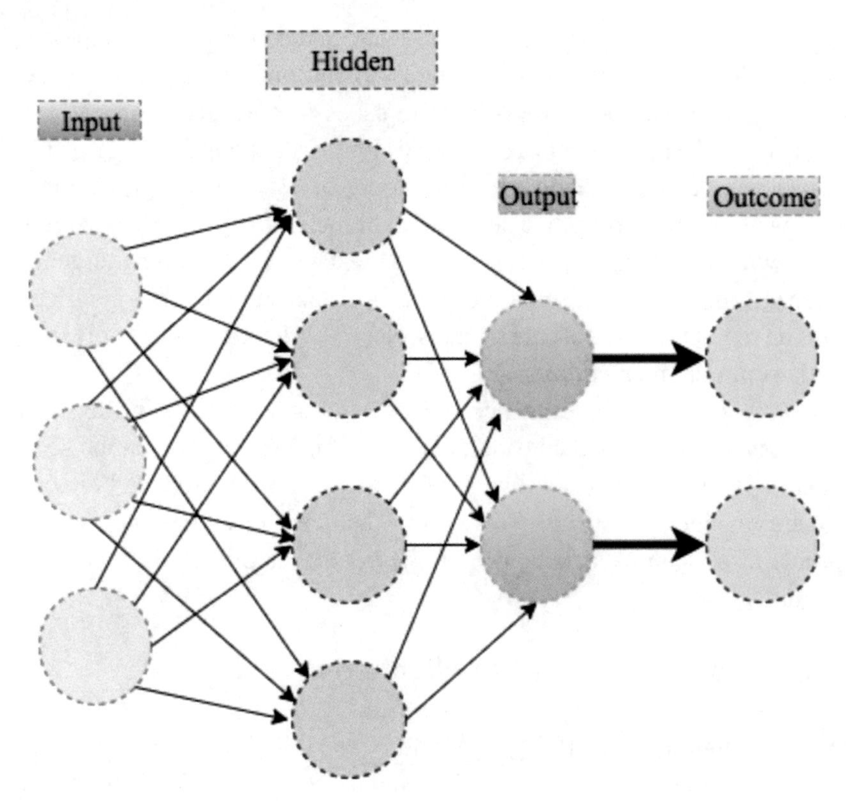

has recently improved recognition accuracy. Learning from a large 'corpus,' or body of language, is required (Davenport & Kalakota, 2019).

NLP systems can transcribe patient interactions, evaluate unstructured patient healthcare data, create reports (for example, on radiological diagnoses), and conduct conversational AI (Davenport & Kalakota, 2019).

AI Applications in Stroke

Atherosclerosis is a frequent and often fatal illness that causes more than 500 million individuals throughout the world. This is China's leading cause of death, and North America's sixth largest cause. Stroke has price the worldwide economy $689 billion in medical expenditures, placing governments and households under hardship. 46 47 As a result, stroke prevention and treatment research is critical. A growing number of stroke-related research have incorporated AI approaches in recent years(Jiang et al., 2017).

AI In Public Healthcare

The application of AI in public healthcare is one of the most promising fields. While acceptance has been slow, usage is steadily rising, thanks in part to the potential cost savings that may be realized if AI replaces face-to-face contacts, which are fundamental to healthcare service delivery (Jung &Padman, 2015). AI is predicted to change the healthcare industry in a variety of ways. This application utilizes both a real and virtual branch. The physical branch mostly intersects with robotics research, which is utilised to assist geriatric patients or accompanying surgeons. Deep learning information management research is a virtual area Artificial intelligence that focuses on regulating patient care systems, electronic health, and actively supporting physicians in treatment choices.

The use of artificial intelligence (AI) technologies to aid clinicians in patient diagnosis has lately gained considerable scientific interest. The public sector's AI research is in early stages, and much of it focuses on the predicted effects of AI, which are mainly theoretical at this point. The need for empirical descriptions of AI problems as seen by stakeholders in the public sector who deal with it (Sun & Medaglia, 2019).

Diagnosis and Treatment Applications

Since its inception in the 1970s at Stanford, MYCIN has been utilized to detect blood-borne bacterial infections. AI has mainly concentrated on illness diagnosis and therapy.8 Despite showing promise in terms of accurately diagnosing and treating sickness, these and other early rule-based systems were not taken into clinical practice. Their methods and medical record systems were inefficient, and they were no better than human diagnosticians.

Watson is a suite of "cognitive services" supplied by application programming interfaces (APIs) that include voice and language, visual, and data-analysis programmers, all of which are based on machine learning. According to most experts, the Watson APIs are theoretically viable, but tackling cancer treatment was an overly ambitious objective. Competition from free "open source" solutions, like as Google's Tensor Flow, has damaged Watson and other commercial programmers (Davenport & Kalakota, 2019).

The IoT idea offers several potentials for remote health monitoring systems. Because they are life- or mission-critical, these systems must provide a high level of access and precision. On the one side, centralized cloud based IoT solutions have issues with punctuality, reliability, and availability (for example, in the event of a delayed or uncertain Internet access), and on the other side, these systems fully outsource data analytics to the network's edge due to insufficient computational capacity in edge nodes, resulting in decreased accuracy and adaptability (Abie, 2019).

Creating a revolutionary computer architecture, a shuttered control strategies enabling of autonomous system changes based on patient condition and implementing machine learning-based data analytics (Abie, 2019).

HiCH provides a customized management technique based on the characteristics available in both fog and cloud computing, as well as for healthcare IoT devices. HiCH's performance was calculated and evaluated in a persistent remote health monitoring case study focusing on arrhythmia detection in patients with cardiovascular diseases (CVDs) (Abie, 2019).

Personalized Healthcare (PH) is a brand-new patient-cantered healthcare strategy that aims to improve the current system. The new development is cantered on the patient information that has been gathered. Electronic health records include Internet of Things (IoT) sensing tools, wearable and mobile devices, web-based information, and social media (EHR). PH analyses data to improve disease progression protocols, illness prognosis, self - regulation and self, and medical treatment using Artificial Intelligence (AI) approaches. Analytic models are typically built using ml techniques. These models are employed in a number of medical judgement systems and healthcare applications. In order to determine the patient's behavioural patterns and clinical concerns, several models evaluate data acquired from these sensor devices and other sources (Ahamed & Farid, 2018).

These models, for example, analyse the collected data to discover changes in the patient's daily routine, habits, and anomalies, as well as changes in sleeping and activity patterns, as well as eating, drinking, and digestion processes. Based on these trends, healthcare apps and decision support tools provide lifestyle counselling, customised therapy, and care plans for patients. Doctors and caregivers may be consulted during the formulation of the treatment regimen to confirm lifestyle recommendations. When ML gets implemented in this environment, however, there are numerous unknowns and grey areas. In nature, clinical, behavioural, and lifestyle data are extremely sensitive. Different forms of bias might be present during the data gathering and interpretation process. It's possible that the dataset used in the training data model is an older version. All of this might lead to the system making an erroneous choice without the user's knowledge (Ahamed & Farid, 2018).

In biomedicine and health-care technologies, the Internet of Things (IoT) and big data analytics revolutions have opened new opportunities. Further developing advances in robotics health care telemedicine employing artificial intelligence techniques have been discussed. The literature shows that AI-based telemedicine's flexibility and adaptability give limitless assistance for health care improvement. The status of the Internet of Robotic Things (IoRT) and the advancement of tele robotic surgery have been debated. In addition, details on wearable devices for biomedical and health-care applications that can gather, evaluate, and anticipate health-related concerns utilizing established procedures and machine intelligence are provided. Finally, beginning with personalized medicine design and progressing to efficient drug delivery and afar, the eventual extension and development of these technologies in the current health-care system and biological research is discussed (Banerjee et al., 2020).

IoT AND AI USED IN COVID-19 PANDEMIC SITUATION

The COVID-19, a pandemic criterion, has sparked widespread concern for mankind. Rather than technological advancement, surgical masks, hand gloves, and antimicrobials are the only existing preventative strategies to curb the transmission of the corona virus. Healthcare professionals and medical personnel are constantly at danger of infection since they are on the front lines interacting with the sick person. The safety of health-care workers is crucial, as the number of targeted health-care workers grows daily basis. A detailed literature assessment on a previous pandemic eruption and COVID-19 was undertaken using suitable resources. Several obstacles were discovered throughout the literature review that limit the operation of health care professionals and pose a risk to their safety. As a result, we must conduct a critical analysis to identify the impediments or challenges that healthcare sectors are encountering in dealing with this pandemic outbreak, and then propose viable alternatives based on popular technologies such as Artificial intelligence and IoT. Physical, operational, resource-based, organizational, technological, and external health-care challenges are all classified as physical, functional, resource-based, organizational, technical, and exterior physical ailments in this study (Kumar et al., 2020).

MACHINE LEARNING AND ITS APPLICATION IN HEALTHCARE

Table 1. Machine Learning and its Application in Healthcare

Automated Diagnosis in Seconds Instead of Days	The image recognition mechanism of Caption Health's machine learning algorithm-based software aids in the proper capture and early interpretations of ultrasound pictures, assisting in the prevention of heart disease in seconds. Paige's machine learning system has been trained to detect cancer diagnoses using previously processed high-resolution pictures of tissue samples kept in a database that is constantly refilling. As a result, clinical decision assistance becomes more efficient and less expensive.
Conversational Interfaces: Intake, Engagement, And Care	In the healthcare business, machine learning use cases include symptom checkers, preliminary diagnoses, intakes, the first point of contact for primary care, waiting list management, and more. The possibility of utilising AI in patient health situations is estimated to result in a 40% increase in outcomes and a 50% decrease in treatment expenditures.
Ml Makes Its Mark with Precision Medicine	Another non-trivial technological adoption is demonstrated by Amplion. Its patented business intelligence engine Dx: Revenue perfectly links test providers and pharmaceutical firms in real-time, using machine learning to analyse over 34 million web sources. This takes precision medicine collaboration to the next level.

ISSUES/CHALLENGES

AI technologies can help with issues including limited data interchange among-s' significant therapeutic, scalability, compliance programs, and standardization. Due of a lack of certainty and trust, patients and healthcare practitioners have readily adopted AI. System failure is one of the trust issues, and it may be devastating. The AI system's capacity replicates the gut sense of a physician and divination is almost incredible, even with fine algorithms and a vast number of computer assets (Jiang et al., 2017).

One of the issues/challenges addressed by IoT is the ability to develop convenient IoT systems that offer cost-effective, appealing resources in each healthcare profession. Defining a worldwide IoT infrastructure for the healthcare business is tough due to the wide range of needs. To serve each resource sector within the healthcare industry, each IoT-based healthcare institution must develop and execute its own unique architecture. Using IoT-based healthcare services presents another set of challenges to achieve integrated data objectives that may agglomerate data from many sources. Data democratization rules and data ownership aggravate the data aggregation challenge (Zeadallyet & Bello, 2021).

Data ownership, correct data storage, production system requirements and operational rules and regulations are all design challenges that must be addressed or stated in order to be implemented. In addition, most wearable technology-based healthcare apps or services will create real-time flowing data, while some may generate data bits as needed. As a result, smart communication protocols that enable the deployment of value-added services inside the network.

Because IoT-related solutions are utilized in virtually every other business, there must be certain obstacles to overcome for IoT-based healthcare solutions to be beneficial. One of these issues is establishing appropriate and associated IoT infrastructures that will provide exceptional, cost-effective healthcare services in each location. Developing a consistent IoT architecture for the healthcare business is tough due to the various requirements and differences in services. As a result, each IoT-based healthcare resource has its own set of challenges, and unique designs are often necessary to satisfy the demands of each service area within the healthcare business. If healthcare stakeholders can view data from the same perspective, it would create an ideal healthcare system that allows for customized solutions to meet their specific wants and expectations. Data bundling is made more difficult by data ownership and data democratization regulations (Zeadallyet & Bello, 2021). When we consider both AI and IOT in healthcare, challenges become complex.

Figure 5. Issues/ Challenges

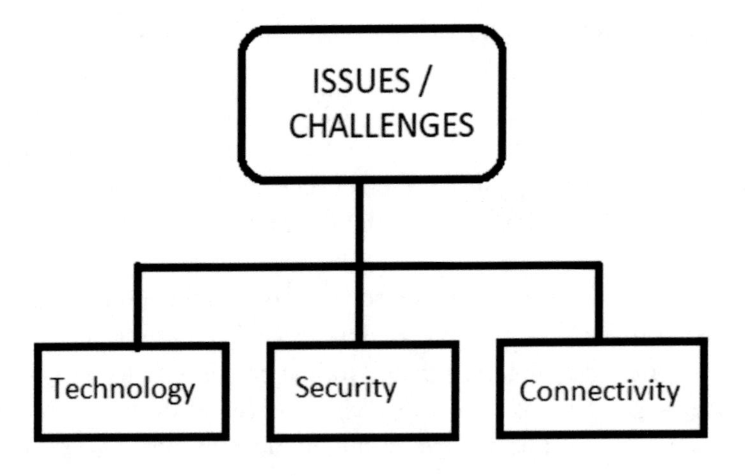

As show in above Figure 5 the major issues addressed are technology, security and connectivity issues.

Security Issues

Security becomes the major issue. As we know AI and IoT collects sensitive data from customers, it's important to keep those data securely. But we don't know when the hackers going to hack.

Disclosure of PHI

Only primary providers should have access to personal health information (PHI) included in medical electronic medical records. It is frequently seen, copied, or modified without the patients' permission. Data from IoT glucose monitors, for example, is easily accessible to other parties and requires additional security.

Privacy Violations

Cybercriminals are interested in highly sensitive information such as demographics, social security numbers, and credit card numbers. They can gain control of patients' personal data, edit it, and misuse it thanks to security flaws. ((Katare et al., 2018))

Technology Issues

The most significant obstacle is technology, which involves competition among all technologies. Giving every technology a chance to compete is not an easy task, as we all know. (Katare et al., 2018) As a result of their nature and features, AI technology was deemed problematic by some Artificial intelligence algorithms lack transparency, and AI systems have trouble processing unstructured data, among other issues. Although government authorities and hospital executives/doctors have raised this technology-related concern, IT professionals think that there are no substantial technological barriers to employing AI in healthcare. In the eyes of government authorities, the most pressing technological issue is the lack of transparency in AI systems. Artificial Intelligence (AI) algorithms convert data inputs into tangible conclusions, which are the patient Companies like IBM mix these algorithms, and no one else knows how they operate. Lack of openness is seen as one of the biggest obstacles in the way of progress. Because AI technology is a "black box," users are unable to evaluate or change its operations in order to deal with future challenges (Sun & Medaglia, 2019).

Connectivity Issues

Using IoT, healthcare providers may link machines to each other, move data, and share information in a way that is highly cost-effective. Due to an increasing number of gadgets, keeping them linked becomes increasingly challenging. Because of this, IoT in healthcare has a problem.

IoT connects and communicates with digital devices over the internet, and communication is effortless in small networks with a few devices. However, when IoT is implemented on a large scale and a large number of devices and sensors are connected and communicating, connection challenges develop. (Katare et al., 2018).

CONCLUSION

The development of new AI-powered applications is gaining popularity in industries like healthcare where human intelligence is crucial. The Internet of Things (IoT), on the other hand, is significantly improving healthcare as its devices may gather entire health data. The healthcare industry can benefit greatly from the combination of these two technologies. The chapter covers the necessity of these two technologies in the healthcare industry as well as applications that use both of them. The methods employed to make this integration possible and the difficulties that can arise. Even though each technology has advantages and disadvantages of its own, integrating these technologies for the healthcare industry may provide a number of implementation challenges.

REFERENCES

Abie, H. (2019, May). Cognitive cybersecurity for CPS-IoT enabled healthcare ecosystems. In *2019 13th International Symposium on Medical Information and Communication Technology (ISMICT)* (pp. 1-6). IEEE.

Ahamed, F., & Farid, F. (2018, December). Applying internet of things and machine-learning for personalized healthcare: Issues and challenges. In *2018 International Conference on Machine Learning and Data Engineering (iCMLDE)* (pp. 19-21). IEEE.

Banerjee, A., Chakraborty, C., Kumar, A., & Biswas, D. (2020). Emerging trends in IoT and big data analytics for biomedical and health care technologies. In *Handbook of data science approaches for biomedical engineering* (pp. 121–152). Academic Press.

Davenport, T., & Kalakota, R. (2019). The potential for artificial intelligence in healthcare. *Future Healthcare Journal*, *6*(2), 94–98. doi:10.7861/futurehosp.6-2-94 PMID:31363513

Froese, T., & Ziemke, T. (2009). Enactive artificial intelligence: Investigating the systemic organization of life and mind. *Artificial Intelligence*, *173*(3-4), 466–500. doi:10.1016/j.artint.2008.12.001

Jiang, F., Jiang, Y., Zhi, H., Dong, Y., Li, H., Ma, S., ... Wang, Y. (2017). Artificial intelligence in healthcare: Past, present and future. *Stroke and Vascular Neurology*, *2*(4).

Jiang, X., Coffee, M., Bari, A., Wang, J., Jiang, X., Huang, J., Shi, J., Dai, J., Cai, J., Zhang, T., Wu, Z., He, G., & Huang, Y. (2020). *Towards an Artificial Intelligence Framework for Data-Driven Prediction of Coronavirus Clinical Severity*. Academic Press.

Katare, G., Padihar, G., & Qureshi, Z. (2018). Challenges in the integration of artificial intelligence and internet of things. *International Journal of System and Software Engineering*, *6*(2), 10–15.

Katare, G., Padihar, G., & Qureshi, Z. (2018). Challenges in the integration of artificial intelligence and internet of things. *International Journal of System and Software Engineering*, *6*(2), 10–15.

Kaur, P., Kumar, R., & Kumar, M. (2019). A healthcare monitoring system using random forest and internet of things (IoT). *Multimedia Tools and Applications*, *78*(14), 19905–19916.

Kumar, S., Raut, R. D., & Narkhede, B. E. (2020). A proposed collaborative framework by using artificial intelligence-internet of things (AI-IoT) in COVID-19 pandemic situation for healthcare workers. *International Journal of Healthcare Management*, *13*(4), 337–345. doi:10.1080/20479700.2020.1810453

Kumari, A., Tanwar, S., Tyagi, S., & Kumar, N. (2018). Fog computing for Healthcare 4.0 environment: Opportunities and challenges. *Computers & Electrical Engineering*, *72*, 1.

Morgan, J. A. (2018). *Yesterday's tomorrow today: Turing, Searle and the contested significance of artificial intelligence*. Academic Press.

Shah, R., & Chircu, A. (2018). IoT and AI in healthcare: A systematic literature review. *Issues in Information Systems*, *19*(3).

Singh, S. K., Rathore, S., & Park, J. H. (2020). Blockiotintelligence: A blockchain-enabled intelligent IoT architecture with artificial intelligence. *Future Generation Computer Systems*, *110*, 721–743. doi:10.1016/j.future.2019.09.002

Sun, T. Q., & Medaglia, R. (2019). Mapping the challenges of Artificial Intelligence in the public sector: Evidence from public healthcare. *Government Information Quarterly*, *36*(2), 368–383.

Vashistha, R., Dangi, A. K., Kumar, A., Chhabra, D., & Shukla, P. (2018). Futuristic biosensors for cardiac health care: an artificial intelligence approach. *Biotech*, *8*(8), 1-11.

Zeadally, S., & Bello, O. (2021). Harnessing the power of Internet of Things based connectivity to improve healthcare. *Internet of Things*, *14*, 100074.

Zhou, J., Wang, Y., Ota, K., & Dong, M. (2019). AAIoT: Accelerating artificial intelligence in IoT systems. *IEEE Wireless Communications Letters*, *8*(3), 825–828. doi:10.1109/LWC.2019.2894703

ADDITIONAL READING

Alshehri, F., & Muhammad, G. (2020). A comprehensive survey of the Internet of Things (IoT) and AI-based smart healthcare. *IEEE Access: Practical Innovations, Open Solutions*, *9*, 3660–3678. doi:10.1109/ACCESS.2020.3047960

Bartoletti, I. (2019, June). AI in healthcare: Ethical and privacy challenges. In *Conference on Artificial Intelligence in Medicine in Europe* (pp. 7-10). Springer. 10.1007/978-3-030-21642-9_2

Kumar, S., Raut, R. D., & Narkhede, B. E. (2020). A proposed collaborative framework by using artificial intelligence-internet of things (AI-IoT) in COVID-19 pandemic situation for healthcare workers. *International Journal of Healthcare Management*, *13*(4), 337–345. doi:10.1080/20479700.2020.1810453

Mathew, P. S., Pillai, A. S., & Palade, V. (2018). Applications of IoT in healthcare. In *Cognitive Computing for Big Data Systems Over IoT* (pp. 263–288). Springer.

Panch, T., Mattie, H., & Celi, L. A. (2019). The "inconvenient truth" about AI in healthcare. *NPJ Digital Medicine*, *2*(1), 1–3. doi:10.103841746-019-0155-4 PMID:31453372

Panesar, A. (2019). *Machine learning and AI for healthcare*. Apress. doi:10.1007/978-1-4842-3799-1

Selvaraj, S., & Sundaravaradhan, S. (2020). Challenges and opportunities in IoT healthcare systems: A systematic review. *SN Applied Sciences*, *2*(1), 1–8. doi:10.100742452-019-1925-y

Shaheen, M. Y. (2021). *AI in Healthcare: medical and socio-economic benefits and challenges. ScienceOpen*. Preprints.

Talukder, A., & Haas, R. (2021, June). AIoT: AI meets IoT and web in smart healthcare. In *13th ACM Web Science Conference 2021* (pp. 92-98). 10.1145/3462741.3466650

Valanarasu, M. R. (2019). Smart and secure IoT and AI integration framework for hospital environment. *Journal of ISMAC*, *1*(03), 172–179. doi:10.36548/jismac.2019.3.004

KEY TERMS AND DEFINITIONS

AI: The theory and creation of computer systems that can carry out tasks that would typically need human intelligence, like speech recognition, visual perception, decision-making, and language translation.

Algorithms: A procedure or set of guidelines to be followed for performing calculations or addressing other problems, particularly by a computer.

Applications: A formal request made to a person in charge, an institution, or an organization asking to be taken into consideration for a position or to be permitted to do or have something.

Deep Learning: A sophisticated form of machine learning with the aim of self-directed information processing that creates nested hierarchical models for data processing and analysis, such as in image recognition or natural language processing.

Design Architecture: In order to construct living spaces, the discipline of architectural design focuses on addressing and meeting requirements and desires while using specific tools and, most importantly, creativity.

Healthcare: The organized provision of medical care to individuals or a community

Internet of Things: Computer equipment integrated into everyday things that communicate to one another through the internet to exchange data.

Neural Network: A computer architecture that can learn through a process of trial and error that connects multiple processors in a way that is like the connections between neurons in the human brain.

Chapter 4
Secure Medical Data Transmission Over Wireless Body Area Network Using Blockchain

Pradeep Bedi
https://orcid.org/0000-0003-1708-6237
Galgotias University, India

S. B. Goyal
https://orcid.org/0000-0002-8411-7630
City University, Malaysia

Jugnesh Kumar
St. Andrews Institute of Technology and Management, India

Anand Singh Rajawat
Sandip University, Nashik, India

ABSTRACT

With the application of wireless body area networks, patients can be remotely monitored by doctors. WBANs collect the medical data and transmit it over the internet for further processing. There is need to ensure security of such highly sensitive data over the network. This has deliberately attracted researcher interest to provide WBAN security by integrating blockchain. This chapter discusses internet of things (IoT) architecture of WBANs and proposes a lightweight secure access control using blockchain to achieve higher performance.

DOI: 10.4018/978-1-6684-4405-4.ch004

INTRODUCTION

Blockchain technology is among the most essential findings and innovative technologies that are playing a critical role in the technical modern world. Blockchain covers the data privacy and keeps assurance among people regardless of their location of access. The growth of blockchain technology has forced researchers and professionals to investigate innovative approaches to utilize blockchain technology in a broad variety of areas over the last couple of years. Blockchain was initially implemented as a tool to power Bitcoin but has now grown to such an extent of being applied to various decentralized implementations as a fundamental technology. Blockchain, specifically, within the medical care, medical experimentation, and insurance sectors, is being considered an important technique for handling confidential information (Fekih and Lahami, 2020). Healthcare could be described as a framework involving three main elements:

- Main suppliers of hospital facilities, such as doctors, nurses, administration of hospitals, and technicians.
- Essential services are linked with medical services, including certain medical research and health insurance.
- Health and health-oriented program recipients, i.e. patients or the people. In an attempt to encourage, preserve or restore the wellbeing of recipients, the healthcare system is considered to be consisting of contact-based and technology-based remote surveillance facilities provided by the constituent service provider

Confidentiality and protection violations are reportedly growing every year in the area of medical care with greater than 300 violations recorded in 2017 and 37 million hospital information compromised between 2010 and 2017. Moreover, the growing digitalization of healthcare also resulted in the identification of issues associated with safe handling, possession, exchange of individual health information, and relevant medical information. Blockchain has been presented as a means of solving crucial healthcare problems, like an encrypted exchange of medical information and enforcement with data protection laws.

The widespread adoption of healthcare digitization has contributed to the production of vast electronic medical databases. Such development raises significant requirements for data security for healthcare when being in use and exchange. As a secure and open platform for storing and sharing information, the emergence of blockchain technology is opening the ways for new opportunities to solve serious healthcare data safety, protection, and integrity problems. Over the past couple of years, blockchain technology has drawn tremendous interest from businesses and also academia. Even so, nearly every other day new blockchain implementations and research studies surface (Yaeger et al., 2019). Blockchain technology is characterized or sometimes may be decentralized network ledger technology for transaction of digital data that can be transmitted to all consumers individually or collectively, enabling secure and verifiable storage of any form of data (Gaggioli, 2018). The smart contract, a legally binding set of policies that comprises a flexible collection of guidelines in which various groups consent to communicate in the context of distributed automated interaction, is also another core principle of the blockchain.

In many fields, blockchain technology has resulted in various smart contract implementations, starting from energy resources, financial services, voting, and healthcare (Li et al.. 2021) (Macrinici et al., 2018). Blockchain technology provides authentication and eliminates the requirement for third-party or intermediary administrators (Omar et al., 2019). In a trustless and insecure atmosphere, it utilizes consensus frameworks and cryptography to check the reliability of a transaction (Gordon and Catalini, 2018). In a decentralized P2P transaction network blockchain, the recipient node examines the message and it retains in a block as the retrieved message is right. To validate the details in each block, "Proof-of-work (PoW)" is used. After the consensus algorithm is executed, the block is introduced to the chain and it is accepted by every node and the chain is continued (Zhang et al., 2017). In healthcare, blockchain can solve the issues relevant to information protection, confidentiality, distribution, and storage. Information sharing is one of the specific needs of the healthcare sector. It is the capability of two or more groups either humans or machines to accurately, effectively, and regularly interchange information and data (Macrinici et al., 2018). Healthcare interoperability aims to promote the sharing of health-related details between healthcare professionals and beneficiaries like electronic health records (EHR) so that the details could be exchanged throughout the system and transmitted by various hospital systems. Besides, interoperability allows service providers to exchange patient health details safely, irrespective of the position of the provider and the trusting relation among them (Zhang et al., 2018). This is especially essential considering that the source of information on health care is complex. This element of information sharing is addressed by the use of blockchain technology that has demonstrated the capability to securely preserve, manage and exchange EHRs across healthcare communities (Casino et al., 2019) . Moreover, rising healthcare services and technology expenses in the market have placed immense pressure on the world's economies (Sharma et al., 2021). Blockchain technology has a beneficial influence on healthcare results for businesses and stakeholders in the healthcare sector to simplify business procedures to help boost patient results, manage patient information, improve compliance, reduce expense and make efficient utilization of healthcare-related data (Mackey et al., 2019). The potential of blockchain technology to affect the movement of medicines and hospital instruments in the complex supply chain of healthcare services is equally significant. Blockchain technology is presently being assessed in different healthcare implementations like information management, storage, accessibility of devices, and internet protection of medical products (IoMT). From the above implementation regions, the majority of benefits offered by blockchain technology have had a positive effect on the quality of experience (QoE) of most investors and enterprise customers, comprising patients, providers, scientists, pharmaceutical firms, and insurance firms. The capability to exchange healthcare information without compromising the confidentiality and information protection of patients is an important course of action towards making the healthcare system smarter and enhancing the quality of healthcare facilities and the satisfaction of consumers.

Application of Blockchain in Healthcare

The blockchain assures the refinement of healthcare application in several ways. This is primarily because of its ability to adapt and willingness to separate, protect, and unprecedentedly exchange medical information and facilities. In the medical care sector, blockchain technology is leading the most important position among the several existing innovations (Gordon and Catalini, 2018). Growing blockchain-based healthcare new technologies, comprising data sources, blockchain technology, medical implementations, and investors, are conceptually categorized into four sections. A detail of the blockchain-based workflow for medical care implementations is shown in fig 1. The workflow consists of four key layers, comprising raw data on healthcare, blockchain technology, implementation of healthcare, and stakeholders. As a decentralized technology, the blockchain allows different stakeholders to get an advantage from various uses of healthcare (Shi et al., 2020).

Previously, all information from medical devices, laboratories, social media, and several other sources are integrated, and new information is collected, which ultimately grows to big data in size. This knowledge is the crucial component of the whole blockchain-based medical care system, and it is the significant element that produces the first layer of the stack. Blockchain technique is at the above all of the raw data layer, which is known to be the central system in search of developing a four-component protected healthcare architecture. There are distinct characteristics in each blockchain network, like consensus mechanisms and procedures. Blockchain systems empower the growth and management of transactions by consumers (Huang, 2019). So many blockchain applications, including Ethereum, Ripple, and Hyperledger Fabric, were developed and are presently being used. Smart contracts, signatures, wallets, activities, membership, and digital property are the important component of the blockchain (Liu et al., 2020). Different types of protocols can be utilized for interacting with many other structures and processes, or even by numerous networks.

Figure 1. Integration and application of block chain in healthcare architecture

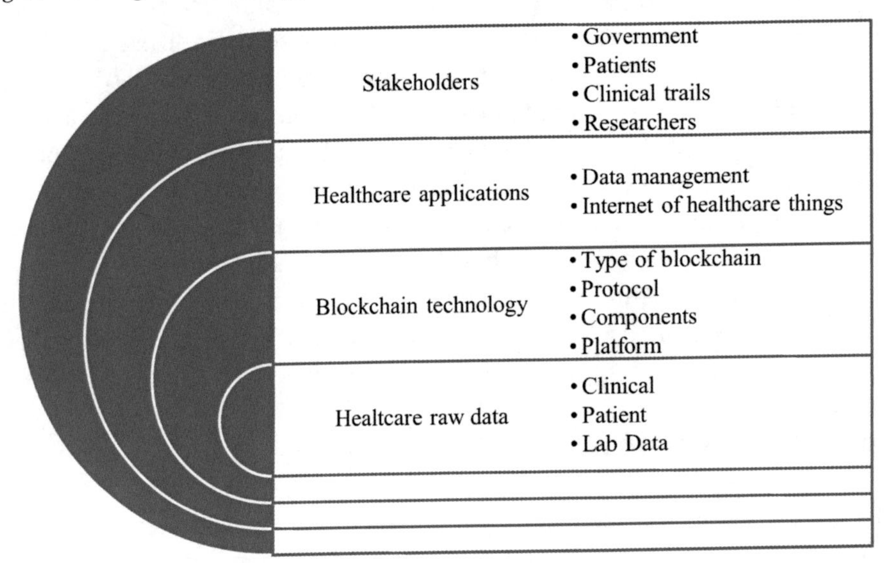

Policymakers may make public, private, or even federal options based on the variety of criteria they needed to fulfill. The next step is to make sure that the applications are compatible with the entire framework once the network is generated by integrating blockchain technology. It is possible to classify blockchain-based healthcare implementations into three broad groups. Information management, namely global scientific data exchange for information management, data storage, and EHRs are represented in the first part. The second level comprising clinical studies and pharmaceuticals represents SCM implementations. Finally, the IoMT added the third level named as a confluence of IoT and medical devices for healthcare, IoT technology and data preservation for medical care, and AI. The key challenges for consumers at this stage are to exchange, process, and handle information efficiently without compromising its protection and confidentiality.

Literature Review

Cheng et al. (2020) presented the blockchain technology to define the security criteria in the verification process, and a blockchain-based network model of MCPS is introduced. It could make sure that information could not be interfered with and untracked by studying the layout of medical data storage. In the protection verification stage, bilinear mapping and intractable challenges may be utilized to resolve the security threat in the verification procedure of medical information providers and users. Then, BAN logic is utilized to evaluate security measures, and security measures are often specifically analyzed and compared. The findings indicate that the blockchain-based MCPS not only embraces the sharing of healthcare information but also fulfills the numerous security needs in the security verification stage. Additionally, the overhead expense of storage and processing is reasonable. The suggested methodology is thus more appropriate for the safe exchange of large-scale medical information.

Griggs et al. (2018) proposed and used the smart contract based blockchain to ensure security on accessing medical sensors. The private blockchain is implemented that interact with smart healthcare devices. By transmitting alerts to patients and healthcare providers, this smart contract system will facilitate real-time patient tracking and medical interventions, while still keeping a secure database of who has started these practices. This will address several security issues related to distant health monitoring and automate the transmission of updates to all concerned groups in a HIPAA compliant way.

Security and privacy of streamed healthcare records from heterogeneously networked systems have been one of the obstacles in healthcare. Omala et al. (2018) initially suggested a heterogeneous signature strategy, in this study where a sender is in a certificate less cryptographic environment (CLC) whereas a recipient is in an identity-based cryptographic environment (IBC). This method is then used to build a heterogeneous protocol for access control. Formal safety evidence for indifferent ability against adaptively selected ciphertext attack and enforceability against adaptively selected message attack In the random oracle model is introduced. This system has lower calculation and communication cost computation compared to some of the established access control methods.

Wang et al. (2019) presented the decentralized blockchain-based security protection architecture differently from conventional centralized systems. Smart contracts, in specific, are exploited to effectively obtain device security, honesty, and authenticity as an advanced application in blockchain technology. In the proposed system, research challenges relating to security and confidentiality concerns are then examined, accompanied by possible alternatives. Eventually, simulations and evaluations of security efficiency are performed to legalize and estimate the usefulness of planned security architecture.

Omar et al. (2019) proposed an information management framework for patient-centric healthcare utilizing blockchain technologies as storage that helps to ensure confidentiality. To encrypt patient information and to make sure pseudonymity, cryptographic methods are utilized. They study the processes for data processing as well as the economic viability of the smart contracts utilized in their system.

Khezr et al. (2019) surveyed the offers a thorough overview of evolving healthcare innovations and relevant implementations focused on blockchain. Researchers bring focus to the research issues in this rapid-growing area in this inquiry, describing them in some depth. They are also showing the capability of blockchain technology to revolutionize the healthcare sector.

McGhin et al. (2019) explored that the blockchain techniques have been adopted by many investigators in both academia and industry have begun to start exploring implementations that are designed for healthcare usage. Smart contracts, scam prevention, and identity confirmation are included in these implementations. There are still problems, even with these changes, since blockchain technology has its unique drawbacks and problems that required to be solved, like mining incentives, mining threats, and important management.

Girardi et al. (2020) addressed several concerns related to health data processing and security shared by new medical or diagnostic devices.

Aguiar et al. (2020) discussed the research into blockchain healthcare implementations. It started by addressing medical information management, and also the exchange of hospital data, the sharing of images, and the management of logs. They also discussed papers that overlap with other fields, like the Internet of Things, identity management, drug monitoring in the supply chain, and protection and confidentiality aspects. They evaluated and compared both the pros and cons of their reports, as they were aware of the other blockchain researches in healthcare. Eventually, by analyzing their advantages and disadvantages and therefore providing direction to other researchers in the field, they aim to explore the concepts of blockchain in the medical field. Besides, the field they outline the strategies utilized in healthcare per implementation and display their advantages and disadvantages.

Pham et al. (2018) suggested a processing method to effectively and carefully store data from the medical equipment in compliance with the patient's health condition. Specifically, before determining whether to write information into the blockchain or not, they filter the sensor readings. By doing so, they could effectively decrease the size of the blockchain and also save the amount of coins for the transaction. Moreover, abnormal sensor data would be instantly written to the blockchain and cause emergency contact with the healthcare provider for on-time care. The presented smart contract for the Ethereum test environment, named TESTRPC, was tested and the system was incorporated with real devices in an experimental atmosphere. On a limited scale, this system functions effectively.

Liu et al. (2020) introduced the Enhanced Biomedical Security Framework (BDL-IBS) for blockchain and Decentralized Ledger-based has been introduced to increase confidentiality and data protection across healthcare implementations. Besides, the aim was to make it easier for patients to utilize the data to improve their treatment as well as provide strong data sharing consent processes between various organizations and implementations, as this comprises handling and accessing a vast volume of medical information, and this technology is capable of storing data to ensure reliability. Eventually, the outcomes showed that the latest digital blockchain-based technologies allow fast, simple, and transparent communications among data providers to improve confidentiality and information protection

Cheng et al. (2019) illustrated the use of blockchain in the security criteria in the procedure of authentication. A blockchain-based MCPS network model is being introduced. Through the study of the design of healthcare data storage, information was assured that it would not be manipulated and discoverable. The security issue has been removed in the authentication procedure of healthcare information users and providers by bilinear mapping. The credibility issue of the trusted third party was eliminated and between the hospital and the blockchain node, the two-way authentication was realized. To check the security and relevant functionality of the authentication method, a security evaluation and effectiveness test was performed. The findings indicate that the blockchain-based MCPS realizes the exchange of healthcare details and satisfies safety criteria in the security authentication process.

Lee et al. (2020) introduced a blockchain-based healthcare information protection system for telecare medical information systems (TMISs) based on the aforementioned functionality and safety criteria, which comprises an authentication method for the medical sensor region and a protocol for the transmission of social network records. To accomplish safe data transmission among human sensors and mobile systems, the former method utilizes elliptic curve point multiplication. The latter method stores information that mobile devices capture and transmit. The system herein is protected from many potential attacks and decreases the number of communication rounds below those of previously existing methods. The information transmission method for the social network, stores records utilizing blockchain technology such that the data owners could allow appropriate people to view data. The suggested methodology thus increases not just the efficiency of computation, but also the protection of earlier studies.

Yang et al. (2019) used blockchain technology's simplicity, security, and productivity to create a collective healthcare decision-making system. This research takes into account the expertise, capacity, and collective rate of success in the healthcare sector of four primary stakeholders (patient, cured patient, healthcare providers, and insurance firm) to introduce a limited reference-based consortium blockchain system and a related algorithm for consensus selection, proof of familiarity (PoF). A straightforward and tenable healthcare decision is made by stakeholders to improve interconnectivity between collaborators through PoF. With multichain 2.0, a blockchain implementation platform, a prototype of PoF is being tested. Besides, two-layer storage, encryption, and a timestamp storing system protect the confidentiality of identities, EMRs, and decisions. Eventually, to enhance personal data privacy and patient-centered outcomes analysis, superiority over existing systems is established.

Xu et al. (2020) presented a blockchain model for sensor systems and the local node should conduct mutual encryption and important consensus before sending information. A stable shared authentication scheme for blockchain-based WBANs is demonstrated in this article. Formal security evaluation and informal security evaluation are utilized to examine the safety of this system, and then the cost of computing and communication is contrasted with that of the existing methods. Similar experimental findings indicate that the current method shows more efficient and promising control over energy usage.

Pawar et al. (2020) studied to use of a wireless internet network as a transmitting and storing system to link the equipment of the patient and the technologies in the blockchain to provide a safe and effective alternative to health care. Potential customers have numerous Wireless Sensor Network problems (WSNs). In WSN, cost efficiency, low power usage, effective data communication among nodes, and security are significant issues. Several WSN issues, including safe data transmission and confidence, etc., can be solved by Blockchain. The survey of the utilization of blockchain technology in the wireless body area network was performed in this study.

Dakhel et al. (2019) used Blockchain technology to sustain patient information and confidentiality, a method to protect patient information was introduced and cryptography algorithms were utilized to protect the channel of data transfer among the patient and the provider of e-health services. The findings indicated that, to preserve the confidentiality of the user, the suggested system satisfied the security goals, including privacy, reliability, security, and non-repudiation, to keep patient information from invasion.

PROBLEM IDENTIFICATION

One of the major concerns in the field of telecommunication is security. A major key issue in body area networks is to securely shared data between source and destination nodes. Due to limited computational resources algorithm needed to be lightweight. As well as while accessing remote data, there is a requirement of high-level security and privacy of sensitive data over remote servers. Some of the security algorithms are used in existing work are illustrated in table 1 that highlights the research direction towards the development of secure and lightweight security algorithm.

PROPOSED METHODOLOGY

Three functions are involved in a stable cloud assisted IoT application: the iot sensors (I), the cloud data center (CDC), the Authenticator (A), and the blockchain. Each

Table 1. Existing security algorithm complexity applied for WBAN

Author	Algorithm Used	Complexity
[30]	ElGamal	$T_{exp}+7T_h+T_m$
[31]	SHA-256 hash functions and bitwise XOR operations	$16T_h$
[32]	AES	$17T_h$
[33]	ECC	$4T_m + 11T_h$

sensor nodes should enroll with the CDC until logging into the system and it will issue a special certificate for accessing WBAN/IoT data files. As a trusted individual, CDC is identified and initializes the device. The data center stores patient health data and diagnostic results from doctors and uploads data transactions. For diagnosis, a client will upload the personal health information encrypted with the customized Elgamal attribute. If a physician fulfills the health data access tree saved on the remote server, the physician can ask for the medical data from the cloud server. The blockchain is organized by Authenticator. The blockchain ledgers can be read by patients and physicians, and the base station can add blocks to the blockchain.

This work proposes a cloud assisted WBAN with blockchain access control to a security authentication system. For health data stored in the cloud server, access control is given using cipher text-policy attribute-based encryption (CP-ABE), and user authentication is accomplished using blockchain.

Figure 2. Comparative Analysis of Existing Techniques

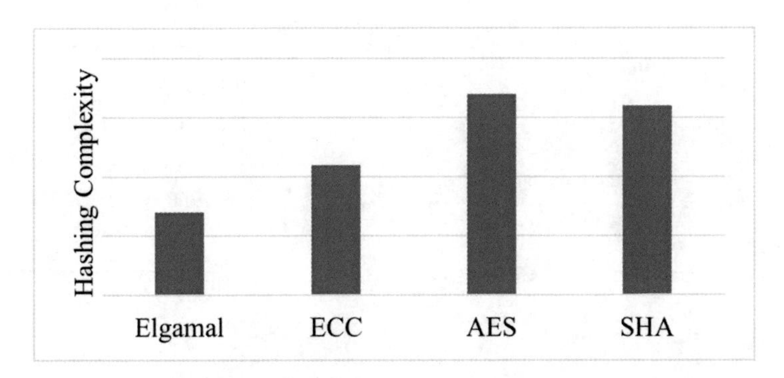

CONCLUSION

In the health sector, WBAN have achieved the revolting future scope for research. Data privacy and security are a crucial concern in the WBAN scenario. A safe structure for addressing these challenges is proposed in this paper. Elgamal security algorithm with attribute-based encryption is used in this context to provide secure access control and to ensure blockchain credibility for low-cost calculation and scalability. In the future, therefore, existing research efforts will be directed towards implementing the secure blockchain-based WBAN framework.

Figure 3. Flow Chart of Proposed Work

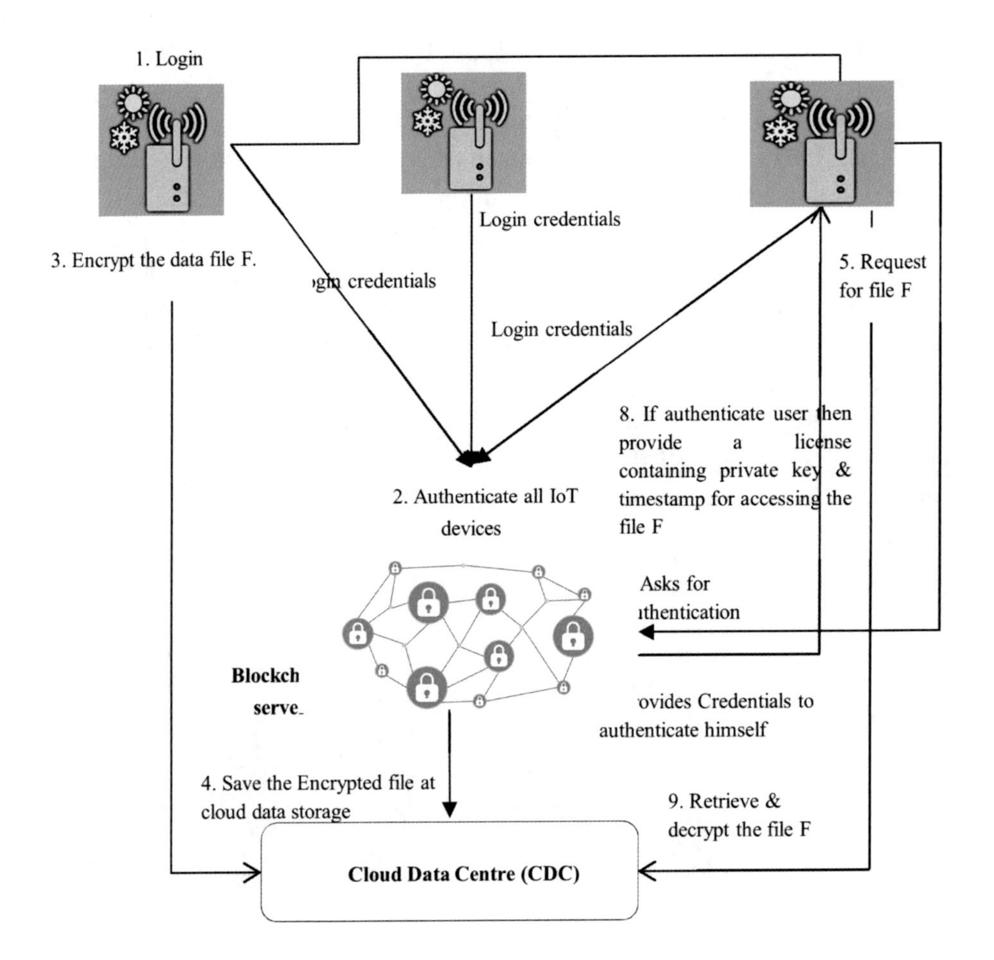

REFERENCES

Al Omar, A., Bhuiyan, M. Z. A., Basu, A., Kiyomoto, S., & Rahman, M. S. (2019). Privacy-friendly platform for healthcare data in cloud based on blockchain environment. *Future Generation Computer Systems*, *95*, 511–521. doi:10.1016/j.future.2018.12.044

Ben Fekih, R., & Lahami, M. (2020). Application of Blockchain Technology in Healthcare: A Comprehensive Study. Lecture Notes in Computer Science, 12157, 268–276. doi:10.1007/978-3-030-51517-1_23

Casino, F., Dasaklis, T. K., & Patsakis, C. (2019). A systematic literature review of blockchain-based applications: Current status, classification and open issues. *Telematics and Informatics*, *36*, 55–81. doi:10.1016/j.tele.2018.11.006

Cheng, X., Chen, F., Xie, D., Sun, H., & Huang, C. (2020). Design of a Secure Medical Data Sharing Scheme Based on Blockchain. *Journal of Medical Systems*, *44*(2), 52. Advance online publication. doi:10.100710916-019-1468-1 PMID:31915982

Cheng, X., Chen, F., Xie, D., Sun, H., Huang, C., & Qi, Z. (2019). Blockchain-Based Secure Authentication Scheme for Medical Data Sharing. *Communications in Computer and Information Science*, *1058*, 396–411. doi:10.1007/978-981-15-0118-0_31

Chenthara, S., Ahmed, K., Wang, H., Whittaker, F., & Chen, Z. (2020). Healthchain: A novel framework on privacy preservation of electronic health records using blockchain technology. *PLoS ONE, 15*(12). doi:10.1371/journal.pone.0243043

Dakhel, M., & Hassan, S. (2020). A Secure Wireless Body Area Network for E-Health Application Using Blockchain. *Communications in Computer and Information Science, 1174*, 395–408. doi:10.1007/978-3-030-38752-5_31

De Aguiar, E. J., Faiçal, B. S., Krishnamachari, B., & Ueyama, J. (2020). A Survey of Blockchain-Based Strategies for Healthcare. *ACM Computing Surveys*, *53*(2), 1–27. Advance online publication. doi:10.1145/3376915

Gaggioli, A. (2018). Blockchain Technology: Living in a Decentralized Everything. *Cyberpsychology, Behavior, and Social Networking*, *21*(1), 65–66. doi:10.1089/cyber.2017.29097.csi

Girardi, F., De Gennaro, G., Colizzi, L., & Convertini, N. (2020). Improving the Healthcare Effectiveness: The Possible Role of EHR, IoMT and Blockchain. *Electronics, 9*(6), 884. doi:10.3390/electronics9060884

Gordon, W. J., & Catalini, C. (2018). Blockchain Technology for Healthcare: Facilitating the Transition to Patient-Driven Interoperability. *Computational and Structural Biotechnology Journal, 16*, 224–230. doi:10.1016/j.csbj.2018.06.003 PMID:30069284

Griggs, K. N., Ossipova, O., Kohlios, C. P., Baccarini, A. N., Howson, E. A., & Hayajneh, T. (2018). Healthcare Blockchain System Using Smart Contracts for Secure Automated Remote Patient Monitoring. *Journal of Medical Systems, 42*(7), 130. Advance online publication. doi:10.100710916-018-0982-x PMID:29876661

Huang, X. (2019). Blockchain in Healthcare: A Patient-Centered Model. *Biomedical Journal of Scientific & Technical Research, 20*(3). Advance online publication. doi:10.26717/BJSTR.2019.20.003448 PMID:31565696

Khezr, S., Moniruzzaman, M., Yassine, A., & Benlamri, R. (2019). Blockchain Technology in Healthcare: A Comprehensive Review and Directions for Future Research. *Applied Sciences, 9*(9), 1736. doi:10.3390/app9091736

Lee, T. F., Li, H. Z., & Hsieh, Y. P. (2021). A blockchain-based medical data preservation scheme for telecare medical information systems. *International Journal of Information Security, 20*(4), 589–601. doi:10.100710207-020-00521-8

Li, H., Xiao, F., Yin, L., & Wu, F. (2021). Application of Blockchain Technology in Energy Trading: A Review. *Frontiers in Energy Research, 9*, 671133. Advance online publication. doi:10.3389/fenrg.2021.671133

Liu, H., Crespo, R. G., & Martínez, O. S. (2020). Enhancing Privacy and Data Security across Healthcare Applications Using Blockchain and Distributed Ledger Concepts. *Healthcare, 8*(3), 243. doi:10.3390/healthcare8030243

Mackey, T. K., Kuo, T. T., Gummadi, B., Clauson, K. A., Church, G., Grishin, D., Obbad, K., Barkovich, R., & Palombini, M. (2019). "Fit-for-purpose?" - Challenges and opportunities for applications of blockchain technology in the future of healthcare. *BMC Medicine, 17*(1), 68. Advance online publication. doi:10.118612916-019-1296-7 PMID:30914045

Macrinici, D., Cartofeanu, C., & Gao, S. (2018). Smart contract applications within blockchain technology: A systematic mapping study. *Telematics and Informatics, 35*(8), 2337–2354. doi:10.1016/j.tele.2018.10.004

McGhin, T., Choo, K. K. R., Liu, C. Z., & He, D. (2019). Blockchain in healthcare applications: Research challenges and opportunities. *Journal of Network and Computer Applications, 135*, 62–75. doi:10.1016/j.jnca.2019.02.027

Omala, A. A., Mbandu, A. S., Mutiria, K. D., Jin, C., & Li, F. (2018). Provably Secure Heterogeneous Access Control Scheme for Wireless Body Area Network. *Journal of Medical Systems, 42*(6), 108. Advance online publication. doi:10.100710916-018-0964-z PMID:29705947

Pawar, R., & Kalbande, D. (2020). Use of blockchain technology in wireless body area networks. *Proceedings of the 3rd International Conference on Intelligent Sustainable Systems, ICISS 2020*, 1333–1336. 10.1109/ICISS49785.2020.9316005

Pham, H. L., Tran, T. H., & Nakashima, Y. (2019). A Secure Remote Healthcare System for Hospital Using Blockchain Smart Contract. *2018 IEEE Globecom Workshops, GC Wkshps 2018 - Proceedings*. doi:10.1109/GLOCOMW.2018.8644164

Sharma, A., Kaur, S., & Singh, M. (2021). A comprehensive review on blockchain and Internet of Things in healthcare. *Transactions on Emerging Telecommunications Technologies*, *32*(10). Advance online publication. doi:10.1002/ett.4333

Shi, S., He, D., Li, L., Kumar, N., Khan, M. K., & Choo, K. K. R. (2020). Applications of blockchain in ensuring the security and privacy of electronic health record systems: A survey. *Computers & Security*, *97*, 101966. Advance online publication. doi:10.1016/j.cose.2020.101966 PMID:32834254

Wang, R., Liu, H., Wang, H., Yang, Q., & Wu, D. (2019). Distributed Security Architecture Based on Blockchain for Connected Health: Architecture, Challenges, and Approaches. *IEEE Wireless Communications*, *26*(6), 30–36. doi:10.1109/MWC.001.1900108

Xu, J., Meng, X., Liang, W., Zhou, H., & Li, K. C. (2020). A secure mutual authentication scheme of blockchain-based in WBANs. *China Communications*, *17*(9), 34–49. doi:10.23919/JCC.2020.09.004

Yaeger, K., Martini, M., Rasouli, J., & Costa, A. (2019). Emerging Blockchain Technology Solutions for Modern Healthcare Infrastructure. *Journal of Scientific Innovation in Medicine*, *2*(1), 1. Advance online publication. doi:10.29024/jsim.7

Yang, J., Onik, M. M. H., Lee, N. Y., Ahmed, M., & Kim, C. S. (2019). Proof-of-Familiarity: A Privacy-Preserved Blockchain Scheme for Collaborative Medical Decision-Making. *Applied Sciences, 9*(7), 1370. doi:10.3390/app9071370

Zhang, P., Schmidt, D. C., White, J., & Lenz, G. (2018). Blockchain Technology Use Cases in Healthcare. *Advances in Computers*, *111*, 1–41. doi:10.1016/bs.adcom.2018.03.006

Zhang, P., White, J., Schmidt, D. C., & Lenz, G. (2017). *Applying Software Patterns to Address Interoperability in Blockchain-based Healthcare Apps*. https://arxiv.org/abs/1706.03700v1

Chapter 5
AI-Enabled Augmented Reality-Based Shared Collaborative Experience

Robin Singh Chouhan
Shri Vaishnav Vidyapeeth Vishwavidyalaya, India

Anand Singh Rajawat
Sandip University, Nashik, India

S. B. Goyal
https://orcid.org/0000-0002-8411-7630
City University, Malaysia

Pradeep Bedi
https://orcid.org/0000-0003-1708-6237
Galgotias University, India

ABSTRACT

The unpopular reality of taxpayers we see in the placement of 3D animations in the real world. The objects used can be viewed and communicated by both individual and multiple users. For example, two users, if they are in the same location, can create a shared experience where both can interact with real-world objects. The real-life experience of unpopular taxpayers we see could improve the efficiency of the education sector as well, as students can have practical experience and visual cues that all students can access using their own learning-enhancing devices.

DOI: 10.4018/978-1-6684-4405-4.ch005

INTRODUCTION

Augmented reality is a dynamic technology that covers three-dimensional objects in the real world. The main purpose of AR is to place 3D objects in a real location so that objects behave as if they are part of the real world and provide a real-life experience for the user you interact with.

With the advancement in technology, the use of unpopular reality for taxpayers we now see is not limited to Head-Mounted displays but is also available on mobile devices (Azuma, 2001). As mobile processors have become very powerful and efficient, they support the unpopular reality of taxpayers that we see to some extent.

AR systems allow users to have in-depth knowledge and make the user feel like 3d objects are real in real life with flexible behavior. The paper discusses resources available that one can use to use and create their own shared personal experiences. This paper also discusses current solutions and applications (Mickael, 2020).

The above figure demonstrates a basic mobile application that uses ARCore to map the table and then place and position a 3d virtual object on top of the flat surface i.e., tabletop.

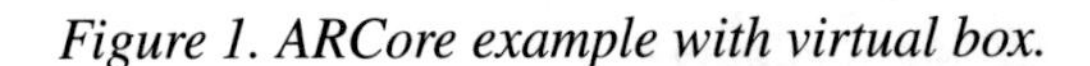

Figure 1. ARCore example with virtual box.

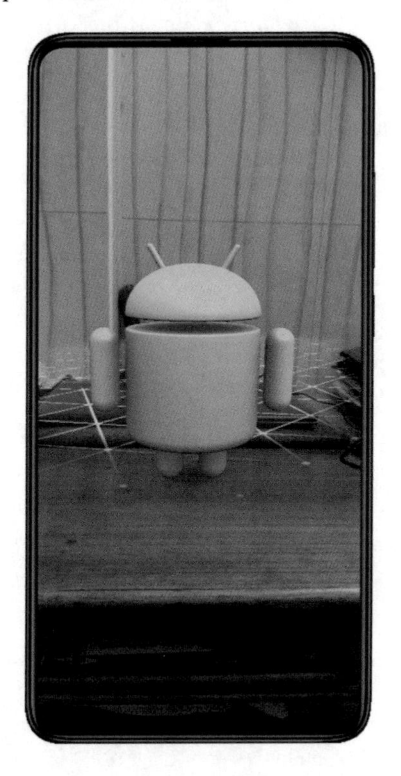

RELATED WORK

The related works include gathering information from previously built projects along with developing basic apps to understand the immersive experiences provided by ARCore, Unity, and Vuforia (Saidin, Nor & Abd halim, 2015).

Just as cell phones do not have as many sensors as head-mounted devices, so cell phones use Google's algorithms to understand the mobile location and to understand the real world as horizontal, precise length distances. of nearby objects. In this google enhanced Google ARCore, ARCore is an advanced google platform to create a real unpopular reality for taxpayers that we see on various android devices running over Android 7 (Nougat). ARCore uses motion tracking to measure phone position and location, and detects flat areas such as floor area, top, walls, etc (Ali, Abdullah & Glackin, 2019).

Motion Tracking: ARCore uses SLAM (simultaneous localization and mapping) to calculate and measure the phone's location in relation to its surroundings. It uses feature points i.e., different features present next to the captured camera image. These unique features are called feature points and these feature points combined with the device IMU together measure the location of the device.

Depth Mapping: ARCore creates in-depth maps using RGB cameras from mobile to define and calculate the depth of the surrounding area and provide real-time information to the user.

Anchors: As the room map continues to update as soon as the user continues to scan around, ARCore needs to keep track of the 3d rendered objects related to the scanned environment.

Augmented Reality in Laboratories

Augmented Reality is an emerging type of experience in which Real World (RW) develops computer-generated content that is tied to specific sites and / or activities (Chang, G, 2011). Over the past few years, AR applications have become portable and widely available on mobile devices (Hsu, 2011). AR is now reflected in our audio and visual media (e.g., news, entertainment, sports) and is beginning to penetrate other aspects of our lives (e.g., online marketing, tourism, marketing) in tangible and exciting ways. To make it easier to read everywhere, AR will provide students with quick access to geographical information collected and provided with multiple sources (2009). Both Horizon Reports 2010 and 2011 predict that AR will see widespread use in US colleges (Alexander T,2017).

Layar (a Netherlands-based company) acquired in 2009, proposes augmented reality browsers and interactive printer tools for mobile devices (Akçayır,2017). Teachers often use Layar to expand posters in a separate lesson. Experts between the ages of 9 and 10, handmade posters depict the functions of the human body. They used Layar creator to develop digital assets in visual posters and helped them understand the basics of biology (C. Cameron, 2014).

A French company called 'Augment' offers a complete solution for setting up, managing and viewing 3D content that is a reality that taxpayers do not like. It has a free license for teaching purposes. The use of 'Climbing' and 3D modeling tools is used to create a detailed historical tour of ancient Rome for students to explore the eternal city. Allows dynamic interaction with the site during field trips instead of viewing study slides.

Latvian Anatomy Next is very useful for medical professionals as it incorporates models with the most accurate 3D anatomy that can be detected by AR and, importantly, accredited and accredited by medical professionals. The authors argue that models can be used to support the curriculum and to develop the skills of academics in the three-dimensional perspective of structural integration. This app can be used as a starting point to train medical students to get more information about surgical procedures (Yeom, S.-J., 2011).

MoleQL is an AR application used to learn and learn chemical concepts and ideas. It helps scientists to overcome the difficulties of studying science by visualizing chemical elements and providing general information about their functioning in the environment. Targeted objects can be digitized separately or integrated into chemical compounds, while they are safer and more economical in educational institutions. The solution has received a lot of feedback from professors and scholars (M. Prensky, 2001).

The list of AR applications listed above in the field of education is far from complete, but it does suggest that the unpopularity of the taxpayers we see makes learning more lively and more convenient and more attractive than the existing curriculum. A major challenge for teachers can be the creation of 3D content in case they want to use completely new models, as this requires more advanced knowledge (Cerqueira, C. S, 2012).

Teaching and learning science is a complex process and its level of inactivity is very high. It is therefore necessary to ensure the effective use of educational resources and to make the selection of additional tools as effective as possible. Chemistry requires familiarity and understanding of complex vocabulary. Sounds and sounds not like something kids have come across before. The style of play can support the seamless development of this important skill (Chang, G., 2011).

As Gee points out, children develop big names while playing Pokémon (not even the real game that tax collectors dislike). They became so absorbed in the field of sports that they soon became proficient in their use of the vernacular. Children build new knowledge based on the knowledge they already have in order to understand new things the old definition of constructivist learning theory (Gutierrez, 2012).

The same straightforward concept can be used in teaching, especially in the study of science and the scholar who has acquired familiarity with common metaphors, the process of building familiarity is very effective. The MoleQL developed by the Estonian company Subatomic OÜ has this idea in mind: the use of AR should be achieved in order to convey a common context to learning, both physical and mental (Martin, S, 2011).

MoleQL operating principles are simple. Initially, the user needs to install the mobile application on a handheld device - a smartphone or tablet. Mole QL operating principles are simple. The first thing you have to do, install the app on a smartphone or tablet (portable device), then print the cards that represent the chemical elements, and then scan the printed cards with the device's camera, and the app will render a 3D object. of chemical compounds that report over the card in the user's natural environment. The main advantage of this application is that it is possible to combine multiple cards, or to change certain conditions such as temperature, it will help the user to see how a particular chemical reaction occurs.

With the aim of investigating the impact (impact) of the popular taxpayer application we see on education for students, a group of 20 participants of first-year electrical engineering specialists, was selected to undertake training using the AR system. 10 of them used a computer screen to visualize 3D computer-generated objects while others used HMD. They were invited to perform the following tasks on the machine with the help of instructions provided by the AR application, and the next day we asked them to perform the same tasks without using the AR application to ensure success, academics were able to work on them without assistance. from a teacher you do not even need to contact, who sees that the procedures are successful. The results show the experts who were able to complete the process in two given sessions

Table 1. AR applications in different fields based on various research.

Heading Level	Day1 Using the AR app	Day 2 Without the use of AR app
Using PC	9	8
Using a head mounted display	10	10

The Satisfaction Survey shows that all academics have expressed an attitude of confidence and optimism in the form of additional facts technology and enhanced content. They feel that the AR application used is strictly configured. A thorough evaluation of the training was intelligent, and many scholars found it extremely useful, very enjoyable and satisfied with the technology and method. All experts considered that the RA system approved for use in education (Singhal, S, 2019).

PROPOSED METHODOLOGY

Simple or basic AR applications often consists of the app scanning the surroundings to understand them and detect unique feature points to make a 3d map, which is then used to place static 3d objects at any position by the user. The objects can then be rotated moved or scaled up or down according to the user. The experience though impressive is limited to the device being used and can't share the information with other devices (Carmigniani J.,2011).

To overcome this problem, cloud anchors come into play. Anchors enable the 3d objects to retain their position and orientation concerning the 3d map to provide a real to life experience. The anchors make it possible to keep sessions available on the same device so that the ar camera can be turned on or off while retaining the information being captured by the ARCore. Cloud anchors are special anchors that by being hosted to ARCore Cloud Anchor API enable the user to share their virtual experience to nearby devices and have a shared experience in real-time.

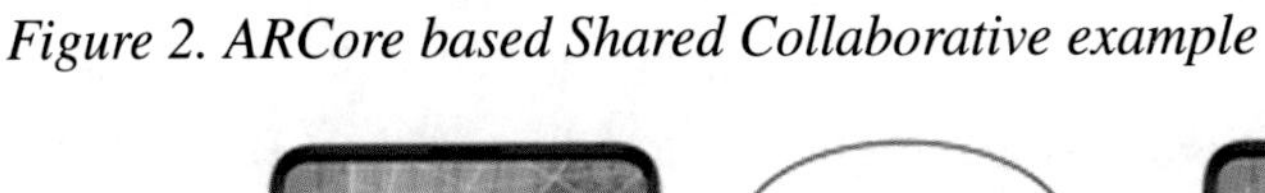

Figure 2. ARCore based Shared Collaborative example

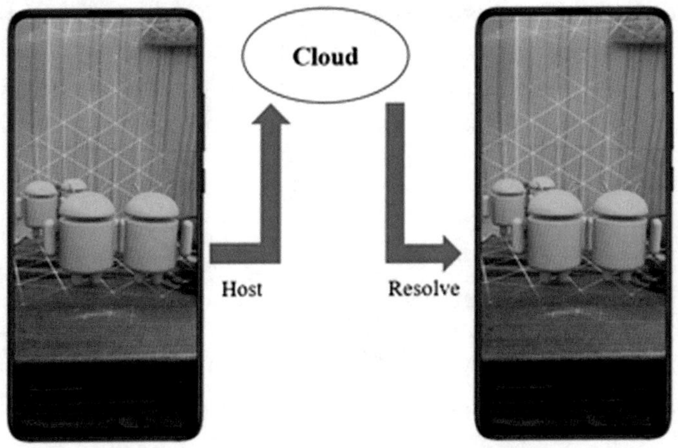

The above figure demonstrates the actual working of the cloud anchors in a mobile application. The steps involved in sharing cloud anchors to share ar information are:

- One user works as a host and scans the surrounding area to build a local anchor.
- When it hosts ARCore using the Google ARCore Anchor API which can be enabled from the Google Cloud Platform, it uploads anchor data to the cloud for a unique id.
- The unique ID can then be shared with other users.
- Some nearby users can solve the anchors by using different ids to recreate the same anchors and the 3d object shape and shape as the host is created in real time.

APPLICATIONS

Augmented reality provides a lot of possible applications in a variety of domains such as medical, entertainment, training, education etc.

Medical: Because of the immersive and interactive experience provided by augmented reality medical students can study the anatomy and other features of animals in a more interactive manner as the students can interact and scale the size of the 3d subjects according to them digitally without actually touching or harming the subject.

Entertainment: Augmented Reality has and can really improve the user experience to provide more entertainment, as instead of just being displayed on a 2d screen, users can get a more immersive 3d experience of the objects they are viewing. For example: in museums people can get a 3d look at the paintings and other artifacts placed in the museum. Also with recent trends AR games have also made their place in the gaming sector of the industry. People can get involved more into the games experience and have a better experience with the AR games (M. Prensky, 2001).

Training: Instead of using screens to provide 2d information to employees or workers, augmented reality can enable the users to get a deeper and more clear understanding of the topics or work areas. For example: Workers or mechanics can get a deeper understanding of the mechanical parts of the vehicle which they can also use to explain and get a deeper understanding of the faults that might have caused the issue in the first place.

Education: AR can majorly benefit and revolutionize the education system, by providing a more immersive and interactive experience to teachers as compared to the one provided by the 2d screens (Singhal, S., 2012). For example: Instead of just looking at images and watching videos about space rockets and solar systems, teachers can use Augmented reality to showcase 3d virtual and interactive space shuttles to students along with a 3d demonstration of the solar system that the students can interact as well using a shared experience and all this can be done using mobile devices thanks to AR Core (Coffin, C., Bostandjiev, 2008).

Table 2. AR applications in different fields based on various research.

Author	Field	Purpose of AR	AR Features Used
Chang et al. (2011)	Medical	Provide training and guide surgical procedures.	AR image guided therapy.
Yeom (2011)	Medical	Teach and test anatomy knowledge.	Interactive 3d anatomy pictures and haptic feedback.
Martin et al. (2011)	History	Gather information to enhance museum experience.	Mobile AR games.
Cerqueira (2012)	Mathematics	Teach geometry using 3d geometry concepts.	Head mounted displays and personal interaction panel.
Fleck & Simon (2013)	Astronomy	Show augmented views of the celestial bodies.	AR learning environment.
Singhal et al. (2012)	Chemistry	Show spatial relation between molecules.	AR for exhibiting the models.
Coffin et al. (2008)	Physics	Overlay graphics on physical props to visualize forces.	Augmented video on physical objects.

LIMITATIONS OF AR

Although having a lot of applications in various domains Augmented Reality often faces certain challenges and limitations. Here are some of the examples:

Realistic Rendering: The current AR solutions are not able to capture enough information in order to render realistic models, due to which even if the system is able to produce realistic models, then also the experience is not fruitful and hence is not favorable. Due to this, developers have started coming to a consensus to develop cartoonist or animated models only so that the interactivity and experience becomes more suitable (L. Kerawalla, 2006).

Estimating Distance: When placing objects in the 3d map, the experience remains intact if the user remains in close proximity to the models. But if there is something in between the user and the model placed after mapping the room then the system is not able update and consider the object in between, which in real case the 3d object should have been behind the object but the model still appears on top of the object. For example: After placing a 3d cube in a room if the person places a chair between the cube and the camera then the cube still appears in front of the chair regardless of the user changing its position.

FUTURE WORK

In order to make sample ARCore applications using java, android studio and ARCore, google had developed an open-source platform named Sceneform. Sceneform is used to convert 3d models from .obj format to .sfb format so that it can be rendered by the use of google arcore in android mobile devices. But in last year's google discontinued its work on project tango as well as sceneform. So now in order to render objects an upgraded version of the sceneform named sceneform maintained is used that instead of converting is directly able to display 3d objects of various formats like .obg, .glb etc.

- Though ARCore has made it easy to use mobile devices to support AR, the mobile devices still lack some important sensors in order to provide better experience, hence more advancements in terms of hardware needs to be made.
- The AR systems need to sense and capture more data relating to the environment instead of just the uyser's position in order to perform effectively.

CONCLUSION

In this paper, we developed basic ar mobile application to place 3d virtual objects on tabletop. We used android studio, java and arcore to build the application. We also used sceneform maintained in order to render the 3d models to android mobile device. We also discussed the concepts behind AR and the applications in which it can be used. We also discussed the limitations and challenged due to which more research and development needs to be done in the field of AR.

REFERENCES

Akçayır, M., & Akçayır, G. (2017). Advantages and challenges associated with augmented reality for education: A systematic review of the literature. *Educational Research Review*, *20*, 1–11. doi:10.1016/j.edurev.2016.11.002

Alexander, T., Westhoven, M., & Conradi, J. (2017). Virtual environments for competency-oriented education and training. In *Advances in Human Factors, Business Management, Training and Education* (pp. 23–29). Springer International Publishing. doi:10.1007/978-3-319-42070-7_3

Ali, A., Glackin, C., Cannings, N., Wall, J., Sharif, S., & Moniri, M. (2019). *A Framework for Augmented Reality Based Shared Experiences*. doi:10.1007/978-3-030-23089-0#about

Azuma, Baillot, Behringer, Feiner, Julier, & MacIntyre. (2001). *Recent Advances in Augmented Reality*. Academic Press.

Cameron, C. (2014). *Spanish students create AR science posters with Layar*. Available: https://www.layar.com/news/blog/2014/12/22/spanishstudents-create-AR-science-posters-with-layar/

Carmigniani, J., & Furht, B. (2011). Augmented Reality: An Overview. In B. Furht (Ed.), *Handbook of Augmented Reality*. Springer. doi:10.1007/978-1-4614-0064-6_1

Cerqueira, C. S., & Kirner, C. (2012). Developing Educational Applications with a Non-Programming Augmented Reality Authoring Tool. *Proceedings of World Conference on Educational Multimedia, Hypermedia and Telecommunications*, 2816-2825.

Chang, G., Morreale, P., & Medicherla, P. (2011). Applications of Augmented Reality Systems in Education. *Proceedings of Society for Information Technology & Teacher Education International Conference*, *2010*, 1380–1385.

Chang, G., Morreale, P., & Medicherla, P. (2011). Applications of Augmented Reality Systems in Education. *Proceedings of Society for Information Technology & Teacher Education International Conference*, *2010*, 1380–1385.

Coffin, C., Bostandjiev, S., Ford, J., & Hollerer, T. (2008). *Enhancing Classroom and Distance Learning Through Augmented Reality*. Academic Press.

Fleck, S., & Simon, G. (2013). *An Augmented Reality Environment for Astronomy Learning in Elementary Grades. An Exploratory Study*. doi:10.1145/2534903.2534907

Gutierrez, M., Guinters, E., & Perez-Lopez, D. (2012). *Improving Strategy of Self-Learning in Engineering: Laboratories with Augmented Reality*. Academic Press.

Hsu, J.-L., & Huang, Y.-H. (2011). *The Advent of Augmented-Learning: A Combination of Augmented Reality and Cloud Computing*. Academic Press.

Kerawalla, Luckin, Seljeflot, & Woolard. (2006). "Making it real": Exploring the potential of augmented reality for teaching primary school science. *Virtual Reality, 10*(3), 163-174.

Martin, S., Diaz, G., Sancristobal, E., Gil, R., Castro, M., & Peire, J. (2011). New technology trends in education: Seven years of forecasts and convergence. *Computer Education, 57*(3), 1893–1906. doi:10.1016/j.compedu.2011.04.003

Prensky, M. (2001). *Digital game-based learning*. McGraw-Hill.

Saidin, N., Abd Halim, N. D., & Yahaya, N. (2015). A Review of Research on Augmented Reality in Education: Advantages and Applications. *International Education Studies, 8*(13). Advance online publication. doi:10.5539/ies.v8n13p1

Sereno, M., Wang, X., Besançon, L., Mcguffin, M., & Isenberg, T. (2020). Collaborative Work in Augmented Reality: A Survey. *IEEE Transactions on Visualization and Computer Graphics*. doi:10.1109/TVCG.2020.3032761

Singhal, S., Bagga, S., Goyal, P., & Saxena, V. (2012). Augmented Chemistry: Interactive Education System. *International Journal of Computers and Applications, 49*(15), 1–5. Advance online publication. doi:10.5120/7700-1041

Yeom, S.-J. (2011). Augmented Reality for Learning Anatomy. Proceedings ASCILITE 2011 Hobart: Concise Paper, 1377-1384.

ADDITIONAL READING

Andone, D., & Frydenberg, M. (2019). Creating Virtual Reality in a Business and Technology Educational Context. In M. tom Dieck & T. Jung (Eds.), *Augmented Reality and Virtual Reality. Progress in IS*. Springer. doi:10.1007/978-3-030-06246-0_11

Baratoff, G., & Regenbrecht, H. (2004). Developing and Applying AR Technology in Design, Production, Service and Training. In S. K. Ong & A. Y. C. Nee (Eds.), *Virtual and Augmented Reality Applications in Manufacturing*. Springer. doi:10.1007/978-1-4471-3873-0_12

Cvetković, D. (Ed.). (2022). *Augmented Reality and Its Application*. IntechOpen. doi:10.5772/intechopen.95165

Haynes, R. (2019). To Have and Vehold: Marrying Museum Objects and Virtual Collections via AR. In M. tom Dieck & T. Jung (Eds.), *Augmented Reality and Virtual Reality. Progress in IS*. Springer. doi:10.1007/978-3-030-06246-0_14

Radu, I. (2014). Augmented reality in education: A meta-review and cross-media analysis. *Personal and Ubiquitous Computing*, *18*(6), 1533–1543. doi:10.100700779-013-0747-y

KEY TERMS AND DEFINITIONS

3D Model Format: Formats used to store and display 3D objects (e.g., .sfb, .obj, etc.).

Anchor: They ensure that the placed objects stay at the same place when user changes its position.

ARCore: Google developed ARCore to support AR applications to mobile devices.

Augmented Reality: Placing of 3D objects into real world environment by the use of ARCore and camera.

Cloud Anchors: Anchors hosted on the cloud ARCore Cloud Anchor API.

Depth Mapping: Scanning and identifying the relative depth of objects with respect to the user.

Feature Points: Unique points in the captured camera image used by the ARCore in addition to device IMU (Inertial Measurement Unit) to provide motion tracking.

Motion Tracking: Tracking the user's position with respect to the tracked real world surrounding.

Rendering: Creating and displaying 3d objects into the augmented reality.

Shared Experience: Sharing the 3D objects and augmented reality experiences among 2 or more devices using cloud.

Chapter 6
A Comparative Study With Linear Regression and Linear Regression With Fuzzy Data for the Same Data Set:
LRFD

Mufala Khan
Lovely Professional University, India

Rakesh Kumar
Lovely Professional University, India

Gaurav Dhiman
Department of Computer Science, Government Bikram College of Commerce, Patiala, India & University Centre for Research and Development, Department of Computer Science and Engineering, Chandigarh University, Gharuan, Mohali, India & Department of Computer Science and Engineering, Graphic Era University (Deemed), Dehradun, India

ABSTRACT

Regression analysis is a quantitative research tool that is used to model and analyse multiple variables in a dependent-independent relationship in order to create the most accurate forecast. These models do not forecast the real value of the data due to uncertainty. As a result, fuzzy regression is critical in overcoming or addressing this type of problem. In this chapter, the authors presented a comparative study of LR models and LR models using fuzzy data and real experimental data. The computational results demonstrate the best linear models for the data set.

DOI: 10.4018/978-1-6684-4405-4.ch006

INTRODUCTION

The collection of statistical methods for evaluating the degree to which one variable is related to another is referred to as regression analysis. It comprises a variety of approaches to demonstrating and assessing multiple variables, with the primary concentration placed on the relationship that exists between dependent variables and one or more independent variables (or "predictors") (Bhoi et al., 2022; Mekala et al., 2022a; Yadav et al., 2022). To be more explicit, regression analysis explains why the average value of the dependent variable, also known as the "criterion variable", shifts when only one of the independent factors is altered while the others remain the same. In the fields of prediction and forecasting, regression analysis is a technique that is frequently utilized. In addition, regression analysis can be used to study the nature of the relationship between an independent variable and the dependent variables, as well as to assess whether or not the independent variable is related to the dependent variables (Sumathy et al., 2022; Alferaidi et al., 2022a; Viriyasitavat et al., 2022; Dhiman et al., 2022a). In the nineteenth century, Francis Galton is credited with coming up with the term "regression" to describe a process that occurs in biological systems. The characteristic observed was that the heights of people whose ancestors had been tall tended to regress towards the normal average as their descendants grew older (a phenomenon that is also k/a regression to the mean). Galton only thought about regression in this biotic way. However, Uday Yule and Karl Pearson later used regression in a more general statistical way in Galton's work. Galton's work inspired them (Gupta et al., 2022; Sharma et al., 2022a; Dinesh Kumar et al., 2022).

Regression can be calculated using the equations Y = a + b or X = a¢ + b¢ Y (depending on whether we're looking at Y on X, where Y depends on X, or X on Y, where X depends on Y). The value of the unknown parameters (***a, b, a', b'***) can be calculated by,

Considering an equation

$$Y = a + bX \tag{1}$$

Where $b=\dfrac{n\left(\sum xy\right)-\left(\sum x\right)\left(\sum y\right)}{n\left(\sum x^2\right)-\left(\sum x\right)^2}$ and a=Y-bX

In an environment characterized by uncertainty, fuzzy regression models are utilized in order to regulate a suitable linear relationship between a dependent variable and a number of independent variables. At first, mathematical programming methods were used to try to figure out what the parameters of an FR model were.

Many years ago, various fields made extensive use of the technique of regression analysis. Tanaka, Uejima, and Asai (1980) were the ones who first presented the concept of fuzzy linear regression. The majority of our lives have been spent playing with crisp sets (Sharma et al., 2022b; Ding et al., 2022; Mekala et al., 2022b). A crisp set is one in which each component is either a member of the set or not. As an illustration, a jellybean is an example of the category of food known as confectionery. Not mashed potatoes, however. On the other hand, fuzzy sets enable elements to only be partially included in a set. The fact that the crisp set-in regression mostly does not convey any idea-related uncertainty is the primary drawback of using this method in regression. In an environment of fuzzy specificity, these kinds of problems can be dealt with in the right way. A piece of information is said to be in a fuzzy state when it does not have a distinct or well-defined border at any point in its presentation (Alferaidi et al., 2022b; Dhiman et al., 2022b; Kanwal et al., 2022).

A fuzzy set's membership function is an oversimplification of the indicator function found in classical sets. As an extension of valuation, it stands for the degree of truth that is represented by fuzzy logic. Although they are conceptually separate from one another, degrees of certainty are frequently confused with probability. This is because "fuzzy fact" denotes membership in loosely defined sets, not the chance of any event or condition. In his first paper, published in 1965, Zadeh was the first person to suggest using a membership function whose range includes the interval [0, 1] when applied to the domain of all possible values (Singh et al., 2022; Swain et al., 2022; Dhiman et al., 2022c; Kour et al., 2022).

When confronted with unpredictability, Lotfi Zadeh's theory proposes that the most effective way to make decisions is to belong to one or more sets. In point of fact, Zadeh stated the following in his important study from the year 1965 (Zeidabadi et al., 2022a, 2022b).

There are many similarities between the framework used in the case of ordinary sets and a fuzzy set, but the fuzzy set concept provides a starting point for a conceptual framework that is more general and capable of improving in order to achieve greater suitability, particularly in the fields of pattern classification and information processing. " Basically, this structure is effective in situations when fuzziness is caused by a lack of clearly defined criteria for belonging to a class rather than random variables (Alharbi et al., 2021; Juneja et al., 2021).

LITERATURE REVIEW

Fuzzy regression models are utilized in a context that is characterized by ambiguity to construct a sufficient linear relationship between a dependent and several independent factors. This relationship is intended to be linear (Kumar and Dhiman, 2021; Vaishnav,

Sharma, and Sharma, 2021). Finding this relationship is important for being able to accurately forecast what will happen in the future. In the beginning, the parameters of the FR model were determined through the use of mathematical programming techniques. This was done to find the model that best corresponds to the data. In the past, researchers working on a wide variety of subjects made substantial use of the approach of regression analysis. This included both quantitative and qualitative researchers. The concept of FLR was proposed by Tanaka, Uejima, and Asai in 1980 (Gupta, Shukla, and Rawat, 2022; Sharma, Nair, and Gomathi, 2022; Shukla et al., 2022). They were the first group of scientists to accomplish this feat. de Andres Sanchez and Terceño Gómez (2003a, 2003b, 2004) and McCauley-Bell et al. (1999), two studies, both used fuzzy regression (FR) in their studies. A non-fuzzy input vector was used in conjunction with a non-fuzzy coefficient matrix, which was based on Tanaka et al. (1989). According to our assumptions, fuzzy numbers are triangular (TFNs). To make the model less fuzzy, support for fuzzy coefficients should be kept to a minimum, but all evidence should still be used (Shapiro, 2005). Up until this moment, the majority of our lives have been spent engaging in the activity of playing with sets that were not soiled. When each of a set's components either belongs or does not belong to the set, we say that the set has crisp components. For example, the category of food known as sweets can be illustrated with a picture such as a jellybean as an example of what constitutes a typical dish from that category. On the other hand, mashed potatoes are not permitted in this context. On the other hand, the inclusion of components is in a set even if they are only present in that set in a limited capacity. This is because fuzzy sets take into account the degree to which a component contributes to the whole. This is because fuzzy sets take into consideration the extent to which a part contributes to the total. The most fundamental disadvantage of doing so is the fact that adopting this strategy in regression rarely communicates any type of idea-related ambiguity. Because of this, it should be avoided because it is one of the fundamental reasons why doing so is a bad idea. In settings with a relatively modest degree of detail, issues of this nature can be resolved in the most time and labor-saving manner possible. It is claimed that a piece of data is in a fuzzy condition whenever it does not, at any point in the presentation of that data, have a clear and well-defined border. This might happen at any time during the display of the data. This is something that could take place at any point throughout the display of the material.

The membership function that is typical of fuzzy sets is built upon the indicator function that is typical of classical sets. This serves as the basis for the membership function that is typical of fuzzy sets. There are many different types of fuzzy regression models, but the most common is the generalized regression model (Gregori et al., 2011). FLR seeks an R-Model that meets a given condition while also fitting all of the data. In this study, nonparametric FR functions with non-fuzzy inputs and

(STF) outputs are studied and predicted using an (ANFIS). To accomplish this, two new hybrid methods have been presented in which FLS and linear programming have been employed for maximizing the secondary weights. The algorithms are employed as part of a multi-layered validation process. Asymmetric trapezoidal fuzzy outputs with crisp inputs and three different nonparametric fuzzy regression methods are also contrasted. There are three nonparametric procedures in statistics (K-NN), (K-S), and TFD, which have been investigated to find the optimal smoothing parameters (Chakravarty et al., 2020). The existence of data outliers is a problem that frequently affects popular regression approaches. The many approaches that have been presented are aimed at minimizing the impact of the outlier on the parameter estimates. In this investigation, an algorithm has been addressed that is based on an (ANBFI) system. The purpose of this method is to define the unknown parameters of a regression model in which the dependent variable contains an outlier. Fuzzy linear programming with (FTN) variable profit optimization (Kumar, 2021) is used. Therefore, three numerical cases are solved to demonstrate the effectiveness of the proposed approach in the estimation of the regression model. In addition to this, the results that were achieved using the various methodologies, such as (LP) and (FWLP), are compared with one another (Chakravarty et al., 2020). A broader version of the indicator function can be found in this membership function. It is a reference to the degree of truth that can be exemplified by fuzzy logic, and in the context of valuation, this term is being used (Hose & Hanss, 2019). The degree of truth and the probability of an event is frequently confused for one another, even though they are conceptually distinct from one another. Even though a lot of people get this wrong, it is nonetheless the case. The term "fuzzy truth" refers to membership in sets that are very loosely specified, which is the source of the misunderstanding that has arisen. It is in no way, shape, or form that refers to the likelihood of any event or condition occurring. In his first article, which dealt with the topic of fuzzy sets and was published in 1965, Zadeh was the first person to suggest membership functions. This paper was also his first publication. This was Zadeh's first time having any of his work published. In his theory of fuzzy sets, Zadeh proposed using a membership function that, when applied to all possible values, has a range that includes the interval [0, 1]. In other words, the membership function would have a range between zero and one. This selection was made available by Zadeh. Lotfi Zadeh's thesis says that the best way to make decisions when things aren't clear is to be a part of one or more sets. This idea is supported by the research that Lotfi Zadeh conducted. This is true, especially in situations where there are several different sets to select from. In his seminal work (Zadeh 1965), he made the subsequent observation about fuzzy sets. "There are many similarities between the outline used in the case of ordinary sets and fuzzy sets, but the framework of fuzzy sets is more general and capable of enhancement to get a broader range of suitability, particularly in fields of pattern recognition," he explains in a statement. (Zadeh, 1965) This structure is ideal for dealing with problems where the source of uncertainty is the lack of well-defined criteria for class membership rather than the absence of random variables. The reason for this is as follows: This is a result of the fact that such a structure provides an efficient method of resolving problems in which the absence of random variables is the primary source of the problem. Because of this, having this kind of framework makes it easy to deal with difficulties, the complexity of which is often brought on by the absence of random variables. This is because having this kind of framework makes it easier to deal with problems.

METHODOLOGY

Linear Regression

Estimating the value of one variable given the values of the other variables and parameters in the data sets is the purpose of the LR analysis. The term "dependent variable" refers to the variable for which the behaviour of which you wish to make a prediction. The variable whose value is being utilized as a basis for making a forecast about another variable is referred to as "independent variable," and this is the meaning of the word "independent variable." In this sort of analysis, the coefficients of the linear equation are found by employing one or more independent variables to determine which ones produce the most accurate predictions of the value of the dependent variable. This can be done with more than one independent variable. Finding a straight line that minimizes the difference between the predictable output values and the actual output value is the objective of linear regression. This can be accomplished by finding the line or surface that best fits the data. There are calculators that can perform simple linear regression, and one of its functions is to use a method k/a "least squares. These calculators are accessible. After that, you must determine, using Y as a starting point, what the value of the X, will be (the independent variable).

Linear regression has an equation of the form $\boldsymbol{Y = a + b\ X}$, where $\boldsymbol{X}$ is the explanatory variable and $\boldsymbol{Y}$ is a dependent variable. The slope of the line is $\boldsymbol{b}$, and $\boldsymbol{a}$ is the intercept (the value of $\boldsymbol{y}$ when $\boldsymbol{x} = 0$).

LR Analysis

The collection of numerical approaches required for simulation, problem resolution, and study into the association between response variables and regressor or predictor ones is the focus of regression assessment. Numerous examples of uses of regression analysis may be found in nearly all areas of applied research, including engineering, chemistry, physics, biology, social science, management, and economics. These applications come in a wide variety of settings. The LR model is one of the most common types, among those that study regression. In addition, the estimate of the model's parameters using probabilistic and linear regression procedures is the primary function of regression models. Certain observations are taken into account when the fuzzy data form is used. As a result, one of the difficulties associated with FLR analysis is figuring out how to estimate coefficients and then proceed to generate a prediction while working within a fuzzy environment.

Fuzzy Regression Analysis

Classical Statistical linear regression takes the form

$$y = a_{0+}a_1x_1 + \ldots + a_nx_n \quad (2)$$

Where y is an output variable, $x_1, x_2, \ldots, x_n$ are input variables, and $y_1, y_2, \ldots, y_n$ are parameters. Problem of regression analysis formulated in terms of this linear form is called linear regression.

Statistical regression offers a wide range of uses, although the following conditions can cause issues:

- This study's sample size is insufficient.
- Verification of the distribution assumptions proves difficult.
- The link between the input and output variables is ill-defined.
- The level of ambiguity of events or their occurrence
- Linearization introduces errors and distortions

This means that statistical regression is hard to do if the data sets are too small, if the linearity assumption is not valid, or if it is not possible to check that the error is normally distributed. When fuzzy regression was first made, this is exactly the kind of problem that was thought to be solved by it.

There are two general ways to develop the FR model:

1. LR with fuzzy Parameters
2. LR with fuzzy Data.

LR with Fuzzy Data

Fuzzy regression uses a form to rapid the relationship between an output variable and its input variables.

$$Y = a_1 X_1 + \ldots\ldots + a_n X_n \tag{3}$$

Where a_1, a_2, …, a_n are real-valued parameters and the values of the I/O variables are likely to be triangular and symmetric.

Let, $X_i = (x_i, s_i)$ for all $i \in N_n$. Then,

$$Y(y) = \begin{cases} 1 - \dfrac{\left|y - a^t X\right|}{a^{t|a|}} & \text{when } a \neq 0 \\ 1 & \text{when } a = 0, y \neq 0 \\ 0 & \text{when } a = 0, y = 0 \end{cases} \tag{4}$$

For all $y \in R$, where

$$a = \begin{bmatrix} a_1 \\ \vdots \\ a_n \end{bmatrix}, \ldots X = \begin{matrix} x_1 \\ \vdots \\ x_n \end{matrix}, \ldots s = \begin{bmatrix} s_1 \\ \vdots \\ s_n \end{bmatrix}$$

Data are given in term of pairs (X^j, Y^j), where X^j is an n-tuple of STFNs, and Y^j is symmetric TFN for $\forall j \in N_n$.

Using these criteria, according to following optimization problem, fuzzy regression problem can be stated in terms of.

Minimize

$$\sum_{j=1}^{m} \left| \int_R Y^j y dy - \int_R Y_j(y) dy \right| \tag{5}$$

s.t. $\min_{j \in N_m} (Y^J, Y_J) \geq h$

let $X_j^i = \left(X_i^j, S_i^j\right)$ for all $i \in N_n$ and $(Y^j = y^j, s^j)$

Then, here's another way you could approach the fuzzy regression problem of this type.

Minimize

$$\sum_{i=1}^{m} | s^{j} - \sum_{i=1}^{n} |a_{i}| s_{j} |$$

$$\text{s.t} \ -\sum_{i=1}^{m} |a_{i}| s^{j} - \sum_{i=1}^{n} a_{i} x_{i}^{j} \leq y^{j} - s^{j}$$

$$\sum_{i=1}^{m} |a_{i}| s^{j} + \sum_{i=1}^{n} a_{i} x_{i}^{j} \geq y^{j} - s^{j}$$

$$a_{i} \in R \ \forall i \in N_{n} \text{ and } \forall j \in N_{m} \quad (6)$$

DATA COLLECTION AND RESULTS

This data is from The Punjab State Cooperative Agricultural Development Bank, Expenditure from 2016-2022 of PSCADB

Table 1. A look at financials from the year 2016-22. (In Crores.)

Credentials	2016-17	2017-18	2018-19	2019-20	2020-21	2021-22
Reserves and other funds	(410.29,0.1015)	(412.63,0)	(408.77,0.2535)	(427.82,0)	(386.58,0.5)	(361.74,0)
Paid-up share capital	(70.91,0.6466)	(71.73,0.8506)	(72.95,0.7286)	(74.52,0.8924))	(75.86,0.7)	(77.16,0.4)
Total own funds	(481.2,0.576)	(484.36,0.26)	(481.73,0.523)	(502.34,0)	(462.44,0.5)	(449.71,0)
Profit	(20.7,0.1015)	(28.77,0)	(25.66,0.4955)	(24.93,0)	(25.42,0.7)	(10.81,0.4)
SADB Level	(487.08,0)	(431.64,0)	(501.11,0)	(506.54,0)	(559.8,0.5)	(490.22,0)
PADBs Level	(513.11,0)	(465.54,0)	(628.07,0)	(646.69,0)	(663.59,0.7)	(488.98,0.4)
Total Loan Outstanding	(2187.95,0)	(2226.66,0)	(2309.87,0)	(2428.86,0)	(2617.95,0.5)	(2704.03,0)
Borrowing Outstanding	(2048.6,0)	(2123.06,0)	(2163.14,0)	(2277.79,0)	(2332.1,0.5)	(2368.63,0.4)
Working capital (Average)	(2783.4, 0.7985)	(2962.53, 0.3945)	(3131.56,0.70)	(3234.98,0.77)	(3210.95,0.5)	(3357,0.4)
SADB	(35.61,0.748)	(54.92,0)	(43.99,0)	(41.09,0)	(21.07,0.7)	(1.9,0)
PABD	(56.31,0.95)	(83.69,0)	(69.65,0)	(66.02,0)	(46.49,0.7)	(12.71,0)

Regression analysis with linear regression and membership function analysis with fuzzy linear regression were both used to solve data from 2020–21 for comparative study of data.

The regression equation is $Y=bX+a$

$b = SP/SSX = 14573593.543/13891598.9957$

$$a = \overline{Y} - b\overline{X} = 938.44 - (1.05 * 945.66) = -53.640706$$

$Y = 1.04909X - 53.64076.$

The equation of simple linear form for the linear regression with fuzzy data is $Y=aX$.

Hence, for the year 2020-21 is

$$Y = 1.02X \tag{7}$$

Figure 1. linear regression graph for the year 2020-21

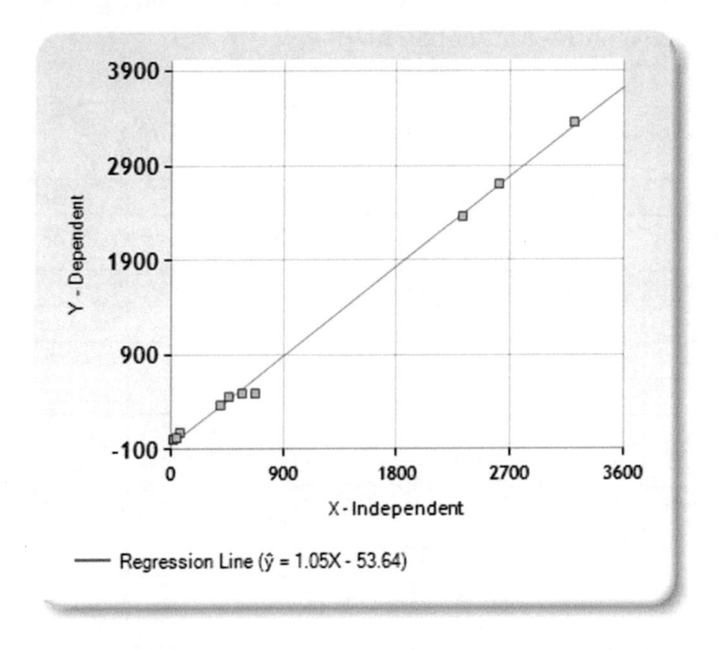

Regression analysis with linear regression and membership function analysis with fuzzy linear regression were both used to solve data from 2019–20

The Regression equation is $Y=bX+a$

$b = SP/SSX = 14173147.536/13158332.6767$

$$a = \overline{Y} - b\overline{X} = 938.44 - (1.08 * 930.14) = -63.4349$$

$$Y = 1.07712X - 63.4349$$

The equation of simple linear form for the linear regression with fuzzy data is $Y=aX$.

Hence, for the year 2020-21 is

$$Y = 19.6X, \quad (8)$$

Figure 2. Linear Regression graph for the year 2019-20

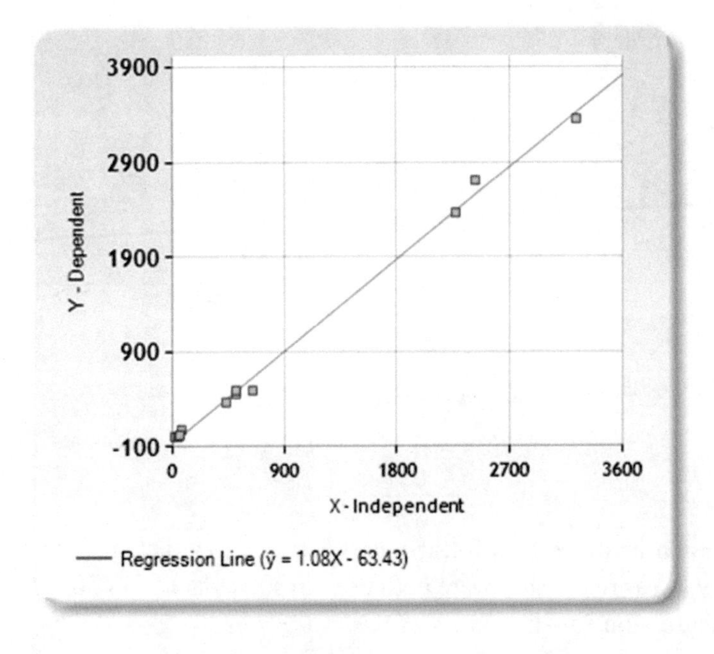

Regression analysis with linear regression and membership function analysis with fuzzy linear regression were both used to solve data from 2018–19

The Regression equation is $Y=bX+a$

$b = SP/SSX = 13575423.3329/12082781.7854$

$$a = \overline{Y} - b\overline{X} = 938.44 - (1.12 * 894.23) = -66.25073$$

$$Y = 1.12353X - 66.25075$$

The equation of simple linear form for the linear regression with fuzzy data is *Y=aX*.

Hence, for the year 20219-20 is

$$Y = 18.73X \quad (9)$$

Figure 3. Linear Regression graph for the year 2018-19

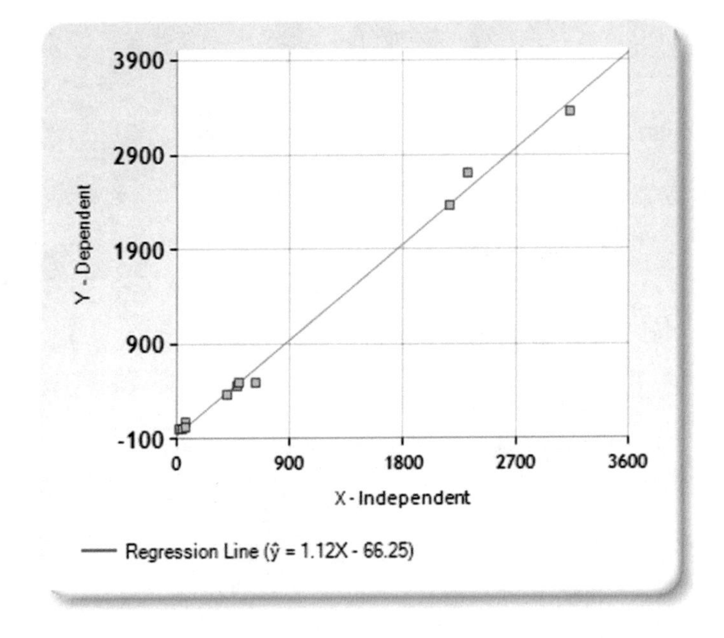

Regression analysis with linear regression and membership function analysis with fuzzy linear regression were both used to solve data from 2017–18

The Regression equation is *Y=bX+a*

$$b = SP/SSX = 13037988.9649/11125981.5397$$

$$a = \overline{Y} - b\overline{X} = 938.44 - (1.17 * 849.59) = -57.15233$$

$$Y = 1.17185X - 57.15233$$

The equation of simple linear form for the linear regression with fuzzy data is $Y=aX$.

Hence, for the year 2020-21 is

$$Y = 17.0X, \tag{10}$$

Figure 4. Linear Regression graph for the year 2017-18

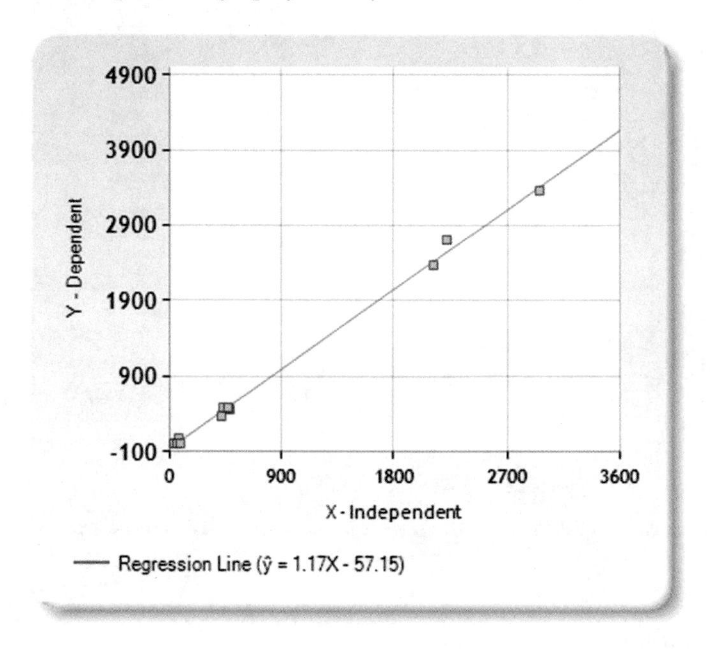

Regression analysis with linear regression and membership function analysis with fuzzy linear regression were both used to solve data from 2016–17

The Regression equation is $Y=bX+a$

$$b = SP/SSX = 12438202.5482/10121342.5036$$

$$a = \overline{Y} - b\overline{X} = 938.44 - (1.23 * 826.83) = -77.6571$$

$$Y = 1.22891X - 77.6571$$

The equation of simple linear form for the linear regression with fuzzy data is $Y=aX$.

Hence, for the year 2020-21 is

$$Y = 23.5X \tag{11}$$

Figure 5. Linear Regression graph for the year 2016-17

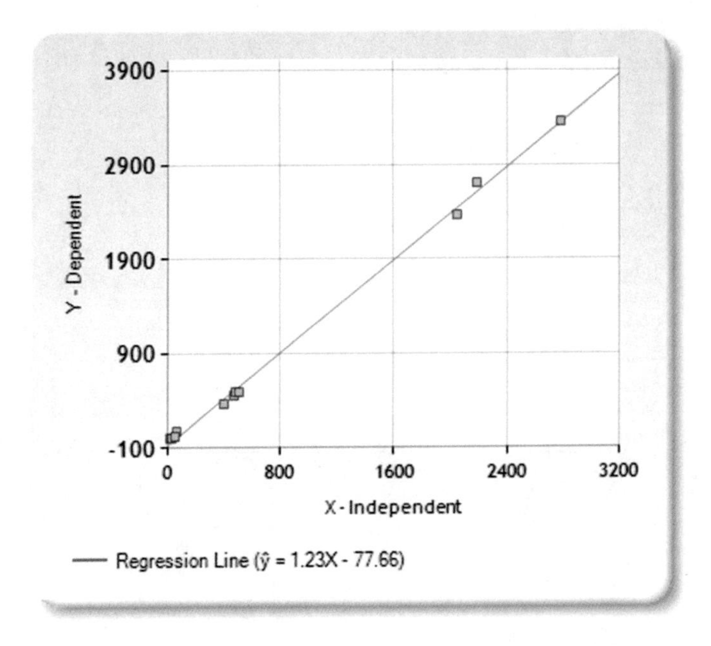

CONCLUSION

In this paper, we undertake a comparative analysis of linear regression models and linear regression models with fuzzy data using actual experimental data from 2016 to 2022. In this research, we have considered the data for the years 2021–22 to be dependent data, whereas the data for the prior years has been considered independent data. The results of the calculations show an example of the best linear model that can be used to describe this set of data.

REFERENCES

Alferaidi, A., Yadav, K., Alharbi, Y., Razmjooy, N., Viriyasitavat, W., Gulati, K., ... Dhiman, G. (2022a). Distributed Deep CNN-LSTM Model for Intrusion Detection Method in IoT-Based Vehicles. *Mathematical Problems in Engineering*.

Alferaidi, A., Yadav, K., Alharbi, Y., Viriyasitavat, W., Kautish, S., & Dhiman, G. (2022b). Federated Learning Algorithms to Optimize the Client and Cost Selections. *Mathematical Problems in Engineering*.

Alharbi, Y., Alferaidi, A., Yadav, K., Dhiman, G., & Kautish, S. (2021). Denial-of-Service Attack Detection over IPv6 Network Based on KNN Algorithm. *Wireless Communications and Mobile Computing*.

Bhoi, A., Balabantaray, R. C., Sahoo, D., Dhiman, G., Khare, M., Narducci, F., & Kaur, A. (2022). Mining social media text for disaster resource management using a feature selection based on forest optimization. *Computers & Industrial Engineering*, 108280.

Chakravarty, S., Demirhan, H., & Baser, F. (2020). Fuzzy regression functions with a noise cluster and the impact of outliers on mainstream machine learning methods in the regression setting. *Applied Soft Computing*, *96*, 106535.

de Andres Sanchez, J., & Gómez, A. T. (2003b). Estimating a term structure of interest rates for fuzzy financial pricing by using fuzzy regression methods. *Fuzzy Sets and Systems*, *139*(2), 313–331.

de Andrés Sánchez, J., & Gómez, A. T. (2004). Estimating a fuzzy term structure of interest rates using fuzzy regression techniques. *European Journal of Operational Research*, *154*(3), 804–818.

de Andres Sanchez, J., & Terceño Gómez, A. (2003a). Applications of fuzzy regression in actuarial analysis. *The Journal of Risk and Insurance*, *70*(4), 665–699.

Dhiman, G., Juneja, S., Mohafez, H., El-Bayoumy, I., Sharma, L. K., Hadizadeh, M., ... Khandaker, M. U. (2022a). Federated learning approach to protect healthcare data over big data scenario. *Sustainability*, *14*(5), 2500.

Dhiman, G., Juneja, S., Viriyasitavat, W., Mohafez, H., Hadizadeh, M., Islam, M. A., ... Gulati, K. (2022c). A novel machine-learning-based hybrid CNN model for tumor identification in medical image processing. *Sustainability*, *14*(3), 1447.

Dhiman, G., Rashid, J., Kim, J., Juneja, S., Viriyasitavat, W., & Gulati, K. (2022b). Privacy for healthcare data using the byzantine consensus method. *Journal of the Institution of Electronics and Telecommunication Engineers*, 1–12.

Dinesh Kumar, R., Golden Julie, E., Harold Robinson, Y., Vimal, S., Dhiman, G., & Veerasamy, M. (2022). Deep convolutional nets learning classification for artistic style transfer. *Scientific Programming*.

Ding, H., Cao, X., Wang, Z., Dhiman, G., Hou, P., Wang, J., ... Hu, X. (2022). Velocity clamping-assisted adaptive salp swarm algorithm: Balance analysis and case studies. *Mathematical Biosciences and Engineering*, *19*(8), 7756–7804.

Gregori, D., Petrinco, M., Bo, S., Desideri, A., Merletti, F., & Pagano, E. (2011). Regression models for analyzing costs and their determinants in health care: An introductory review. *International Journal for Quality in Health Care*, *23*(3), 331–341.

Gupta, N., Gupta, K., Gupta, D., Juneja, S., Turabieh, H., Dhiman, G., ... Viriyasitavat, W. (2022). Enhanced virtualization-based dynamic bin-packing optimized energy management solution for heterogeneous clouds. *Mathematical Problems in Engineering*.

Gupta, V. K., Shukla, S. K., & Rawat, R. S. (2022). Crime tracking system and people's safety in India using machine learning approaches. *International Journal of Modern Research*, *2*(1), 1–7.

Hose, D., & Hanss, M. (2019). Fuzzy linear least squares for the identification of possibilistic regression models. *Fuzzy Sets and Systems*, *367*, 82–95.

Juneja, S., Juneja, A., Dhiman, G., Jain, S., Dhankhar, A., & Kautish, S. (2021). computer Vision-Enabled character recognition of hand Gestures for patients with hearing and speaking disability. *Mobile Information Systems*.

Kanwal, S., Rashid, J., Kim, J., Juneja, S., Dhiman, G., & Hussain, A. (2022). Mitigating the coexistence technique in wireless body area networks by using superframe interleaving. *Journal of the Institution of Electronics and Telecommunication Engineers*, 1–15.

Kour, K., Gupta, D., Gupta, K., Dhiman, G., Juneja, S., Viriyasitavat, W., ... Islam, M. A. (2022). Smart-hydroponic-based framework for saffron cultivation: A precision smart agriculture perspective. *Sustainability*, *14*(3), 1120.

Kumar, R., Chandrawat, R. K., Sarkar, B., Joshi, V., & Majumder, A. (2021). An advanced optimization technique for smart production using α-cut based quadrilateral fuzzy number. *International Journal of Fuzzy Systems*, *23*(1), 107–127.

Kumar, R., & Dhiman, G. (2021). A comparative study of fuzzy optimization through fuzzy number. *International Journal of Modern Research*, *1*(1), 1–14.

McCauley-Bell, P. R., Crumpton-Young, L. L., & Badiru, A. B. (1999). Techniques and applications of fuzzy theory in quantifying risk levels in occupational injuries and illnesses. In *Fuzzy Theory Systems* (pp. 223–265). Academic Press.

Mekala, M. S., Dhiman, G., Srivastava, G., Nain, Z., Zhang, H., Viriyasitavat, W., & Varma, G. P. S. (2022a). *A DRL-Based Service Offloading Approach Using DAG for Edge Computational Orchestration. IEEE Transactions on Computational Social Systems.*

Mekala, M. S., Srivastava, G., Lin, J. C. W., Dhiman, G., Park, J. H., & Jung, H. Y. (2022b). An efficient quantum based D2D computation and communication approach for the Internet of Things. *Optical and Quantum Electronics, 54*(6), 1–19.

Shapiro, A. F. (2005). Fuzzy regression models. *Article of Penn State University, 102*(2), 373–383.

Sharma, S., Gupta, S., Gupta, D., Juneja, S., Gupta, P., Dhiman, G., & Kautish, S. (2022a). Deep Learning Model for the Automatic Classification of White Blood Cells. *Computational Intelligence and Neuroscience.*

Sharma, S., Gupta, S., Gupta, D., Juneja, S., Singal, G., Dhiman, G., & Kautish, S. (2022b). Recognition of Gurmukhi Handwritten City Names Using Deep Learning and Cloud Computing. *Scientific Programming.*

Sharma, T., Nair, R., & Gomathi, S. (2022). Breast cancer image classification using transfer learning and convolutional neural network. *International Journal of Modern Research, 2*(1), 8–16.

Shukla, S. K., Gupta, V. K., Joshi, K., Gupta, A., & Singh, M. K. (2022). Self-aware Execution Environment Model (SAE2) for the Performance Improvement of Multicore Systems. *International Journal of Modern Research, 2*(1), 17–27.

Singh, N., Houssein, E. H., Singh, S. B., & Dhiman, G. (2022). HSSAHHO: A novel hybrid Salp swarm-Harris hawks optimization algorithm for complex engineering problems. *Journal of Ambient Intelligence and Humanized Computing*, 1–37.

Sumathy, B., Chakrabarty, A., Gupta, S., Hishan, S. S., Raj, B., Gulati, K., & Dhiman, G. (2022). Prediction of Diabetic Retinopathy Using Health Records With Machine Learning Classifiers and Data Science. *International Journal of Reliable and Quality E-Healthcare, 11*(2), 1–16.

Swain, S., Bhushan, B., Dhiman, G., & Viriyasitavat, W. (2022). Appositeness of Optimized and Reliable Machine Learning for Healthcare: A Survey. *Archives of Computational Methods in Engineering*, 1–23.

Tanaka, H., Hayashi, I., & Watada, J. (1989). Possibilistic linear regression analysis for fuzzy data. *European Journal of Operational Research, 40*(3), 389–396.

Tanaka, H., Uejima, S., & Asai, K. (1980). *Fuzzy linear regression model*. Presented at the *International Congress on Applied Systems Research and Cybernetics*, Acapulco, Mexico.

Vaishnav, P. K., Sharma, S., & Sharma, P. (2021). Analytical review analysis for screening COVID-19 disease. *International Journal of Modern Research*, *1*(1), 22–29.

Viriyasitavat, W., Xu, L. D., Sapsomboon, A., Dhiman, G., & Hoonsopon, D. (2022). Building trust of Blockchain-based Internet-of-Thing services using public key infrastructure. *Enterprise Information Systems*, 1–24.

Yadav, K., Jain, A., Osman Sid Ahmed, N. M., Saad Hamad, S. A., Dhiman, G., & Alotaibi, S. D. (2022). Internet of Thing based Koch Fractal Curve Fractal Antennas for Wireless Applications. *Journal of the Institution of Electronics and Telecommunication Engineers*, 1–10.

Zadeh, L. A. (1965, June). Fuzzy sets. *Information and Control*, *8*(3), 338–353. doi:10.1016/S0019-9958(65)90241-X

Zeidabadi, F. A., Doumari, S. A., Dehghani, M., Montazeri, Z., Trojovsky, P., & Dhiman, G. (2022a). MLA: A new mutated leader algorithm for solving optimization problems. *Computers. Materials & Continua*, *70*(3), 5631–5649.

Zeidabadi, F. A., Doumari, S. A., Dehghani, M., Montazeri, Z., Trojovsky, P., & Dhiman, G. (2022b). AMBO: All members-based optimizer for solving optimization problems. *CMC-Comput. Mater. Contin*, *70*, 2905–2921.

ADDITIONAL READING

Azadeh, A., Seraj, O., & Saberi, M. (2011). An integrated fuzzy regression–analysis of variance algorithm for improvement of electricity consumption estimation in uncertain environments. *International Journal of Advanced Manufacturing Technology*, *53*(5), 645–660. doi:10.100700170-010-2862-5

Azadeh, A., Sohrabi, P., & Ebrahimipour, V. (2013). A fuzzy regression approach for improvement of gasoline consumption estimation with uncertain data. *International Journal of Industrial and Systems Engineering*, *13*(1), 92–109. doi:10.1504/IJISE.2013.050547

Baser, F., & Apaydin, A. (2010). Calculating insurance claim reserves with hybrid fuzzy least squares regression analysis. *Gazi University Journal of Science*, *23*(2), 163–170.

Chandrawat, R. K., & Joshi, V. (2020, May). Profit Optimization of products at different selling prices with fuzzy linear programming problem using situational based fuzzy triangular numbers. *Journal of Physics: Conference Series*, *1531*(1), 012085.

Chen, F., Chen, Y., Zhou, J., & Liu, Y. (2015). Optimizing h value for fuzzy regression with asymmetric triangular coefficient. *Engineering Applications of Artificial Intelligence*, 1–9.

Dubois, D., & Prade, H. (1978). Operations on fuzzy numbers. *International Journal of Systems Science*, *9*(6), 613–626. doi:10.1080/00207727808941724

Dubois, D., & Prade, H. (1980). Systems of linear fuzzy constraints. *Fuzzy Sets and Systems*, *3*(1), 37–48. doi:10.1016/0165-0114(80)90004-4

Huang, C. Y., & Tzeng, G. H. (2008). Multiple generation product life cycle predictions using a novel two-stage fuzzy piecewise regression analysis method. *Technological Forecasting and Social Change*, *75*(1), 12–31.

Ishibuchi, H., & Nii, M. (2001). Fuzzy regression using asymmetric fuzzy coefficients and fuzzified neural networks. *Fuzzy Sets and Systems*, *119*(2), 273–290.

Kao, C., & Chyu, C. L. (2002). A fuzzy linear regression model with better explanatory power. *Fuzzy Sets and Systems*, *126*(3), 401–409. doi:10.1016/S0165-0114(01)00069-0

Kao, C., & Chyu, C. L. (2003). Least-squares estimates in fuzzy regression analysis. *European Journal of Operational Research*, *148*(2), 426–435. doi:10.1016/S0377-2217(02)00423-X

Kim, B., & Bishu, R. R. (1998). Evaluation of fuzzy linear regression models by comparing membership functions. *Fuzzy Sets and Systems*, *100*(1-3), 343–352. doi:10.1016/S0165-0114(97)00100-0

Kumar, R., Dhiman, G., Kumar, N., Chandrawat, R. K., Joshi, V., & Kaur, A. (2021b). A novel approach to optimize the production cost of railway coaches of India using situational-based composite triangular and trapezoidal fuzzy LPP models. *Complex & Intelligent Systems*, *7*(4), 2053–2068.

Prade, H. M. (1980). Operations research with fuzzy data. In *Fuzzy Sets* (pp. 155–170). Springer. doi:10.1007/978-1-4684-3848-2_14

Pushpa, B., & Vasuki, R. (2013). A least absolute approach to multiple fuzzy regression using Tw-norm based operations. *International Journal of Fuzzy Logic Systems*, *3*(2), 73–84. doi:10.5121/ijfls.2013.3206

Tanaka, H. (1992). Possibilistic regression analysis based on linear programming. *Fuzzy Regression Analysis*.

Tanaka, H., & Asai, K. (1981). Fuzzy linear programming based on fuzzy functions. *IFAC Proceedings Volumes, 14*(2), 785-790.

Wang, H. F., & Tsaur, R. C. (2000). Resolution of fuzzy regression model. *European Journal of Operational Research, 126*(3), 637–650.

Yager, R. R. (1979). On solving fuzzy mathematical relationships. *Information and Control, 41*(1), 29–55. doi:10.1016/S0019-9958(79)80004-2

Chapter 7
A Comparative Study of Fuzzy Linear and Multi-Objective Optimization

Pinki Gulia
Lovely Professional University, India

Rakesh Kumar
Lovely Professional University, India

Amandeep Kaur
Chandigarh University, India

Gaurav Dhiman
Department of Computer Science, Government Bikram College of Commerce, Patiala, India & University Centre for Research and Development, Department of Computer Science and Engineering, Chandigarh University, Gharuan, Mohali, India & Department of Computer Science and Engineering, Graphic Era University (Deemed), Dehradun, India

ABSTRACT

A new paradigm for the solution of problems involving single- and multi-objective fuzzy linear programming is presented in this chapter. As opposed to complex arithmetic and logic for intervals, the method offered uses basic fuzzy mathematical operations for fuzzy integers instead. Using fuzzy numbers to express variables and parameters in a fuzzy linear programming issue (FLPP) is common. However, the authors only talked about FLPP with fuzzy parameters here. Triangular fuzzy numbers are used as fuzzy parameters. Ranking functions are used to convert fuzzy problems into clear ones. Crisp optimization techniques have been used. The proposed solution is tested on a variety of real-world examples that address both of these concerns.

DOI: 10.4018/978-1-6684-4405-4.ch007

INTRODUCTION

The acceptance value of elements in fuzzy logic can range from 0 to 1, making it a type of many-valued logic (*Zadeh 1988*, n.d.) When dealing with the concept of incomplete truth, it is utilised. In Boolean logic, however, elements can only accept the exact values 0 and 1. Fuzzy sets are comparable to sets in which the elements have varying degrees of membership (Goguen, 1973), but they are not identical. In an attempt to expand the concept of accumulation, Dieter Klaua and Lotfi A. Zadeh created Fuzzy Sets in 1965.

The use of operational research has already been formally accepted as a means of enhancing optimization. LPPs aid in the efficient utilisation of existing mechanisms. In this way, we can better respond to the existing environment. Profitability is the key issue here. Optimization is a method of analysis in the field of optimization. Optimization is a mathematical technique used to achieve an objective function. It is a scientific idea that has emerged since World War 2, when a number of factors had to be maximised based on a set of challenges. Transporting large amounts of materials is a serious concern for him. Optimization is a theoretical strategy for resolving specific problems within a system of equations (Sharma et al., 2022a), (Kumar et al., 2022), (Sharma et al., 2022b), (Ding et al., 2022), (Kanwal et al., 2022), (Alferaidi et al., 2022).

Management can make better decisions with the help of linear programming. Operational research employs this method frequently. Using this mathematical method, a company can make the best use of its limited resources. The following terms are commonly used in linear programming: In order to make a decision, we need to know what variables we need to look for. Decision variables must meet certain constraints before they can be used. The term "objective function" refers to a process in which we must strive to improve. Linear relationship situations in which the optimization problem and the constraints are expressed mathematically. A workable solution in which the variables meet the criteria (Zeidabadi et al., 2022), (Yadav et al., 2022), (Swain et al., 2022), (Viriyasitavat et al., 2021), (Prasanna et al., 2021), (Oliva et al., 2021). The best feasible value for the goal function represents the ideal solution. A simple LPP can

$$\text{maximum or minimum } Z = \sum_{k=1}^{n} \mathrm{C_k\, D_k} \quad (1)$$

be represented as:

$$\text{Subject to } \sum_{k=1}^{n} x_{p,k} D_k \leq y_p \text{ for p= 1, 2, ...m,} \tag{2}$$

A fuzzy technique was used to resolve LPP concerns when the data was unknown. The Fuzzy Linear Programming Problem is the name given to this group of problems (FLPP) (Bellman & Zadeh, 1970). A wide range of decision-making processes are required to address these concerns. According to (Ghanbari et al., 2020) when solving a problem involving fuzzy linear programming, variables and parameters are regarded as fuzzy numbers. FLPP can be put into three groups: variables treated as fuzzy numbers (FVLPP), parameters treated as fuzzy numbers (FNLPP), and both variables and parameters (FFLPP). We simply talked about FNLPP in terms of the solution approach (Kumar and Dhiman, 2021), (Vaishnav et al., 2021), (Chatterjee, 2021), (Gupta et al., 2022). This model's assumptions are tested using real-world examples. Depending on the nature of fuzzy numbers, there are a variety of different types of difficulties. Only triangular fuzzy numbers were employed in the suggested study. The best strategy for solving a problem depends on the number of objective functions it contains. Problem types and solution models are covered in detail in the manuscript under consideration. The LPP technique is used to solve FLPP that have been transformed into simpler ones (Alferaidi et al., 2022), (Puti et al., 2022), (Viriyasitavat et al., 2022), (Dhiman et al., 2022), (Gupta et al., 2022).

Literature Review

Optimization for linear objective functions, as well as systems of inequalities and equations, can be accomplished using technique of optimization(Kuschel & Rackwitz, 1997). Constraints are linear inequalities or equations that must be met. The objective function describes the quantity that has to be increased or decreased (optimised) (Sharma et al., 2022), (Shukla et al., 2022). The linear programming model searches for optimal values to find the optimal (maximum or minimum) values for the variables. LPP designs can be used to model a wide range of real-world issues. This method will not work for all issues, however, unless additional "arbitrary" constraints are applied, in which case the objective function will not be completely unique. There are LP models that necessitate several concurrent goal functions that will be identified using MOLP models (Multi-Objective Linear Programming) (or more briefly, "objectives") (Marler & Arora, 2010). Linear programming problems are known as imprecise linear programming problems if their participant ranks increase or decrease over a certain duration of time, which is why they are called fuzzy linear programming problems. This enrollment role can produce the best results across the bottom and top limits of the linear programming issue's scope. As a result, our initial problem would be transformed into a single, clear question (Tanaka & Asai, 1984).

Linear Programming problems with many objectives can be solved using a new technique described in this (Benayoun et al., n.d.)study. "Best compromise" is a more appropriate term for this kind of dilemma. A systematic investigation of solutions is used instead of a prior distribution of weighted sums of the goal measures in the procedure presented. Goal programming is given a weighted makeover based on a new model centred on the principle of decreasing the distances between ideal goals and realistic ones in (Kamal et al., 2018) . Multi-Objective Linear Programming problems can be solved with this method. The suggested model solves MOLPP by handling a sequence of single-goal subproblems where the objectives are turned into constraints. In everyday life, finding the perfect place to launch a new business or office is the toughest challenge. Problems like these are known as facility location issues, or FLOs. These issues have spawned a number of algorithms. In (R. Kumar et al., 2017), (Mekala et al., 2022), (Yadav et al., 2022), (Sumathy et al., 2022), (Nair et al., 2022) we examine five strategies that have been used to solve the problem of finding a facility. Same strategy of distance is used for clustering in (Chandrawat et al., 2019).

TFN1 shows the many possible ways that different companies' products could be sold, and TFN2 is made by using TFN1 as a starting point. TFN2 shows all the ways that an industry that uses multiple sell prices could make money(R. Kumar et al., 2020). Using combined triangular fuzzy plus trapezoidal FLPP, the study (R. Kumar, Dhiman, et al., 2021) compares and contrasts the best ways to maximise manufacturing costs while minimising waste. Several different situations of volatility are described, and practical models for reducing production costs are provided as well. In (R. Kumar, Chandrawat, et al., 2021) paper demonstrates a strategy for optimizing a FLPP using fuzzy integers to represent the right-side variables. Improvements to quadrilateral fuzzy numbers centred on a-cuts are suggested to solve any fuzzy mathematical programming and also the required activities on the suggested number. In (Deep et al., 2017) Triangular fuzzy programming problem (s, l, r) models are used to manufacture products since the total costs of the various constraints fluctuate or are unpredictable. For various constraints, the actual cost of manufacturing leads to destruction because of unpredictable increments. The work (A. Kumar et al., 2011) proposes a book method for solving the same type of fuzzy linear programming problems with a fuzzy optimization algorithm. The suggested method is easier to use to solve FFLP problems with equality restrictions that come up in real life.

PRELIMINARIES

Basic Definitions

Definition 1: Let U be the universe of discourse. A fuzzy set $\tilde{F}$ is denoted by the pair (U, f) where $f_{\tilde{F}}$ is the membership value function from U to [0,1]. For every value of x ∈. U, there exist a membership value $f_{\tilde{F}}(x)$ which belongs to [0,1]. So, a fuzzy set $\tilde{F}$ is denoted by

$$\tilde{F} = \{(U, f): \forall\, x \in U\}, \tag{3}$$

where the membership function is given as

$$f_{\tilde{F}};\ U \rightarrow [0.1] \tag{4}$$

Definition 2: Triangular fuzzy numbers $\tilde{F}$= (g, h, i) are those whose membership function is defined as

$$f_{\tilde{F}} = \begin{cases} \dfrac{x-g}{h-g}, & g \le x \le h \\ \dfrac{x-i}{h-i}, & h \le x \le i \\ 0, & \text{otherwise} \end{cases}. \tag{5}$$

Definition 3: Let $\tilde{F}$= (g, h, i) be a triangular fuzzy number. Then $\tilde{F}$ is non-negative fuzzy number if $g \geq 0$.

Definition 4: Let $\tilde{F}$(g, h, i) and $\tilde{G}$(l, m, n) are the fuzzy numbers which are triangular. Then $\tilde{F}$ and $\tilde{G}$ are equal if and only if g= l, h= m, i= n.

Definition 5: If the height of a fuzzy set which is the maximum membership value in that set is 1, then the fuzzy set is called normal fuzzy set.

Definition 6: Let R be a function defined by:

R: F(R)→R;

where R is real number and F(R) is a set of fuzzy numbers.

As R is function which transform every fuzzy number to a real number into a natural order, so R is called a ranking function. Let $\tilde{F}(g, h, i)$ be a fuzzy number then $R(\tilde{F}) = \frac{g+2h+i}{4}$.

Arithmetic Operations

Let us take $\tilde{F}(g, h, i)$ and $\tilde{G}(l, m, n)$; two fuzzy numbers which are triangular. Then

Addition

$\tilde{F} \oplus \tilde{G} = (g, h, i) \oplus (l, m, n) = (g + l, h + m, i + n)$

Subtraction

$\tilde{F} \ominus \tilde{G} = (g, h, i) \ominus (l, m, n) = (g - l, h - m, i - n)$

Negation

$-\tilde{F} = -(g, h, i) = (-g, -h, -i)$

A SINGLE-OBJECTIVE FUZZY LINEAR PROGRAMMING PROBLEM (FLPP) WITH PARAMETERS REPRESENTED BY TRIANGULAR FUZZY NUMBERS

Construction of FLPP

It consists of two steps:

I. Formulate LPP
II. Mathematical model formation

Formulation of FLPP

After gathering information from various sources, build the problem by defining its boundaries.

Mathematical Model Formation

Formulate the problem into mathematical form

I. **Decision variable**: These are the variables which we have to find out. Let x_1, $x_2 \ldots x_n$ are 'n' number of unknown variables.

II. **Objective Function**: It is the function which we have to optimize. Let $\tilde{d}_1$, $\tilde{d}_2 \ldots \tilde{d}_n$ (triangular fuzzy number) are cost/ profit coefficients corresponding to decision variables given above. Then objective function can be expressed as

$$\text{Maximum/Minimum } \tilde{Z} = d\Delta_1 x_1 + d\Delta_2 x_2 + \ldots + d\Delta_n x_n \tag{6}$$

III. **Constraints:** They represents the limitations on variables. They can be formulated as

$$b\Delta_{11}x_1 + b\Delta_{12}x_2 + \ldots + b\Delta_{1n}x_n \le a\Delta_1$$

$$b\Delta_{21}x_1 + b\Delta_{22}x_2 + \ldots + b\Delta_{1n}x_n \le a\Delta_2$$

$$b\Delta_{m1}y_1 + b\Delta_{m2}y_2 + \ldots + b\Delta_{m2n}y_n \le a\Delta_m$$

$$x_1, x_2, \ldots, x_n \ge 0 \tag{7}$$

Simply the problem can be represented as

$$\text{Max/Min } \tilde{Z} = \sum_{j=1}^{n} d\Delta_j x_j , \tag{8}$$

$$\text{Subject to } \sum_{j=1}^{n} b\Delta_{ij} x_j = a\Delta_i \,; \forall \text{ i} = 1, 2, \ldots \text{m}, \tag{9}$$

Here $\tilde{a}_i$ and $\tilde{b}_{ij}$ are triangular fuzzy numbers.

Solution Method

Step 1: convert the fuzzy parameters into crisp parameters in objective function by the help of ranking function. For example-

Max $[(1,3,5)\ x_1 + (2,3,4)\ x_2]$ converted to Max $[3x_1 + 3x_2]$ (10)

Step 2: convert the fuzzy parameters into crisp parameters in constraints by the equality/ inequality of left and right sides. For example –

Subjected to: $(1,2,3)x_1 + (4,5,6)x_2 \leq (5,6,7)$ (11)

converted to

subjected to: $x_1 + 4x_2 \leq 5$

$2x_1 + 5x_2 \leq 6$

$3x_1 + 6x_2 \leq 7$ (12)

Step 3: Now the new crisp LPP formed. Existing LPP approaches can be used to solve linear programming issues. Two methods of their solution are given below:

Graphical Method

a) Define the LPP (Linear programming problem) challenge.
b) Create a graph and draw the lines of constraint.
c) Each constraint line should have a valid side, so find it.
d) Highlight the areas where a solution is possible.
e) The goal function should be plotted on a graph.
f) Locate the ideal location.

Simplex Method

Slack variables are introduced in the proper format, and the table is created. The pivot variables are also introduced. Then, the new tableau is created and checked for optimal solutions. The optimal values are identified.

Numerical Example 1

Assume that FNLPP

Maximum $\Omega = (1,2,3)y_1 + (2,2.5,3)y_2$ (13)

Subjected to $(3,4,5)y_1 + (2,5,6)y_2 \leq (5,6,8)$

$(1,7,8)y_1 + (1,2,3)y_2 \leq (2,5,4)$

$y_1,y_2 \geq 0$ (14)

Solution:

Step1: Maximum $\Omega= 2y_1 + 2.5y_2$ (15)

Step2: Subjected to $3y_1 + 2y_2 \leq 5$ (16)

$1y_1 + 1y_2 \leq 2$ (17)

Similarly other inequalities are given by:

$4y_1 + 5y_2 \leq 6,$ (18)

$7y_1 + 2y_2 \leq 5,$ (19)

$5y_1 + 6y_2 \leq 8,$ (20)

$8y_1 + 3y_2 \leq 4,$ (21)

$y_1,y_2 \geq 0,$ (22)

Step 3: As the decision variables are two graphical methods can be applied'

Graph of the problem is given by Figure 1.

The extreme points are the points which bound to the common region at which the value of objective function is given in the table 1.

The maximum value of the objective function Z=3 occurs at 2 extreme points. Hence, problem has multiple optimal solutions and max Z=3.

Figure 1. The area defined by the six inequalities of numerical experiment 1

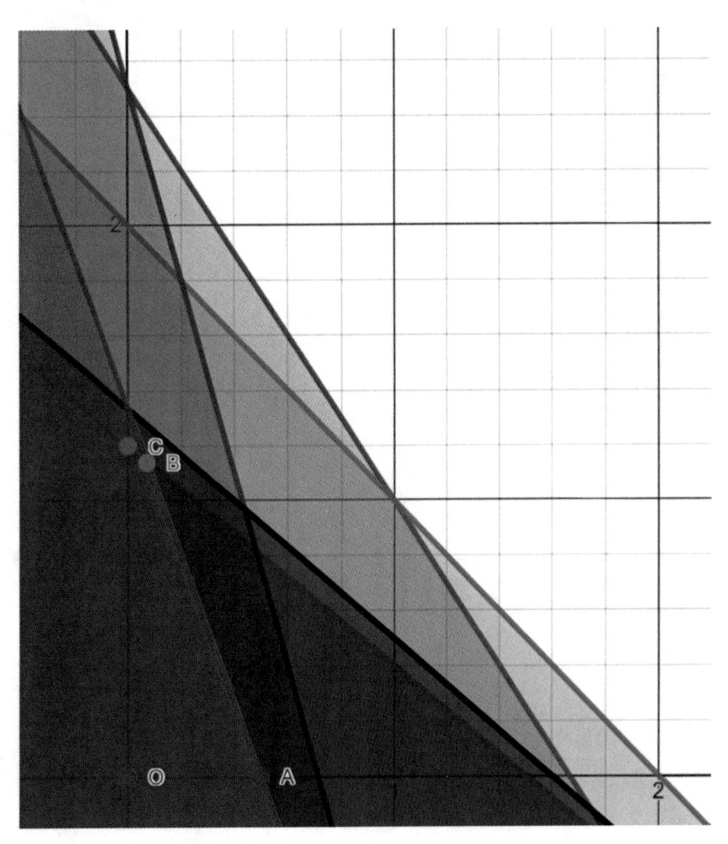

Table 1. Feasible Solution at corner points of feasible region from figure 1

Corner points of feasible region (y_1, y_2)	Lines whose intersection points are these corner points	Feasible solution $Z=2y_1+2.5y_2$
O = (0,0)	$7 \rightarrow y_1 \geq 0$ $8 \rightarrow y_2 \geq 0$	2(0) + 2.5(0) = 0
A = (0.5,0)	$6 \rightarrow 8y_1+3y_2 \leq 4$ $8 \rightarrow y_2 \geq 0$	2(0.5) + 2.5(0) = 1
B = (0.07,1.14)	$3 \rightarrow 4y_1+5y_2 \leq 6$ $6 \rightarrow 8y_1+3y_2 \leq 4$	2(0.07) +2.5(1.14) = 3
C = (0,1.2)	$3 \rightarrow 4y_1+5y_2 \leq 6$ $7 \rightarrow y_1 \geq 0$	2(0) +2.5(1.2) = 3

MULTI-OBJECTIVE FUZZY LINEAR PROGRAMMING PROBLEM (FLPP) USING FUZZY TRIANGULAR NUMBER PARAMETERS

It consists of two things:

1) construction of multi-objective FLPP
2) solution methods

Construction of FLPP

Formulate multi- objective FLPP
Mathematical model formation of multi-objective FLPP

Formulation of FLPP

To begin solving the problem, get information from diverse sources and then establish the issue's boundaries.

Mathematical Model Formation for Multi- Objective FLPP

Mathematically express the issue:

i. **Decision variable**: Those are the things that we need to figure out right now. Let x_1 be the first unknown, x_2 the second, and so on until x_n is the nth unknown.
ii. **Objective Function**: These also defined same as single objective function. Here number of objective functions are more than 1.

Maximum/Minimum $Z_1 = d\Delta_1 x_1 + d\Delta_2 x_2 + \ldots + d\Delta_n x_n$

Maximum/Minimum $Z_2 = c\Delta_1 x_1 + c\Delta_2 x_2 + \ldots +_n c\Delta x_n$

iii. **Constraints:** They represents the limitations on variables same as single objective problems. Simply the problem can be represented as

Max/Min $Z_1 = \sum_{j=1}^{n} d\Delta_j x_j$

$$\text{Max/Min } \tilde{Z}_2 = \sum_{j=1}^{n} c\Delta_j x_j$$

$$\text{Subject to } \sum_{j=1}^{n} b\Delta_{ij} x_j = a\Delta_i \text{; } \forall i = 1, 2, \ldots m$$

Here $\tilde{d}_j$, $\tilde{c}_j$, $\tilde{a}_i$ and $\tilde{b}_{ij}$ are triangular fuzzy numbers.

Method of Solution

Step1: To begin, you will utilize the ranking function to assist you in transforming fuzzy parameters in the optimization problem into crisp parameters for every objective function, just like for single objective issues.

Step2: Then put limits on the fuzzy parameters by converting them into crisp parameters based on their left-to-right equality and inequality.

Step3: The new crisp multi-objective linear programming issue can now be solved using the previous LPP methods. For a method for LPP with several objectives, see the following:

Weighed Sum Method

There are varying weights associated with the many objective functions based on the relative importance of each, and all multi-objective functions are summed up to create a single objective function. It is possible to use a predetermined sequence of goals or weight each individual goal in order to minimize the weighted sum of target deviations.

Predetermined Sequence of Weight

Step 1: Multiply the objective functions with their corresponding weights and then sum up to convert the multiple functions into a single function. For example:

Let Z_1, Z_2 are two objective function which we have to maximize under same conditions. Let w_1 and w_2 are the weights corresponding to both objectives. Then the conversion of multi-objective situation into single objective situation is as follows:

$$\left.\begin{array}{l}\max Z_1 \\ \max Z_2\end{array}\right\} \text{ is converted to } \max\{(w_1Z_1)+(w_2Z_2)\}$$

The condition on w_1 and w_2 is that their sum should be equal to 1 i.e. $w_1, w_2 \in [0,1]$ and $w_1+w_2=1$

Step2: Now the problem will look like a single objective linear programming problem which can be solved by the above methods already given.

Weight Each Individual Goal in Order to Minimize the Weighted Sum of Target Deviations

Step 1: Find the ideal (optimum) solution for every objective individually.

Step2: Then convert the multiple objectives into a single objective of distance which is defined below:

$$D_{ideal} = \sum_{i=1}^{n} \left|Z_i - Z_i^{ideal}\right|(1-w_i)d, \tag{25}$$

where Z_i are n number of objective functions, d is the minimum of the deviational distances of ideal solution to the different optimal solution corresponding to different weight function and w_i are the weights corresponding to objective function Z_i. So,

$$d = \sqrt{\sum_{i=1}^{n} \left|Z_i - Z_i^{ideal}\right|^2}, \tag{26}$$

Step 3: Now the problem will be a single objective linear programming problem. Solve it by using existing methods.

Numerical Example 2

Assume that we have two objectives whose preference weights are given as: $w_1 = 0.5$ and $w_2 = 0.5$ corresponding to Z_1 and Z_2 respectively. The multi-objective FNLPP is given as

$$\text{Maximum } Z_1 = (1,2,3)y_1 + (2,2.5,3)y_2 \tag{27}$$

$$\text{Maximum } Z_2 = (2,3,4)y_1 + (6,8,10)\, y_2 \tag{28}$$

$$\text{Subjected to } (3,4,7)y_1 + (2,5,8)y_2 \leq (5,6,8) \tag{29}$$

$$(1,5,8)y_1 + (1,2,3)y_2 \leq (2,5,4) \tag{30}$$

$$y_1, y_2 \geq 0 \tag{31}$$

Solution:

Step1: Maximum $Z_1 = 2y_1 + 2.5y_2$ (32)

$$\text{Maximum } Z_2 = 3y_1 + 8y_2 \tag{33}$$

Step2: Subjected to $3y_1 + 2y_2 \leq 5$ (34)

$$1y_1 + 1y_2 \leq 2 \tag{35}$$

$$4y_1 + 5y_2 \leq 6 \tag{36}$$

$$5y_1 + 2y_2 \leq 5 \tag{37}$$

$$7y_1 + 8y_2 \leq 8 \tag{38}$$

$$8y_1 + 3y_2 \leq 4 \tag{39}$$

$$y_1, y_2 \geq 0$$

Step3: Maximum $Z = 2.5y_1 + 5.25y_2$ (41)

$$\text{Subjected to } 3y_1 + 2y_2 \leq 5 \tag{42}$$

$$1y_1 + 1y_2 \leq 2 \tag{43}$$

$$4y_1 + 5y_2 \leq 6 \tag{44}$$

$$5y_1 + 2y_2 \leq 5 \tag{45}$$

$$7y_1 + 8y_2 \leq 8 \tag{46}$$

$$8y_1 + 3y_2 \leq 4 \tag{47}$$

$$y_1, y_2 \geq 0$$

Figure 2. The area defined by the six inequalities of numerical experiment 2

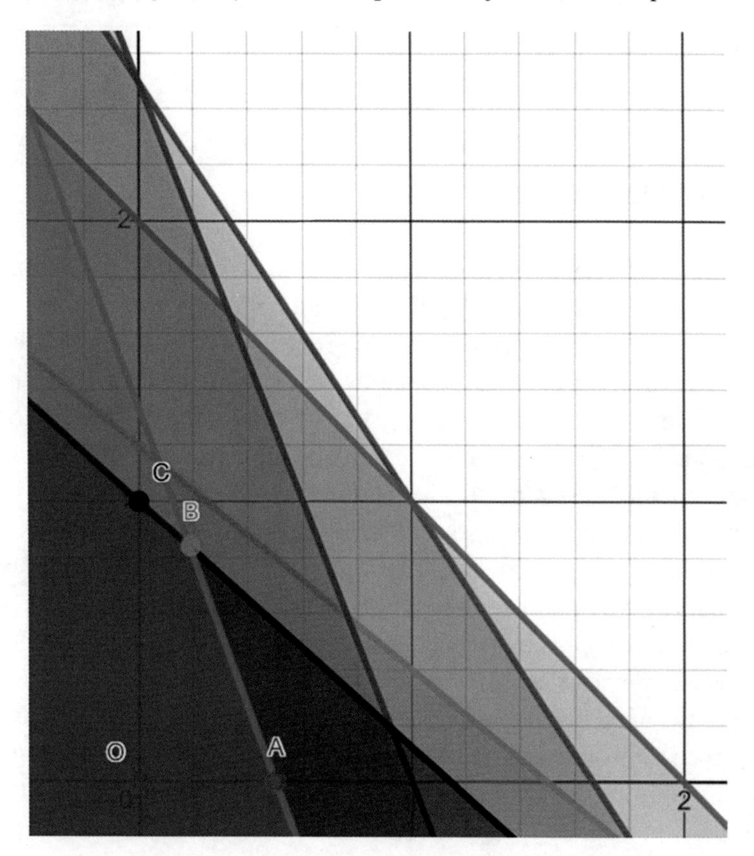

The extreme points are the points which bound to the common region at which the value of objective function is given in the table 2.

The maximum value at extreme points from the feasible solutions is Z=5.25 which is at (0,1). Accordingly, y_1=0, y_2=1, and max Z = 5.25 are the best solutions to the presented LPP issue.

Table 2. Feasible Solution at corner points of feasible region from figure 2

Corner points of feasible region (y_1, y_2)	Lines whose intersection points are these corner points	Feasible solutions $Z=2.5y_1+5.25y_2$
O (0,0)	$7 \rightarrow y_1 \geq 0$ $8 \rightarrow y_2 \geq 0$	2.5(0) + 5.25(0) = 0
A (0.5,0)	$6 \rightarrow 8y_1+3y_2 \leq 4$ $8 \rightarrow y_2 \geq 0$	2.5(0.5) + 5.25(0) = 1.25
B (0.19,0.84)	$5 \rightarrow 7y_1+8y_2 \leq 8$ $6 \rightarrow 8y_1+3y_2 \leq 4$	2.5(0.19) + 5.25(0.84) = 4.86
C (0,1)	$5 \rightarrow 7y_1+8y_2 \leq 8$ $7 \rightarrow y_1 \geq 0$	2.5(0) + 5.25(1) = 5.25

CONCLUSION

Benefits of FLPP System

Parameters and right-hand halves must be clearly described in classical mathematical optimization models. A wide range of information must be gathered and processed in order to avoid a dissatisfactory model. Some model parameters can only be calculated loosely in real-world situations. Although “average data” is used to represent “uncertain information” in existing theories, fuzzy models allow for the accurate modeling of the personal thoughts of the decision maker as a decision maker can explain it. As a result, the likelihood of choosing solutions that aren’t in line with the true nature of the problem is significantly reduced. It takes a lot of computing power to use random and fixed models to simulate real-world issues. As opposed to the above statement, we know that an optimal solution can be described with only a few constraints in the end. After the fact, especially with larger systems, we find that a large portion of the data is completely pointless. Because we should first analyze the approach to determine whether or not well-defined information is required, processing of data is beset by a conundrum. Using real-world programming issues with multiple criteria, it should be shown that the challenge of data analysis can be properly managed by representing the issues as fuzzy systems and addressing them interactively.

REFERENCES

Alferaidi, A., Yadav, K., Alharbi, Y., Razmjooy, N., Viriyasitavat, W., Gulati, K., Kautish, S., & Dhiman, G. (2022). Distributed Deep CNN-LSTM Model for Intrusion Detection Method in IoT-Based Vehicles. *Mathematical Problems in Engineering*.

Alferaidi, A., Yadav, K., Alharbi, Y., Viriyasitavat, W., Kautish, S., & Dhiman, G. (2022). Federated Learning Algorithms to Optimize the Client and Cost Selections. *Mathematical Problems in Engineering*.

Bellman, R. E., & Zadeh, L. A. (1970). Decision-Making in a Fuzzy Environment. *Management Science*, *17*(4), B-141–B-164. doi:10.1287/mnsc.17.4.B141

Benayoun, R., Tergny, J., & Laritchev, O. (n.d.). *Mathematical Programming*. North-Holland Publishing Company.

Chandrawat, R. K., Kumar, R., Makkar, V., Yadav, M., & Kumari, P. (2019). A comparative fuzzy cluster analysis of the Binder's performance grades using fuzzy equivalence relation via different distance measures. *Communications in Computer and Information Science*, *955*, 108–118. doi:10.1007/978-981-13-3140-4_11

Chatterjee, I. (2021). Artificial intelligence and patentability: Review and discussions. *International Journal of Modern Research*, *1*(1), 15–21.

Deep, K., Bansal, J. C., Das, K. N., Lal, A. K., Garg, H., Nagar, A. K., & Pant, M. (Eds.). (2017). *Proceedings of Sixth International Conference on Soft Computing for Problem Solving* (*Vol. 546*). Springer Singapore. 10.1007/978-981-10-3322-3

Dhiman, G., Juneja, S., Mohafez, H., El-Bayoumy, I., Sharma, L. K., Hadizadeh, M., Islam, M. A., Viriyasitavat, W., & Khandaker, M. U. (2022). Federated learning approach to protect healthcare data over big data scenario. *Sustainability*, *14*(5), 2500.

Dinesh Kumar, R., Golden Julie, E., Harold Robinson, Y., Vimal, S., Dhiman, G., & Veerasamy, M. (2022). Deep Convolutional Nets Learning Classification for Artistic Style Transfer. *Scientific Programming*.

Ding, H., Cao, X., Wang, Z., Dhiman, G., Hou, P., Wang, J., Li, A., & Hu, X. (2022). Velocity clamping-assisted adaptive salp swarm algorithm: Balance analysis and case studies. *Mathematical Biosciences and Engineering*, *19*(8), 7756–7804.

Ghanbari, R., Ghorbani-Moghadam, K., Mahdavi-Amiri, N., & de Baets, B. (2020). Fuzzy linear programming problems: Models and solutions. *Soft Computing*, *24*(13), 10043–10073. doi:10.100700500-019-04519-w

Goguen, J. A. (1965). Fuzzy sets. *Information and Control*, *8*, 338–353.

Gupta, N., Gupta, K., Gupta, D., Juneja, S., Turabieh, H., Dhiman, G., Kautish, S., & Viriyasitavat, W. (2022). Enhanced virtualization-based dynamic bin-packing optimized energy management solution for heterogeneous clouds. *Mathematical Problems in Engineering*.

Gupta, V. K., Shukla, S. K., & Rawat, R. S. (2022). Crime tracking system and people's safety in India using machine learning approaches. *International Journal of Modern Research*, *2*(1), 1–7.

Kamal, M., Jalil, S. A., Muneeb, S. M., & Ali, I. (2018). A Distance Based Method for Solving Multi-Objective Optimization Problems. *Journal of Modern Applied Statistical Methods; JMASM*, *17*(1), 2–23. doi:10.22237/jmasm/1532525455

Kanwal, S., Rashid, J., Kim, J., Juneja, S., Dhiman, G., & Hussain, A. (2022). Mitigating the coexistence technique in wireless body area networks by using superframe interleaving. *Journal of the Institution of Electronics and Telecommunication Engineers*, 1–15.

Kumar, A., Kaur, J., & Singh, P. (2011). A new method for solving fully fuzzy linear programming problems. *Applied Mathematical Modelling*, *35*(2), 817–823. doi:10.1016/j.apm.2010.07.037

Kumar, R., Chandrawat, R. K., Garg, B. P., & Joshi, V. (2017). Comparison of optimized algorithms in facility location allocation problems with different distance measures. *AIP Conference Proceedings*, *1860*, 020041. Advance online publication. doi:10.1063/1.4990340

Kumar, R., Chandrawat, R. K., & Joshi, V. (2020). Profit Optimization of products at different selling prices with fuzzy linear programming problem using situational based fuzzy triangular numbers. *Journal of Physics: Conference Series*, *1531*(1), 012085. Advance online publication. doi:10.1088/1742-6596/1531/1/012085

Kumar, R., Chandrawat, R. K., Sarkar, B., Joshi, V., & Majumder, A. (2021). An Advanced Optimization Technique for Smart Production Using α-Cut Based Quadrilateral Fuzzy Number. *International Journal of Fuzzy Systems*, *23*(1), 107–127. doi:10.100740815-020-01002-9

Kumar, R., & Dhiman, G. (2021). A comparative study of fuzzy optimization through fuzzy number. *International Journal of Modern Research*, *1*(1), 1–14.

Kumar, R., Dhiman, G., Kumar, N., Chandrawat, R. K., Joshi, V., & Kaur, A. (2021). A novel approach to optimize the production cost of railway coaches of India using situational-based composite triangular and trapezoidal fuzzy LPP models. *Complex & Intelligent Systems*, *7*(4), 2053–2068. doi:10.100740747-021-00313-0

Kuschel, N., & Rackwitz, R. (1997). Two Basic Problems in Reliability-Based Structural Optimization. In Mathematical Methods of Operations Research (Vol. 46). doi:10.1007/BF01194859

Marler, R. T., & Arora, J. S. (2010). The weighted sum method for multi-objective optimization: New insights. *Structural and Multidisciplinary Optimization*, *41*(6), 853–862. doi:10.100700158-009-0460-7

Mekala, M. S., Dhiman, G., Srivastava, G., Nain, Z., Zhang, H., Viriyasitavat, W., & Varma, G. P. S. (2022). A DRL-Based Service Offloading Approach Using DAG for Edge Computational Orchestration. *IEEE Transactions on Computational Social Systems*.

Nair, R., Soni, M., Bajpai, B., Dhiman, G., & Sagayam, K. M. (2022). Predicting the Death Rate Around the World Due to COVID-19 Using Regression Analysis. *International Journal of Swarm Intelligence Research*, *13*(2), 1–13. doi:10.4018/IJSIR.287545

Oliva, D., Esquivel-Torres, S., Hinojosa, S., Pérez-Cisneros, M., Osuna-Enciso, V., Ortega-Sánchez, N., Dhiman, G., & Heidari, A. A. (2021). Opposition-based moth swarm algorithm. *Expert Systems with Applications*, *184*, 115481.

Prasanna, K., Ramana, K., Dhiman, G., Kautish, S., & Chakravarthy, V. D. (2021). PoC Design: A Methodology for Proof-of-Concept (PoC) Development on Internet of Things Connected Dynamic Environments. *Security and Communication Networks*.

Puri, T., Soni, M., Dhiman, G., Ibrahim Khalaf, O., & Raza Khan, I. (2022). Detection of emotion of speech for RAVDESS audio using hybrid convolution neural network. *Journal of Healthcare Engineering*.

Sharma, S., Gupta, S., Gupta, D., Juneja, S., Gupta, P., Dhiman, G., & Kautish, S. (2022). Deep Learning Model for the Automatic Classification of White Blood Cells. *Computational Intelligence and Neuroscience*.

Sharma, S., Gupta, S., Gupta, D., Juneja, S., Singal, G., Dhiman, G., & Kautish, S. (2022). Recognition of Gurmukhi Handwritten City Names Using Deep Learning and Cloud Computing. *Scientific Programming*.

Sharma, T., Nair, R., & Gomathi, S. (2022). Breast Cancer Image Classification using Transfer Learning and Convolutional Neural Network. *International Journal of Modern Research*, *2*(1), 8–16.

Shukla, S. K., Gupta, V. K., Joshi, K., Gupta, A., & Singh, M. K. (2022). Self-aware Execution Environment Model (SAE2) for the Performance Improvement of Multicore Systems. *International Journal of Modern Research*, *2*(1), 17–27.

Sumathy, B., Chakrabarty, A., Gupta, S., Hishan, S. S., Raj, B., Gulati, K., & Dhiman, G. (2022). Prediction of Diabetic Retinopathy Using Health Records With Machine Learning Classifiers and Data Science. *International Journal of Reliable and Quality E-Healthcare, 11*(2), 1–16. doi:10.4018/IJRQEH.299959

Swain, S., Bhushan, B., Dhiman, G., & Viriyasitavat, W. (2022). Appositeness of Optimized and Reliable Machine Learning for Healthcare: A Survey. *Archives of Computational Methods in Engineering*, 1–23.

Tanaka, H., & Asai, K. (1984). Fuzzy linear programming problems with fuzzy numbers. *Fuzzy Sets and Systems, 13*(1), 1–10. doi:10.1016/0165-0114(84)90022-8

Vaishnav, P. K., Sharma, S., & Sharma, P. (2021). Analytical review analysis for screening COVID-19 disease. *International Journal of Modern Research, 1*(1), 22–29.

Viriyasitavat, W., Da Xu, L., Dhiman, G., Sapsomboon, A., Pungpapong, V., & Bi, Z. (2021). Service Workflow: State-of-the-Art and Future Trends. *IEEE Transactions on Services Computing.*

Viriyasitavat, W., Xu, L. D., Sapsomboon, A., Dhiman, G., & Hoonsopon, D. (2022). Building trust of Blockchain-based Internet-of-Thing services using public key infrastructure. *Enterprise Information Systems*, 1–24.

Yadav, K., Alshudukhi, J. S., Dhiman, G., & Viriyasitavat, W. (2022). iTSA: An improved Tunicate Swarm Algorithm for defensive resource assignment problem. *Soft Computing, 26*(10), 4929–4937.

Yadav, K., Jain, A., Osman Sid Ahmed, N. M., Saad Hamad, S. A., Dhiman, G., & Alotaibi, S. D. (2022). Internet of Thing based Koch Fractal Curve Fractal Antennas for Wireless Applications. *Journal of the Institution of Electronics and Telecommunication Engineers*, 1–10. doi:10.1080/03772063.2022.2058631

Zadeh. (1971). Similarity relations and fuzzy orderings. *Information Sciences, 3*, 177–200.

Zeidabadi, F. A., Dehghani, M., Trojovský, P., Hubálovský, Š., Leiva, V., & Dhiman, G. (2022). Archery algorithm: A novel stochastic optimization algorithm for solving optimization problems. *Computers, Materials and Continua, 72*(1), 399–416.

Chapter 8
Clustering and Regression Analysis on COVID-19 in India Using Python

Uma Bhattacharya
Lovely Professional University, India

Rakesh Kumar
Lovely Professional University, India

Amandeep Kaur
Chandigarh University, India

Gaurav Dhiman
Department of Computer Science, Government Bikram College of Commerce, Patiala, India & University Centre for Research and Development, Department of Computer Science and Engineering, Chandigarh University, Gharuan, Mohali, India & Department of Computer Science and Engineering, Graphic Era University (Deemed), Dehradun, India

ABSTRACT

Since 2019, the world has been dealing with an outbreak of the COVID-19 virus. A highly transmissible new coronavirus causes a severe acute respiratory illness. Every country, including India, took steps to battle the virus, such as announcing a phased lockdown. The COVID-19 pandemic has wreaked havoc on India. In reality, the third COVID-19 wave has already begun. The development of COVID-19 vaccinations aided in the healing of the planet. Multiple nations are conducting clinical tests on potential COVID-19 vaccines. India initiated the world's largest vaccination campaign on January 16, 2021. The Indian government has made significant progress in both vaccinating everyone and developing the COVID-19 vaccine. The use of Covaxin and Covishield dosages in different Indian states is investigated in this chapter.

DOI: 10.4018/978-1-6684-4405-4.ch008

INTRODUCTION

The first coronavirus case was discovered two years ago, and the entire globe has been in a state of terror since then. The coronavirus is thought to have originated in the city of Wuhan, China, with the first case recorded in December 2019. The COVID-19 virus quickly spread over the world. On January 30, 2020, the World Health Organization (WHO) declared the outbreak a Public Health Emergency of International Concern, and on March 11, 2020, it was declared a pandemic. In India, the first case of COVID was discovered in Kerala in January 2020. The number of new cases in India increased from 88,600 to 88,600 in just nine months, with a week average of 84,559. The initial wave of the Corona virus was discovered to have a greater impact on the health of the elderly (Dai et al., 2020). With their own processes, all countries proclaimed a lockdown. The world came to a halt. The second wave of the Corona virus swept the world soon after, and this strain was found to be lethal. It was also discovered that the virus attacked children and adults more aggressively. To prevent the virus from spreading, those who were infected were isolated for at least 14 days. It's very contagious and can strike at any time (Elimat et al., 2021). The world had never been prepared for a pandemic of this magnitude, and we were racing to produce a vaccine to stop it from spreading. The world appears to have gone insane in its search for a treatment for the coronavirus, an extremely hazardous disease that has engulfed the planet in panic. Medical researchers must produce a vaccine that will provide acquired immunity against the coronavirus 2 (SARS-CoV-2) that causes severe acute respiratory illness (Forni et al., 2021).

The first COVID vaccination, the Pfizer-BioNTech COVID-19 vaccine, was licenced by the US Food and Drug Administration for people aged 16 and up. Countries such as China, Russia, and the United States of America, for instance. On January 16, 2021, India launched the world's largest vaccination campaign. Considering India's large population, importing vaccines would have been prohibitively expensive. Furthermore, because the Indian government wanted to vaccinate every citizen, it was ideal to manufacture the COVID-19 vaccines in India (Elimat et al., 2021). India also planned to export vaccines to countries that couldn't afford the more expensive vaccines. The goal of manufacturing COVID vaccines in India is to ensure that each citizen in the country receives all of the required doses, as well as to make them affordable to the world's poorest countries. Covishield and Covaxin are mostly used in India at the moment. There were also rumours about the COVID vaccinations' ineffectiveness. Some of them include the following: they are unsafe, they induce infertility, they modify DNA, they are unsafe for persons with allergies, vaccines are not thoroughly evaluated, and so on. All of these, however, turned out to be rumours. All of the COVID-19 vaccines that have been licenced for use have been thoroughly evaluated, are entirely safe, and appropriately trigger the COVID virus, according to studies (Joshi et al., 2019). Furthermore, the race to develop a powerful cure (vaccine) for the sickness drove them to develop and release the most effective vaccine, which might potentially trigger the symptoms of any future form of the Corona Virus.

We wanted to study how the COVID-19 vaccinations, which were created in many places throughout the world, impacted people's health and immunity. Our primary goal is to investigate how the two COVID-19 vaccines now in use in India, Covishield and Covaxin, affect health. Another goal of this research is to determine which of the two COVID vaccines is superior in terms of providing robust immunity and having the least negative impact on people's health.

RELATED WORKS

Ever since the SARS-CoV2 Virus has struck the world, there is a constant urge and interest of people to know, to find out and research about it. What is this Corona Virus? From where and how did this even originated? Why is this virus so dangerous to people? How is the world handling it? What precautions do we need to take to curb its growth? Is there a requirement for a vaccine? If yes, will the vaccine be able to provide shield to us from the virus? All these questions led people and researchers to dive into this topic and bring into light the cause, effect and remedies of this SARS-CoV 2. V.M. Kumar *et al.* (2021) in Strategy for COVID-19 vaccination in India: the country with the second highest population and number of cases, has vividly described each and every Covid Vaccine manufactured in India, explained their trial phase along with the strategy adopted by India for Covid-19 vaccination. H. Dai *et al.* (2020) in their editorial Who is running faster, the virus or the vaccine? has described about the pros and cons of the virus as well as the vaccine. They have explained how the pace of people being vaccinated is getting affected. Also, what measures are taken for vaccinating the mass. J. Connor *et al.* (2020) in their review article Health risks and outcomes that disproportionately affect women during the Covid-19 pandemic: A review has brought out the risk factors that affected women during the Covid pandemic. The article concluded that Gender differences in health risks and implications are likely to be expanded during the Covid-19 pandemic. We wanted to study how the COVID-19 vaccination drives throughout India was carried out. Our primary goal is to investigate how the two COVID-19 vaccines now in use in India, Covishield and Covaxin, affect the survival rate. Another goal of this research is to determine which of the two COVID vaccines is superior in terms of providing robust immunity and having the least negative impact on people's health.

MATERIALS AND METHODS

There are three types of data in the dataset used for this investigation. The initial set of data pertains to COVID-19 cases that have been detected, cured, and died across India's states and union territories. It takes place between January 30, 2020, and August 11, 2021. The second type of information is state-by-state testing information for COVID-19 cases found, including the number of positive and negative cases. From April 17, 2020, to August 10, 2021, it was recorded. The third kind has the combined data of Covid-19 vaccinations, which distinguishes between Covishield and Covaxin doses. The dataset is also segmented by the Indian government's age-group slabs. From January 16, 2021, to August 9, 2021, it was recorded. This entire dataset was taken from Kaggle's official website (https://www.kaggle.com/) (https://www.kaggle.com/sudalairajkumar/covid19-in-india). Tableau and MS Excel were used to conduct the analysis.

COVID VACCINATION IN INDIA

The Indian government took significant measures to respond to the worldwide pandemic and began preparing the health system to handle all elements of COVID-19 management. As a result, India was able to maintain the lowest mortality rate and the highest recovery rate in the world during the pandemic. On January 16, 2021, free immunisation against SARS-CoV-2 began. Vaccinating a large portion of the population during the COVID epidemic and its variants was a big task for the Indian government. According to the most recent statistics, India has a population of 1.39 billion people (Kaplan et al., 2021). As a result, mass vaccination faced a significant challenge, but the current government's management was able to overcome it. The following vaccinations are produced in India:

- Covaxin by Bharat Biotech International Limited in collaboration with National Institute of Virology of ICMR. It is the first domestic covid vaccine manufactured in India.
- Covishield by Serum Institute of India (Pune).
- ZyCoV-D by Cadila Healthcare (Ahmedabad)
- Sputnik-V by Dr. Reddy's Laboratories (Hyderabad), originally developed by Gamaleya National Center of Epidemiology and Microbiology of Moscow, Russia.
- mRNA vaccine by Gennova Biopharmaceuticals Ltd (Pune) in collaboration with HDT Biotech Corporation (USA).

The Indian government established the NEGVAC (National Expert Group on Vaccine Administration) for COVID-19. It was designed specifically to provide guidelines covering all aspects for the Covid Vaccine Administration in India. According to NEGVAC, it was determined that the COVID vaccines would be distributed initially to frontline workers, health personnel, and those over the age of 60. Several centres were established around India to make the vaccine more accessible. Vaccines were next made available to adults between the ages of 45 and 60, and then to those between the ages of 18 and 44(Robert et al., 2021).

EXPLORATORY DATA ANALYSIS

Following are the analysis of the dataset taken for this study using the software Tableau & MS Excel.

Figure 1 depicts the total dosages provided in India's various states and union territories from January to August 2021, which shows that the Andaman and Nicobar Islands have the fewest vaccination doses delivered, while Maharashtra has the most, followed by Uttar Pradesh and Gujarat.

Figure 1. Doses of Vaccines Administered In States/UTs of India

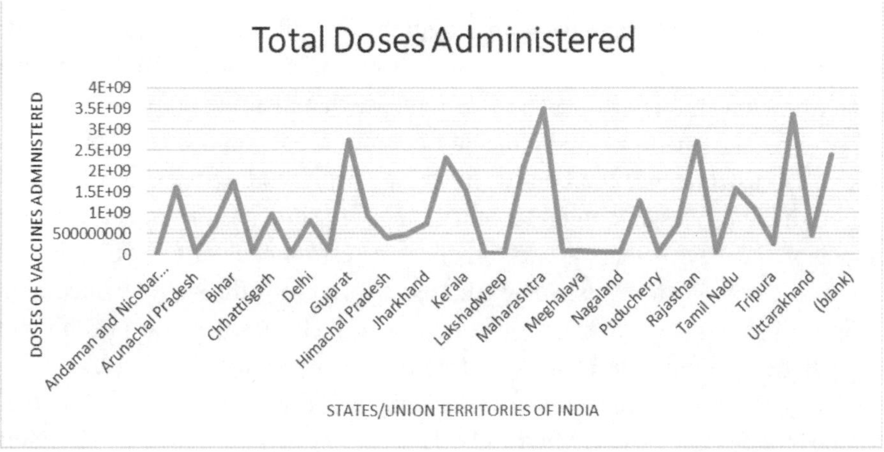

Figure 2 shows a 3-D representation of the state-by-state distribution of total doses separated into first and second doses in India from January to August 2021. The sum of total doses administered in the particular state or UT is represented by the blue bar; the sum of the first dose administered in the particular state or UT is represented by the grey bar; and the sum of the second dose administered in the particular state or UT is represented by the orange bar. This graph depicts the total number of immunizations given vs. the first and second doses.

Figure 2. State wise doses administered

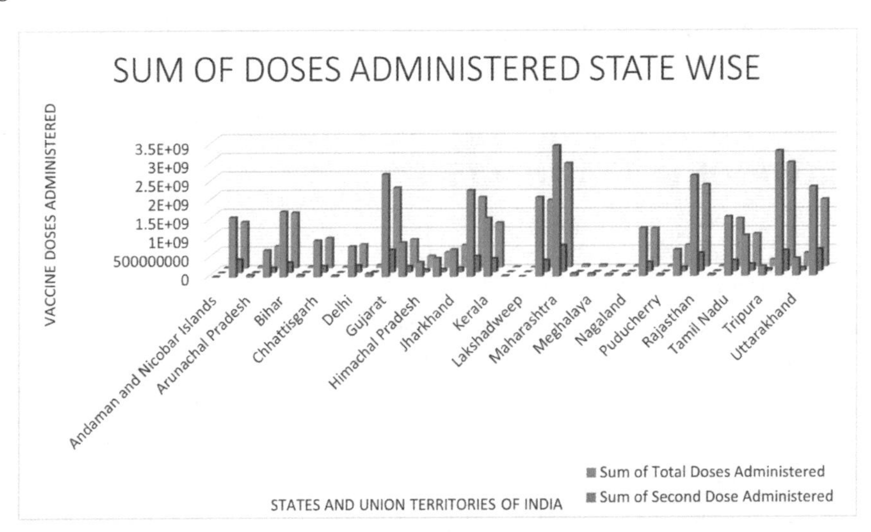

Figure 3 provides a graphical representation of confirmed Covid cases and cured cases among those confirmed patients in various Indian states, with data spanning January to August 2021. A clustered column graph and a line graph are combined in Figure-3. The green-colored clustered column graph depicts confirmed Covid Positive cases, while the blue-colored line graph depicts the Cured Covid Patients in different Indian states and union territories. Maharashtra has the largest confirmed number of COVID patients as well as the greatest number of COVID cases that have been cured. With the use of Treemaps, this figure is further explained below.

Figure 4 shows a tree map of confirmed COVID-19 positive cases from various Indian states and union territories. A tree map is a way for showing hierarchical data that uses nested objects, usually rectangles, to display it. We can see that Maharashtra has the most verified COVID cases, with 19, followed by Karnataka, Uttar Pradesh, and so on, by comparing the sizes of the rectangles. Similarly, the number of verified COVID positive cases is lowest in Daman and Diu.

Figure 5 shows a tree map of treated COVID patients from the confirmed COVID-19 cases depicted in Figure 4. We may predict that the state of Maharashtra has the greatest number of healed COVID cases based on the sizes of the rectangles in the preceding graphic.

Figure 3. State wise Confirmed vs Cured cases

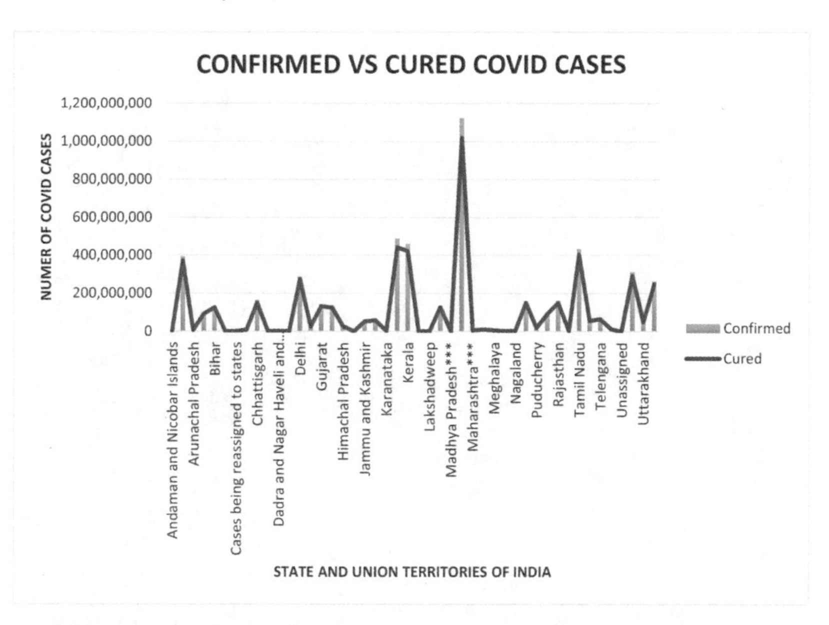

Figure 4. Confirmed Covid Positive Cases

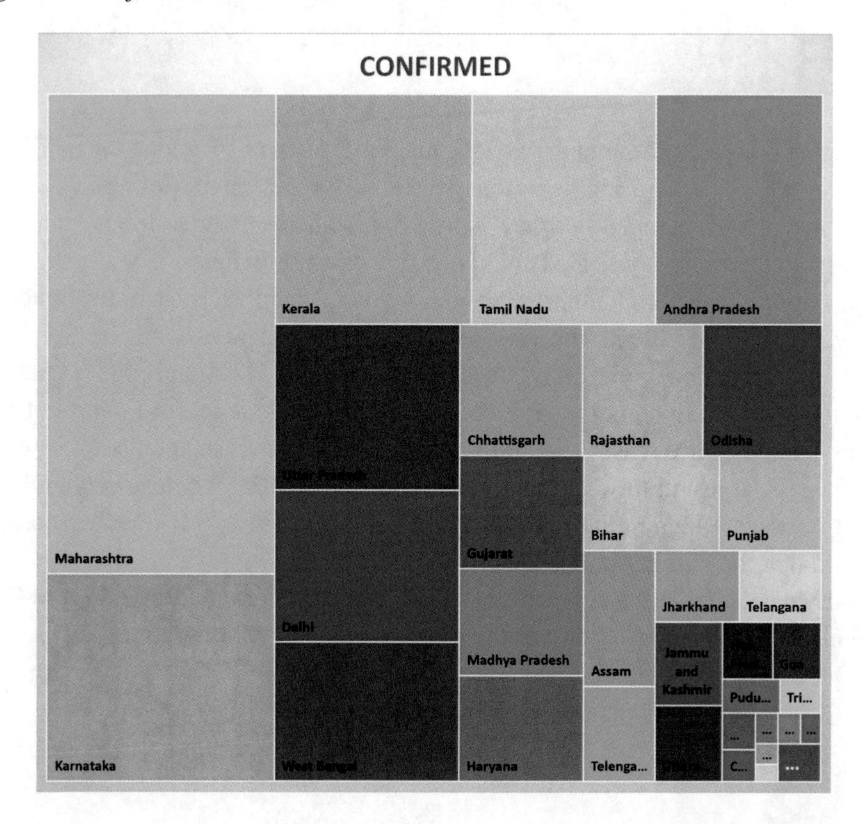

Figure 5. Number of Cured Covid Cases

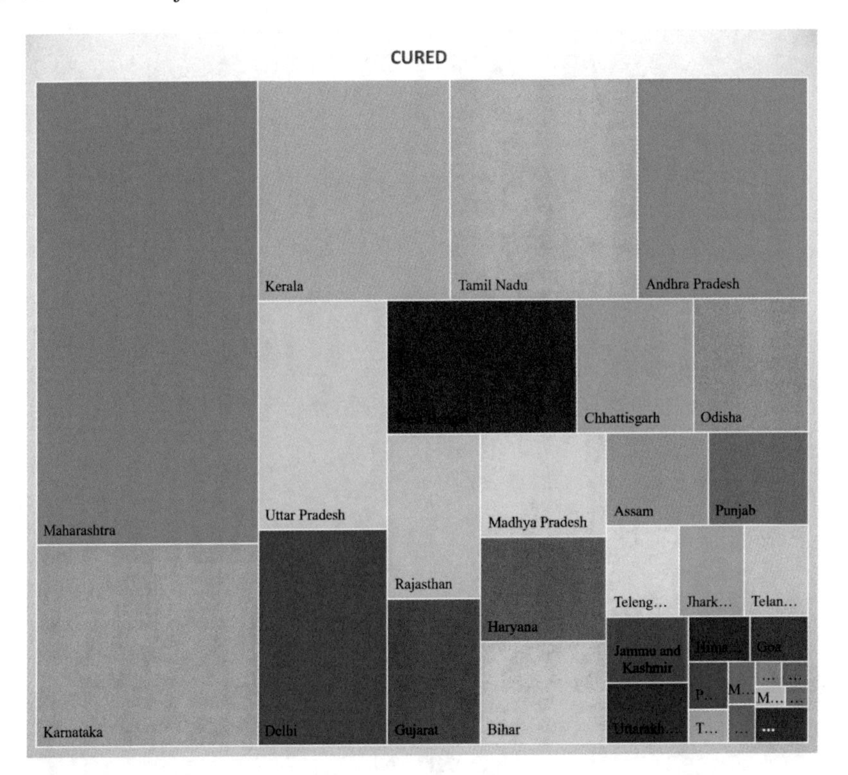

Figure 6 depicts the number of deaths caused by Covid 19 among the confirmed cases of Covid 19 in India's various states and union territories. Based on the diameters of the rectangles, we may deduce that Maharashtra has the largest number of deaths among the confirmed covid positive cases in India.

In Figure 7, the orange bar represents the total number of samples collected, the yellow bar represents the number of positive instances, and the green bar represents the number of negative cases from April 2020 to August 2021. It depicts a comparison study that compares the number of total samples to the number of positive and negative cases. According to the graph above, the number of positive instances is largest in July 2020 and lowest in August 2021, whereas the number of negative cases is highest in May 2020 and lowest in August 2021. Furthermore, we can see that the number of positive cases in 2021 is lower than in 2020 due to the Covid Vaccination Drive. Table 1 contains a tabular representation of Figure 4 that provides a detailed perspective of the above graphical representation.

Figure 6. Number of Deaths of Covid Cases

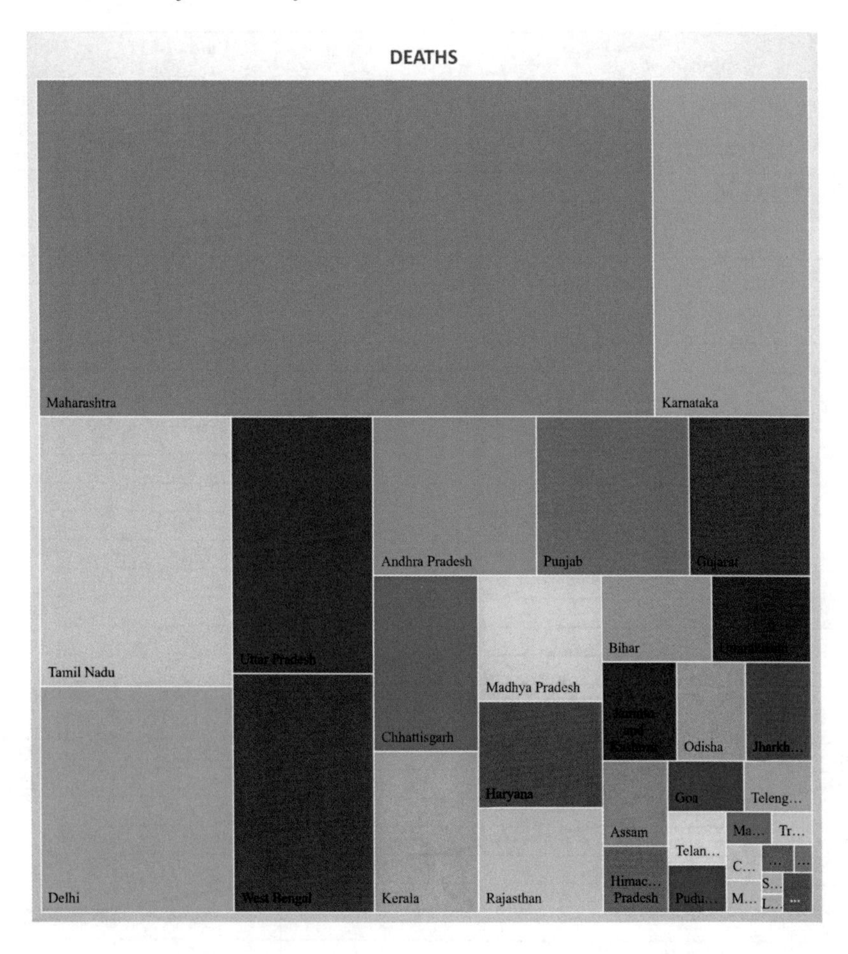

Figure 7. Count of Total Samples vs Count of Positive & Count of Negative Cases

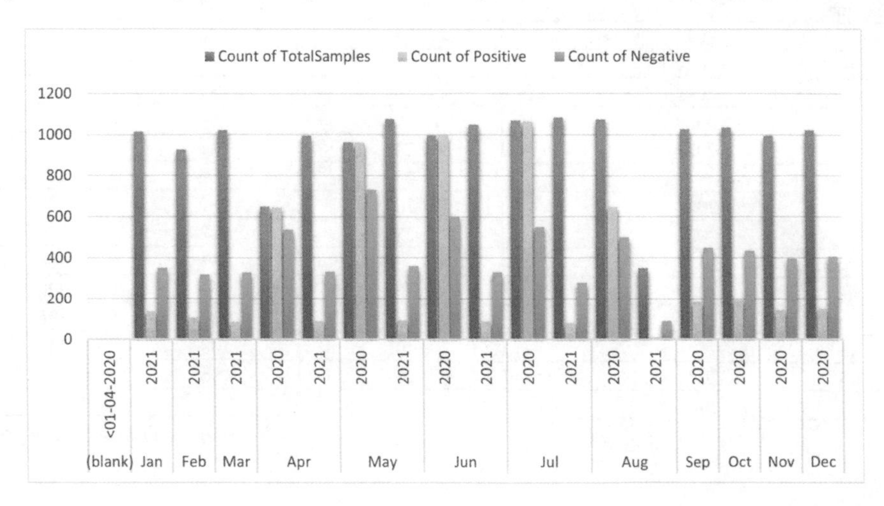

Table 1. Tabular Representation of Figure 5

Row Labels	Count of Total Samples	Count of Negative	Count of Positive
Andaman and Nicobar Islands	453	1	430
2020	232	1	231
2021	221		199
Andhra Pradesh	488	436	123
2020	266	237	123
2021	222	199	
Arunachal Pradesh	477	428	116
2020	255	254	116
2021	222	174	
Assam	469	48	114
2020	247	48	114
2021	222		
Bihar	489	1	126
2020	267	1	126
2021	222		
Chandigarh	479	478	127
2020	264	264	127
2021	215	214	
Chhattisgarh	482	63	126
2020	260	63	126
2021	222		
Dadra and Nagar Haveli and Daman and Diu	170	170	151
2020	170	170	151
Delhi	489	22	123
2020	267	22	123
2021	222		
Goa	483	2	125
2020	261	2	125
2021	222		
Gujarat	487	95	171
2020	267	95	171
2021	220		
Haryana	492	341	148
2020	270	270	147
2021	222	71	1
Himachal Pradesh	488	487	128
2020	266	266	128
2021	222	221	
Jammu and Kashmir	489	489	129
2020	267	267	129
2021	222	222	
Jharkhand	484	483	416
2020	263	263	220
2021	221	220	196
Karnataka	491	108	131
2020	269	108	131
2021	222		

continued on following page

Table 1. Continued

Row Labels	Count of Total Samples	Count of Negative	Count of Positive
Kerala	497	73	307
2020	275	73	275
2021	222		32
Ladakh	294	249	93
2020	175	161	93
2021	119	88	
Lakshadweep	195		
2021	195		
Madhya Pradesh	492	411	140
2020	270	270	130
2021	222	141	10
Maharashtra	488	195	196
2020	266	195	196
2021	222		
Manipur	406		80
2020	193		80
2021	213		
Meghalaya	409	346	106
2020	212	150	106
2021	197	196	
Mizoram	465	2	125
2020	260	2	125
2021	205		
Nagaland	484	69	130
2020	264	69	130
2021	220		
Odisha	492	13	142
2020	270	13	142
2021	222		
Puducherry	478	464	276
2020	257	257	223
2021	221	207	53
Punjab	491	51	132
2020	269	51	132
2021	222		
Rajasthan	491	263	134
2020	269	263	134
2021	222		
Sikkim	413	64	93
2020	229	64	93
2021	184		
Tamil Nadu	491	83	135
2020	269	83	135
2021	222		
Telangana	419	30	75
2020	200	30	75
2021	219		

continued on following page

Table 1. Continued

Row Labels		Count of Total Samples	Count of Negative	Count of Positive
Tripura		447	444	431
	2020	248	245	237
	2021	199	199	194
Uttar Pradesh		490	69	121
	2020	268	68	121
	2021	222	1	
Uttarakhand		491	490	132
	2020	269	269	132
	2021	222	221	
West Bengal		493	1	130
	2020	271	1	130
	2021	222		
<01-04-2020				
Grand Total		16336	6969	5662

The Table show the Count of Total Samples, Count of Negative and Count of Positive Samples in different States and Union Territories of India divided into two parts. The first is from April 2020 to December 2020 and the second part is from January 2021 to August 2021. This is the Tabular representation of the figure we described above on Figure 5.

Figure 8 displays the monthly sum of Covaxin and Covishield dosages given from January to August 2021.

Figure 8. Monthly Sum of doses Administered of Covishield & Covaxin

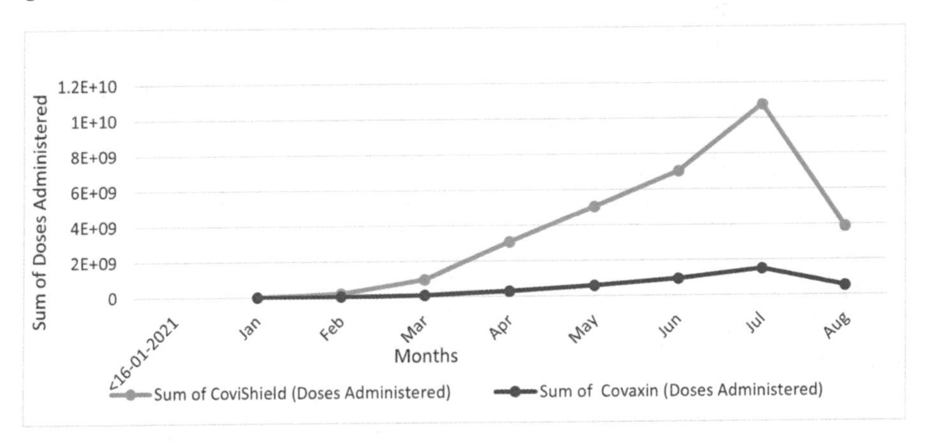

The green line graph indicates the total number of Covishield vaccine doses administered, whereas the blue line graph depicts the total number of Covaxin doses administered. It is a comparison of the two doses provided. The aggregate of each dose grows from January to July, then declines in August. The figure above shows that the total number of Covishield vaccine doses administered is more than the total number of Covaxin doses administered. Furthermore, we can forecast that the month of July would have the highest total of all doses provided.

The Government of India announced age slabs for the smooth movement of vaccination drive. The age slabs were 60+ Years, 45-60 Years, and 18-44 Years. Based on this, Figure 6 shows the graphical representation of individuals vaccinated from January 2021 to August 2021. The Green bar shows vaccination of individuals aged 60+ years; Blue bar shows vaccination of individuals aged 45-60 years; and the yellow bar shows the vaccination of individuals aged 8-44 years. We can see from the representation that maximum number of individuals were vaccinated in the month of June. If we look deeper into the representation, we can see that the maximum number of individuals vaccinated are of the age group 45- 60. One point to note here is that, since the vaccination drive in India started in phases and that the vaccination of individuals aged between 18-44 years were at the last, the number of individuals vaccinated is therefore less.

Figure 9. Sum of Individuals Vaccinated based on Age Groups

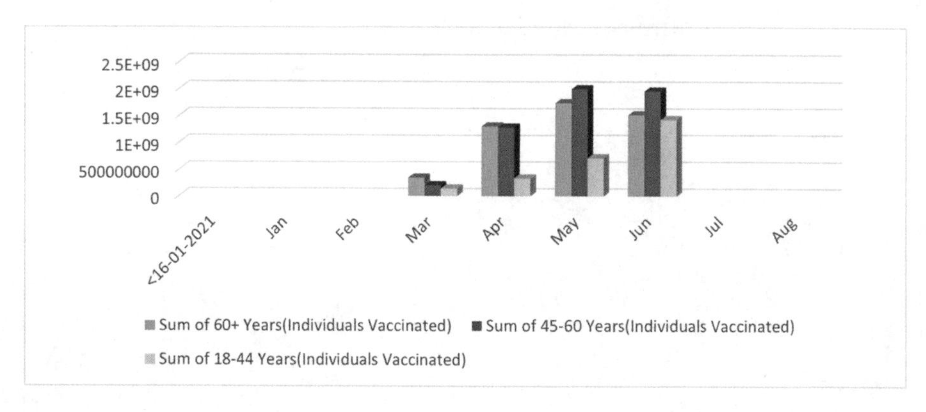

Figure 10 illustrates the total number of people vaccinated and differentiated by gender, i.e., male and female, from January 2021 to August 2021. The blue bar represents the total number of males vaccinated, whereas the orange bar represents the total number of females immunised. We can infer from the preceding figure that the number of males vaccinated is greater than the number of females.

Figure 10. Individuals Vaccinated based on Gender

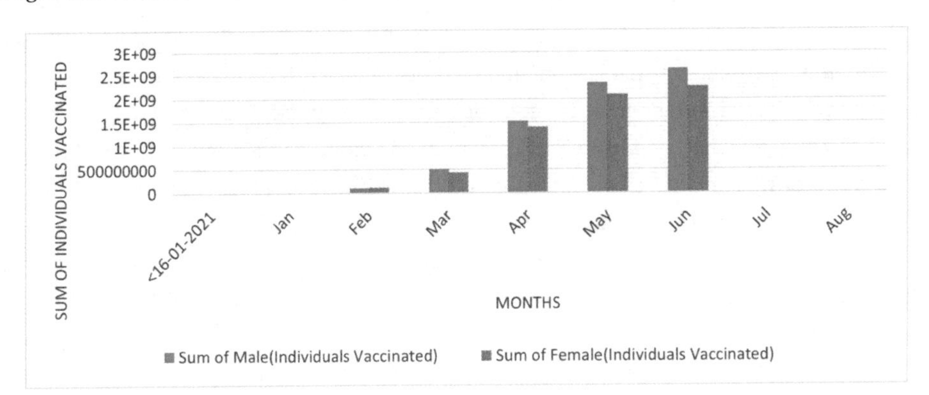

CLUSTERING ANALYSIS

The clustering of State/Union Territory can be done considering different features. Here we are trying to cluster different State/Union Territory based on the Mortality and Recovery rate of individual State/Union Territory.

As we all are well aware that COVID-19 has different Mortality Rate among different States/Union Territories based on different factors and so does the individual State/Union Territory follow the Recovery Rate because of pandemic controlling practices. Also, Mortality Rate and Recovery Rate both together takes into account all types of cases Confirmed, Cured and Deaths.

Figure 11. Number of Clusters using The Elbow Method

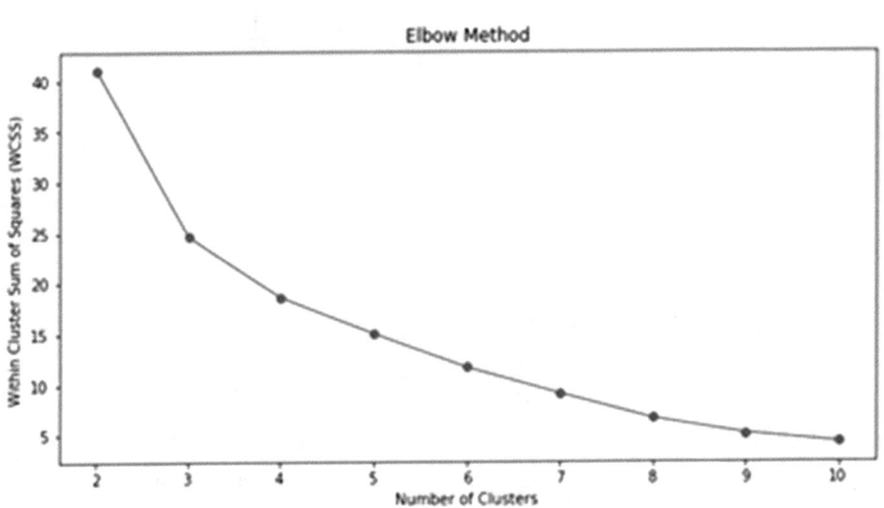

From Figure 11, we can clearly see that the Elbow is formed at the value 3. Hence, k=3 where k is the optimal number of clusters. This method is known as k-means clustering.

Another well-known approach for predicting optimal number of clusters is the Hierarchical method. Figure 12 is the representation of the same and the figure is called Dendrogram. From the above Dendrogram, we can see that optimal number of clusters is three.

Figure 12. Dendrogram for finding optimal number of Clusters

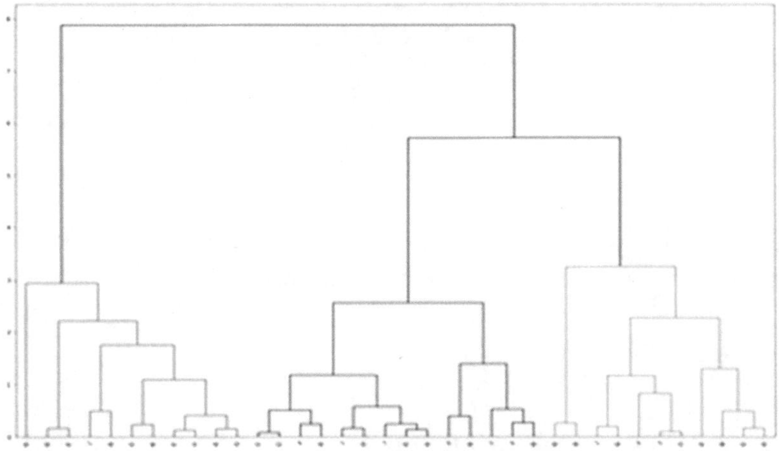

REGRESSION ANALYSIS

- Linear Regression Model for Confirm Cases Prediction

Figure 13. Linear Regression Best Fit Line

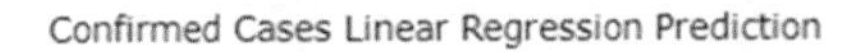

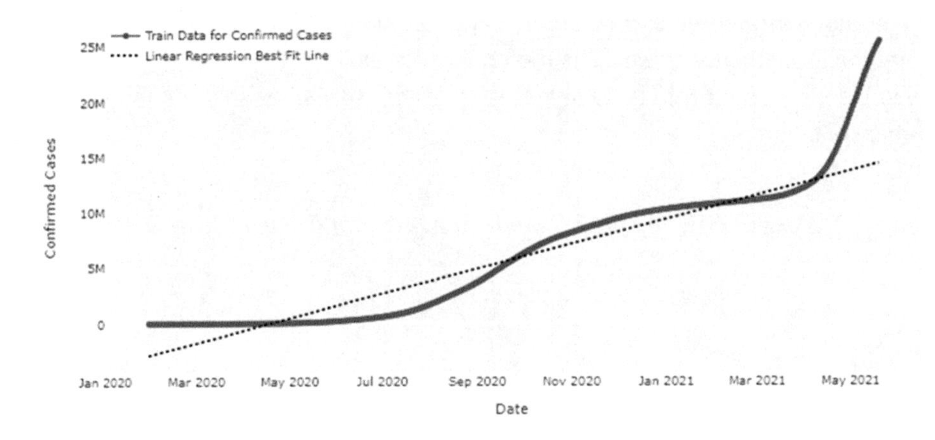

The Linear Regression Model is absolutely falling apart. As it is clearly visible, the trend of Confirmed Cases in absolutely not Linear.

- Polynomial Regression for Prediction of Confirmed Cases

Figure 14. Polynomial Regression Best Fit

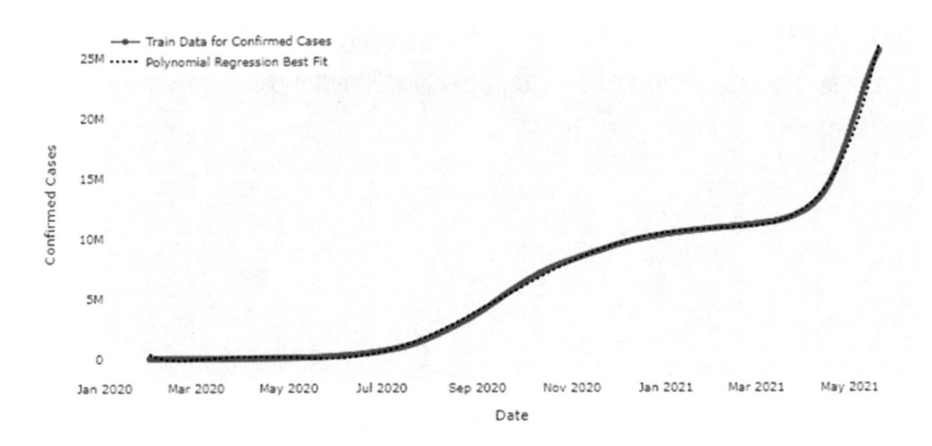

- Support Vector Machine for Prediction of Confirmed Cases

Figure 15. Support Vector Machine Best fit Kernel

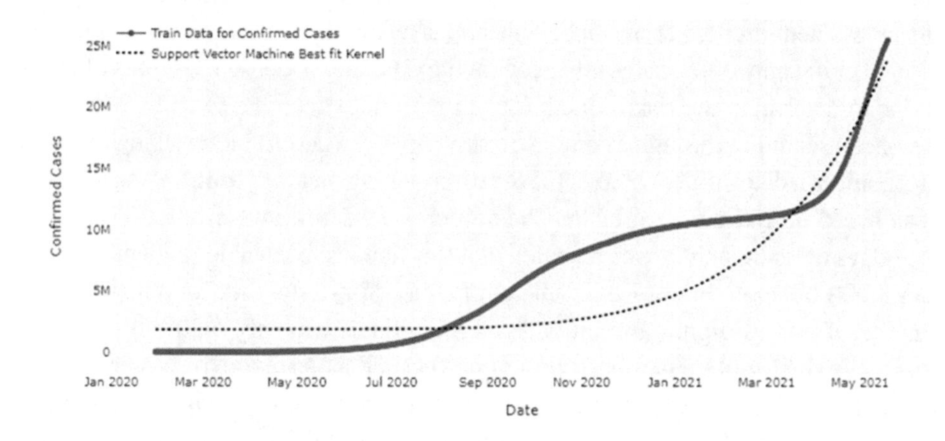

From Figure 15, we can infer that Support Vector Machine model isn't providing great results now, the predictions are either overshooting or really lower than what's expected.

DISCUSSION

Implementing mass vaccination in a country with a large population, such as India, is undoubtedly a difficult assignment for the government. India, on the other hand, was able to overcome the obstacle by efficiently managing the immunisation drives. The federal government directed those states begin teaching worried healthcare workers in the correct use of vaccines. Groups were constituted and established for the scientific guidance on the vaccination programme. National Expert Group on Vaccine Administration for COVID-19 (NEGVAC) was constituted in August 2020, to formulate comprehensive action plan for vaccine administration. National Task Force for Focused Research on Corona Vaccine was established in April 2020 to guide the process for coronavirus vaccine development, encourage domestic Research & Development of Drugs, Diagnostics and Vaccines. An Empowered Group on Vaccine Administration for COVID-19 (EGVAC) has also been constituted in January 2021, to facilitate optimal utilization of technology so as to make COVID vaccination all inclusive, transparent, simple and scalable, headed by CEO, National

Health Authority. National Technical Advisory Group on Immunization (NTAGI), through its Standing Technical Sub-Committee (STSC) and COVID-19 Working Group, has been providing advice on technical matters with respect to COVID-19 vaccination. The National Informatics centre under the Ministry of Electronics and Information Technology developed a mobile application named Aarogya Setu on 6 July 2020. It is an Indian COVID-19 contact – tracing, syndromic mapping and self-assessment digital service app. This app is available in 12 different languages. It is a tracking app which takes into account the GPS and Bluetooth features of one's device to determine the risk if one has been within six feet of a Covid-19-infected person, by scanning through a database of known cases across India. Using location information, it determines whether the location one is in belongs to one of the infected areas based on the data available. The app crossed 5 million installations within three days of its launch. It was revealed that this app has been able to identify more than 3,000 hotspots in 3-17 days ahead of time. Similarly, the Co-Win Software is a one-of-a-kind digital app that allows individuals to apply online for vaccine slots using their mobile number and unique ID such as Aadhar No., Voter ID, and so on, and book the closest place accessible to them without having to drive far to obtain the vaccine. It is an Indian government web portal for Covid-19 vaccination registration, owned and operated by India's Ministry of Health and Family Welfare. It is available in 12 different languages. It was launched on 16 January 2021. The platform has been integrated in the Aarogya Setu App. After successfully receiving the vaccine, the individual could download the vaccination certificate, which included information such as the name of the vaccine taker, the name of the vaccine giver, the location and date on which the individual received the vaccine dose (first/second), and the date on which the individual is eligible to receive the next dose. As of now, three vaccines can be registered on the platform Covishield, Covaxin and Sputnik V. Currently, two doses of each vaccine, Covaxin and Covishield, are administered. Individuals aged 18 and up are successfully receiving free vaccinations at various vaccination centres. Trials for vaccine candidates for people under the age of 18 are currently underway, so that children under the age of 18 can receive the vaccination without losing their immunity. From the cluster analysis, we can find out the Average Mortality and Average Recovery Rate for all three clusters. The table below is the calculated values for all the three clusters.

- Few States belonging to Cluster 0: ('Kerala', 'Andhra Pradesh', 'Rajasthan', 'Bihar', 'Odisha', 'Telangana', 'Assam', 'Arunachal Pradesh', 'Dadra and Nagar Haveli and Daman and Diu', 'Mizoram')
- Few States belonging to Cluster 1: ('Karnataka', 'Punjab', 'Uttarakhand', 'Jammu and Kashmir', 'Himachal Pradesh', 'Goa', 'Puducherry', 'Manipur', 'Meghalaya', 'Nagaland')

- Few States belonging to Cluster 2: ('Maharashtra', 'Tamil Nadu', 'Uttar Pradesh', 'Delhi', 'West Bengal', 'Chhattisgarh', 'Gujarat', 'Madhya Pradesh', 'Haryana', 'Jharkhand')

Table 2. Average Recovery Rate for all Three Clusters

STATE/UNIONTERRITORY	Confirmed	Cured	Deaths	Mortality	Recovery	Clusters
Karnataka	2272374.00	1674487.00	22838.00		73.69	
Punjab	511652.00	427058.00	12317.00			
Uttarakhand	295790.00	214426.00	5132.00		72.49	
Jammu and Kashmir	251919.00	197701.00	3293.00		78.48	
Himachal Pradesh	166678.00	129330.00	2460.00		77.59	
Goa	138776.00	112633.00	2197.00			
Puducherry	87749.00	69060.00	1212.00	1.38	78.70	
Manipur	40683.00	33466.00	612.00	1.50		
Meghalaya	24872.00	19185.00	355.00		77.13	
Nagaland	18714.00	14079.00	228.00	1.22	75.23	
Sikkim	11689.00	8427.00	212.00	1.81	72.09	
Maharashtra	5433506.00	4927480.00	83777.00	1.54		2.00
Tamil Nadu	1664350.00	1403052.00	18369.00			
Uttar Pradesh	1637663.00	1483249.00	18072.00			
Delhi	1402873.00	1329899.00	22111.00			
West Bengal	1171861.00	1026492.00	13576.00			
Chhattisgarh	925531.00	823113.00	12036.00			
Gujarat	766201.00	660489.00	9269.00			
Madhya Pradesh	742718.00	652612.00	7139.00	0.96		
Haryana	709689.00	626852.00	6923.00			
Jharkhand	320934.00	284805.00	4601.00	1.43		
Chandigarh	56513.00	48831.00	647.00			
Tripura	42776.00	36402.00	450.00	1.05		
Ladakh	16784.00	15031.00	170.00	1.01		
Andaman and Nicobar Islands	6674.00	6359.00	92.00	1.38		
Kerala	2200706.00	1846105.00	6612.00	0.30		0.00
Andhra Pradesh	1475372.00	1254291.00	9580.00	0.65		0.00
Rajasthan	879664.00	713129.00	7080.00	0.80	81.07	0.00
Bihar	664115.00	595377.00	4039.00	0.61		0.00
Odisha	633302.00	536595.00	2357.00	0.37		0.00
Telangana	536766.00	485644.00	3012.00	0.56		0.00
Assam	340858.00	290774.00	2344.00	0.69		0.00
Arunachal Pradesh	22462.00	19977.00	88.00	0.39		0.00
Dadra and Nagar Haveli and Daman and Diu	9652.00	8944.00	4.00	0.04	92.66	0.00
Mizoram	9252.00	7094.00	29.00	0.31	76.68	0.00
Lakshadweep	5212.00	3915.00	15.00	0.29	75.12	0.00

Table 3. Average Mortality Rate

Average Mortality Rate of Cluster 0	0.4562051389936401
Average Recovery Rate of Cluster 0	84.86585221363326
Average Mortality Rate of Cluster 1	1.5325799965110962
Average Recovery Rate of Cluster 1	77.48213037005056
Average Mortality Rate of Cluster 2	1.2108853861677105
Average Recovery Rate of Cluster 2	88.88347505518554

Figure 16.

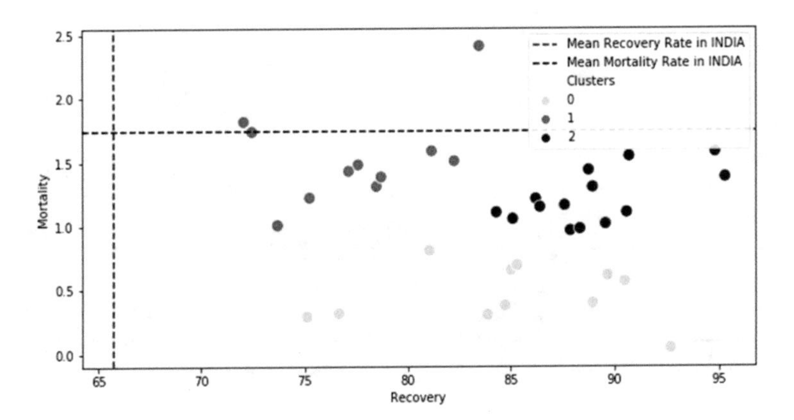

Under the Regression Analysis,

- Root Mean Square Error for Linear Regression is calculated to be 7898554.466441718.
- Root Mean Squared Error for Polynomial Regression is calculated to be 920247.1555306285.
- Root Mean Square Error for Support Vector Machine is calculated to be 1041554.641824152.

CONCLUSION

The purpose of this research is to examine the COVID vaccination in India. According to the graphs we utilised, Madhya Pradesh has the maximum total doses provided with Uttar Pradesh at second number and Gujarat at third number of maximum of Total Doses administered., while Lakshadweep has the lowest of total doses administered.

Furthermore, Uttar Pradesh has the most number first dosages administered with Maharashtra at second position and Gujarat at third. Maharashtra has the highest number of second doses administered. Maharashtra has the most verified positive COVID cases, as well as the most cured patients. It is observed from our EDA that approximately 91% of the patients who tested positive for Covid-19 virus were cured after taking precautionary measures like being in quarantine for at least fourteen days, adopting a better lifestyle for boosting immunity, wearing masks properly, sanitising regularly etc. Due to proper implementation of the Covid guidelines, the death rate recorded is roughly ranges from 1.12% to 2.12%, in different states of India. Moreover, July 2021 has recorded the highest numbers of total samples collected. Of these total samples collected, the positivity rate is roughly recorded as 51.44% whereas the negativity rate has been recorded as roughly 39.95%. From Figure 8 we conclude that the doses of Covishield vaccine administered are significantly higher than the doses of Covaxin vaccine administered. The July month has been recorded with highest number of both Covaxin and Covishield vaccine administered. Another result drawn from our data analysis is that people aged between 45-60 years were more likely to get themselves vaccinated as compared to individuals aged between 18-44 years and 60+ years or we can say that maximum number of vaccinations given to people are of age group 45-60. In addition to this, the number of Male genders vaccinated are more than the Females. The purpose of this analysis is to highlight the vaccination strategy adopted by the Government in the midst of the Covid pandemic that too in a densely populated country, India where the novel Corona Virus can be easily transmitted from one person to another. India's vaccination campaign is the fastest to reach 10 million vaccines. The drives have been supervised at the national, state, and district levels to ensure that they run smoothly. People who have received both doses of the COVID vaccination, whether Covishield or Covaxin, are protected from the COVID virus, according to the government, but they must continue to follow COVID guidelines for best outcomes. Our analysis showed that people who got themselves vaccinated with both the doses have lesser chances of death, maximum people come under the age group of 45-60 years.

From Clustering Analysis, we can conclude that:

- Cluster 2 is a set of States which have really Low Mortality Rate and Highest Recovery Rate. Basically, few States among these clusters have seen already the worst of this pandemic but are now recovering with healthy Recovery Rate.
- Cluster 0 is set of States which have Lowest Mortality Rate and considerably Good Recovery Rate. These are the set of States which has been able to control the COVID-19 by following pandemic controlling practices rigorously.

- Cluster 1 is set of States which have Highest Mortality Rate and Least Recovery Rate. These States/UTs need to pace up their Recovery Rate to get out it, Some of these States/UTs have really high number of Infected Cases but Low Mortality, is positive sign out of it.

From Regression Analysis, we can conclude that the Polynomial Regression Model is best fit model for prediction of Confirmed Cases.

REFERENCES

Clemente-Suárez. (2020). Dynamics of population immunity due to the herd effect in the COVID-19 pandemic. *Vaccines, 8*(2), 236.

Dai, H., Han, J., & Lichtfouse, E. (2020). Who is running faster, the virus or the vaccine? *Environmental Chemistry Letters*, *18*(6), 1761–1766. doi:10.100710311-020-01110-w PMID:33082737

El-Elimat. (2021). Acceptance and attitudes toward COVID-19 vaccines: a cross-sectional study from Jordan. *Plos one, 16*(4), e0250555.

Forni, G., & Mantovani, A. (2021). COVID-19 vaccines: Where we stand and challenges ahead. *Cell Death and Differentiation*, *28*(2), 626–639. doi:10.103841418-020-00720-9 PMID:33479399

Joshi, V., & Chandrawat, R. K. (2019). Comparative Analysis of Different Structure of the Crisp and Fuzzy Regression Equations Using Realistic Data. *Think India Journal*, *22*(37), 1288–1303.

Kaplan, R. M., & Milstein, A. (2021). Influence of a COVID-19 vaccine's effectiveness and safety profile on vaccination acceptance. *Proceedings of the National Academy of Sciences*. 10.1073/pnas.2021726118

Kumar, R. (2017). Comparison of optimized algorithms in facility location allocation problems with different distance measures. AIP Conference Proceedings, 1860(1). doi:10.1063/1.4990340

Kumar, R., Chandrawat, R. K., Sarkar, B., Joshi, V., & Majumder, A. (2021). An advanced optimization technique for smart production using α-cut based quadrilateral fuzzy number. *International Journal of Fuzzy Systems*, *23*(1), 107–127. doi:10.100740815-020-01002-9

Kumar, R., & Dhiman, G. (2021). A comparative study of fuzzy optimization through fuzzy number. *International Journal of Modern Research*, *1*(1), 1–14.

Kumar, R., Dhiman, G., Kumar, N., Chandrawat, R. K., Joshi, V., & Kaur, A. (2021). A novel approach to optimize the production cost of railway coaches of India using situational-based composite triangular and trapezoidal fuzzy LPP models. *Complex & Intelligent Systems*, *7*(4), 2053–2068. doi:10.100740747-021-00313-0

Kumar, R., Joshi, V., Dhiman, G., & Viriyasitavat, W. (2021). An improved exponential metric space approach for C-mean clustering analysing. *Expert Systems: International Journal of Knowledge Engineering and Neural Networks*, e12896. doi:10.1111/exsy.12896

Kumar, V. M. (2021). Strategy for COVID-19 vaccination in India: The country with the second highest population and number of cases. *NPJ Vaccines*, *6*(1), 1–7. PMID:33398010

OECD. (2021). *Coronavirus (COVID-19) vaccines for developing countries: An equal shot at recovery, OECD policy responses to coronavirus (COVID-19)*. OECD.

Samaddar, A., Gadepalli, R., Nag, V. L., & Misra, S. (2020). The enigma of low COVID-19 fatality rate in India. *Frontiers in Genetics*, *11*, 854. doi:10.3389/fgene.2020.00854 PMID:32849833

Sharma, O., Sultan, A. A., Ding, H., & Triggle, C. R. (2020). A Review of the Progress and Challenges of Developing a Vaccine for COVID-19. *Frontiers in Immunology*, *11*, 2413. doi:10.3389/fimmu.2020.585354 PMID:33163000

Su. (2021). COVID-19 Vaccine Donations—Vaccine Empathy or Vaccine Diplomacy? A Narrative Literature Review. *Vaccines, 9*(9).

Vaghela. (2021). World's largest vaccination drive in India: Challenges and recommendations. *Health Science Reports, 4*(3).

Wang, J., Peng, Y., Xu, H., Cui, Z., & Williams, R. O. III. (2020). The COVID-19 vaccine race: Challenges and opportunities in vaccine formulation. *AAPS PharmSciTech*, *21*(6), 1–12. doi:10.120812249-020-01744-7 PMID:32761294

World Health Organization. (2021). *Cohort study to measure COVID-19 vaccine effectiveness among health workers in the WHO European Region: Guidance document*. Author.

ADDITIONAL READING

Kumar, R., Chandrawat, R., & Joshi, V. (2020). Profit Optimization of products at different selling prices with fuzzy linear programming problem using situational based fuzzy triangular numbers. *Journal of Physics: Conference Series*, *1531*(1), 12085. doi:10.1088/1742-6596/1531/1/012085

Kumar, R., & Gupta, S. (2013). Application of Fuzzy c- means clustering for Facility location and Transportation problems. *International Transactions in Applied Sciences*, *5*, 35–42.

Kumar, R., & Joshi, V. (2020). A New Approach to Optimize the Membership Grade in Fuzzy Linear Programming Problem. *European Journal of Molecular & Clinical Medicine*, *7*(7), 3774–3786.

Kumar, R., Khepar, J., Yadav, K., Kareri, E., Alotaibi, S. D., Viriyasitavat, W., Gulati, K., Kotecha, K., & Dhiman, G. (2022). A Systematic Review on Generalized Fuzzy Numbers and Its Applications: Past, Present and Future. *Archives of Computational Methods in Engineering*, (Jul). Advance online publication. doi:10.100711831-022-09779-8

KEY TERMS AND DEFINITIONS

Clustering: The task of grouping a set of objects in such a way that objects in the same group are more similar to each other than to those in other groups.

Dendrogram: A type of tree diagram showing hierarchical clustering-relationships between similar sets of data.

Hierarchial Clustering: A method of cluster analysis which seeks to build a hierarchy of clusters.

Pandemic: An epidemic of an infectious disease that has spread across a large region.

Regression: Regression analysis is a set of statistical processes for estimating the relationships between a dependent variable and one or more independent variables.

Robust: Something that is able to withstand or overcome adverse conditions.

Treemap: A diagram representing hierarchical data in the form of nested rectangles, the area of each corresponding to its numerical value.

Chapter 9
A Comprehensive Study of Various Fuzzy C-Means Clustering Algorithms

Pooja Sangwan
Lovely Professional University, India

Rakesh Kumar
Lovely Professional University, India

Amandeep Kaur
Chandigarh University, India

Gaurav Dhiman
Department of Computer Science, Government Bikram College of Commerce, Patiala, India & University Centre for Research and Development, Department of Computer Science and Engineering, Chandigarh University, Gharuan, Mohali, India & Department of Computer Science and Engineering, Graphic Era University (Deemed), Dehradun, India

ABSTRACT

Digital image processing is becoming another ever-growing yet popular field of demands for daily life, ranging from medicine, room evaluation, security, support, and security of the automotive community, among many others. The proposed framework focuses mostly on fuzzy logic structures somewhere in optical image processing. The main goal of most of this work is to demonstrate how fuzzy logic is implemented in image processing with little more than a quick introduction of fuzzy logic and optical image processing. Fuzzy logic, one of those artificial intelligence decision-making approaches, provides even greater room for use. When everything that would also

DOI: 10.4018/978-1-6684-4405-4.ch009

have been allowed access to declarations at all since birth, particularly concerning in popularity in recent years, fuzzy logic as a whole has been proven to be true in virtually all systemic fields. Furthermore, the implications continue to suggest that the previously presented technique is worthy of attention in image processing software systems with the appropriate expansion.

INTRODUCTION

In 1965 Lotfi A. Zadeh and Dieter Klaus developed Fuzzy sets independently as an enhancement of both the traditional instance of collection. Fuzzy relations are increasingly employed in a range of areas, including language studies, decision-making, and clustering. Fuzzy logic has been extended to a wide range of disciplines ranging from control theory to artificial intelligence. Fuzzy relations were designed to enable the machine to decide the distinctions that are neither right nor wrong between data.

The clustering algorithm separates a data collection into classes/clusters, with related data objects allocated to the same clusters. When the boundary between clusters is ill-defined, resulting in circumstances where the same data object belongs to more than one class, the concept of fuzzy clustering comes into play.

Clustering or cluster analysis have the steps like handing over of data points to clusters such that items in the same cluster are as analogous as possible, otherwise clusters are contradictory as possible.

BACKGROUND

The Fuzzy C-means clustering model (FCM) was first developed by Dunn in 1974(Informa et al., 2008)and was subsequently expanded and understood by Bezdek in 1983. Since then, some discrepancies of this method and models improvements are recommended in the writings by few researchers. In (Pal et al., 2005), Pal and Bezdek introduced a diverse fuzzy-possibilistic clustering, which is primarily an amalgamation of fuzzy and possibilistic clustering models, in disagreement that FPCM elucidates the FCM's noise sensitivity defect and solves the PCM's previous conterminous clusters challenging problem. They also provide first order necessary conditions for the extremes of the PFCM objective function and use them as the foundation for an average interchanging optimization algorithm for locating the confined minima. Here, two of the numerical examples have been mentioned for FCM and PCM. Also, there were a few studies done on the linguistic variables in FCM, such as the effort of Auephanwiriyakul and Keller (Auephanwiriyakul & Keller, 2002) in where there were a well-organized method based upon the fuzzy arithmetic and optimization has been technologically advanced and investigated in demand to deal with the linguistic vector that has an enormous computational complication. Pedrycz and Vukovich in(Pedrycz & Vulkovich, 2004) have also anticipated a method that supplements the customary fuzzy c-means algorithm by the encompassing of the unusual objective function by the administration constituent (labeled patterns). Investigational consequences demonstrate that the overseen clustering suggested in the study, which further helps in efficiently to reunite the fundamental and the cataloguing statistics about the given data. In addition to this, they have also deliberated the use of this kind of clustering in the vector quantization of being observed as the standard method of the data compression. The contemporary work of Lazaro in(Rodríguez Ramos et al., 2017), the fresh description of the procedure was technologically advanced letting it a great amount of parallelism, which makes the hardware execution well-matched for the actual time video presentation. When allocating through the noise in the fuzzy c-means clustering, a researcher proposed upgrades to the system's toughness or robustness. Certainly, Dave's proposed robust version of fuzzy C-means (robust-FCM) is one of the most well-known robust fuzzy clustering techniques. In robust-FCM, noise is considered as another further cluster, a noise cluster. A moment ago, Cimin has presented an extension in(Cimino & Frosini, 2007) which leads to the robust-FCM as a innovative technique destined to figure out the optimum expanse which further representing the state line of the noise cluster established upon the investigation of the scattering of the proportion of the objects. In (Kumar, 2021) it presents a rule-based technique for exactly calculating all of the biggest collections of fuzzy contextual disparities. As an extension to fuzzy relational coefficients, fuzzy relational inequalities may be expanded to additional fuzzy logic fields. In(Chandrawat et al., 2017) the situational based Fuzzy model is being expressed to mitigate the destruction in the cost optimization and examining the credibility of optimized value. It describes a strategy for obtaining optimization using a fuzzy linear programming problem in(Kumar et al., 2021) in which fuzzy integers represent the right-side parameters. To answer the fuzzy linear programming problem, a comparative examination of modelling and optimizing creation cost using a novel α-cut based quadrilateral fuzzy number is presented. Rakesh Kumar in (Chandrawat et al., 2019) uses fuzzy equivalence clustering to identify the performance grades of binders for NCHRP 90-07 utilizing the Minkowski, Mahalanobis, Cosine, Chebychev, and Correlation distance functions.

The application of the fuzzy c-means clustering extended a widespread series from image processing, data mining, biomedical statistics handling for the communication and for the mechanism engineering presentations. The utmost common applications you will bring into being in literature are the image processing tasks, such as the thresholding of the image or segmentation of the image. Chi, Yan, and Pham(Del Moral, 2020) covered a wide range of FCM applications in their book, including the characterization of tissues seen in Magnetic Resonance Imaging (MRI) pictures and the segmentation of natural color images. In their study, a novel spatially weighted fuzzy c-means clustering method for picture thresholding the authors argue that the suggested model is extra resistive to noise due to the neighborhood model demonstrated by Yang in(Yang et al., 2004). Similar researchers extended the given approach by adding a fresh consequence term to FCM for the picture separation procedure. Srinivasa proposed a systematic extraction of the characteristic for categorization in(Srinivasa & Medasani, 2004). He discovered that the classification accuracy gained by fuzzy c-means clustering is quite close to the classification accuracy obtained using problem-specific extraction features. As a result, it is feasible to build a standard, simpler and more generic extraction mechanism for the function. Fuzzy C-Means clustering is frequently used to separate Electromagnetic Emission signals from other signal sources. Omkar in(Senthilnath et al., 2011) presented a study that suggests that FCM has been used as an efficient methodology in Pseudo-Destructive Testing for unaccompanied signaling recognition. Furthermore, uses of FCM in biomedical evidence may be seen in(Chankong et al., 2014) Theera-Umpon's (2005) study, in which his scholar proposed a methodology for segmenting single-cell pictures of lymphocytes across the bone marrow into specified locations, namely nucleus and non-nucleus. The findings of this study showed significant segmentation and encouraging success throughout classification compared with real world data of an expert.

MAIN FOCUS OF THE CHAPTER

Fuzzy Clustering Model

Clustering is amongst the most significant natural language processing processes as it plays a key role in identifying data configurations. In considering the fact that modern world problems in pattern recognition involve processing of mathematical data, fuzzy clustering method would be seen to serve the best. Fuzzy clustering can indeed be categorized into two specific classes, which include: Fuzzy point prototype and Fuzzy nonpoint prototype, dependent on Fuzzy partition, and Fuzzy hierarchical clustering system based on Fuzzy equivalence comparisons.

The performance of a certain clustering model and algorithm that optimizes it is a data set "X", c-partition 'u' as well as vector sets $v=\{v_1,v_2,v_3\}$ translated as a reference point (cluster center) for cluster points. Next let us discuss similar clustering models across.

1) Fuzzy C-Means

Among the clustering point-prototype models, C-Means models are generally the most developed. The Fuzzy C-Means clustering technique is an iterative clustering approach that produces the suitable 'c' divisions by lowering the Function Jury object. The standard FCM framework is proposed as follows: Fuzzy Clustering Models as well as Algorithm through contrasting with those of the crisp c-partitions, components could correspond to the several clusters and to differing degrees in a blurry case. Requirements provided in formulas that may include normalization of either the total membership of each data function vector to 1 and therefore that variable can't fully belong to much more clusters than it exists. The fuzzifier 'm', need to be more than 1, because the problem of optimization is a crisp case when m=1. In the literature, m = 2 is the frequently used value for the fuzzifier.

Let's explain the discrepancy between smooth and fuzzy c-means that used a favorite illustration throughout the research. It can indeed be demonstrated that somehow the fuzzy case of clustering provides a much better explanation of the needle point as it allocates its membership almost equally for each cluster. Fuzzy cluster which are further categorized as smooth clustering, also recognized as the soft k-means to which each data point will care what happens to additional clusters than one. Clustering or Cluster assessment involves the measures of handing across pieces of information to clusters in this kind of way which objects in much the same cluster are almost as consistent as possible, therefore clusters would be inconsistent.

Essentially, FCM is an over provisioning algorithm. In terms of image analysis, the operation space will be partitioned into the collection of clusters that the consumer specifies. It is unaffected by the number of clusters currently existing in the data collection. It is mostly related to the probabilistic constraint on either the membership interest or the membership interest. The acquired membership value, together with the usage of FCM, delivers the pixel's "degree of sharing" far into the function space of the various clusters. In other words, it appears to represent the extent to which clusters will share a pixel.

a) Algorithm for FCM

Here is the algorithm which is thoroughly based upon the assumptions that any arbitrary no. of clusters (say q) has given a real number (say m) which belongs to the positive natural numbers i.e. m ϵ (1, ¥).

Here, the algorithm will continuously compute the value until and unless any stopping or terminating condition will not apply. Here, the terminating conditions depend upon the ε, which is very small positive number.

Here, let t=0 for the initial fuzzy pseudo partition P^t.

After that compute q clusters $Z_1+Z_2+Z_3+\ldots+Z_q$ for P^t and for the value of m.

Keep on updating the value of P^t to P^{t+1} until the condition of termination comes i.e.

$$P^t - P^{t+1} < \Delta$$

So, the given algorithm after the pseudo partition is;

$$Ai^{t+1}\left(Y_K\right) = \left(\left[\sum_{j=1}^{q} \frac{Y_k - Z_i}{Y_k - Z_i}\right]^{\frac{1}{m-1}}\right)^{-1}, \tag{1}$$

This algorithm is further modified as;

$$\mathrm{D}[\mathrm{i}] = Y_k - Z_i^{\frac{2}{m-1}}, \tag{2}$$

$$\mathrm{D}[\mathrm{j}] = Y_k - Z_j^{\frac{2}{m-1}}, \tag{3}$$

After putting equation (2) and (3) in equation (1), we get;

$$A_i^{t+1} = \left[\sum_{j=1}^{q} \frac{D[i]}{D[j]}\right]^{-1}, \tag{4}$$

Now we need to check the terminating condition, i.e.

$$P^t - P^{t+1} \leq \Delta, \tag{5}$$

if terminating condition is satisfied then the partition has been done else get back to the equation (4) where we define the membership function and amend it accordingly to the given algorithm and iterate it until the terminating condition is fulfilled that is equation (5).

b) Advantages of FCM

i) Any such approach provides a strong superimposed set of data outcome as well as being comparatively smoother from those of the clustering k-means.

ii) The data point will provide their position throughout at least single region, while each data collection in k-means clustering corresponds to one cluster only.

c) Disadvantages of FCM

i) Number of groups should always be predefined.

ii) Uneven distribution of important weight factors.

2) Possibilistic C-Means

This section discusses the 'what' and 'why' of PCM. 'What' refers to what PCM is, while 'Why' explains why it was chosen over FCM.

What is PCM?

Possibilistic C-Means is a specific application of the possibility theory developed by Krishnapuram and Keller (PCM). It is a clustering algorithm that modifies the FCM goal function. As a result, comprehension is interwoven into the 'what' and 'how' of PCM, and the mathematical limitation addressed by PCM is all about 'breaking boundaries'.

Why PCM?

Unlike FCM, PCM membership value can be understood as "degree of belongingness, compatibility". The degree of belongingness denotes the degree to which the points are members of a class. The degree of compatibility is the degree to which the points in the cluster and the cluster mean are compatible. All of the above allow a point to belong to a class. This is in contrast to FCM, where it is the "degree of sharing." As PCM reduces the constraint on FCM, the above-mentioned variation in the interpretation of membership values is noticed.

a) Possibilistic C-Mean algorithm:

The distinction between PCM and FCM was established in the previous section. It was demonstrated that PCM works by loosening the limitation on FCM. However, applying this reduction of restriction to the original objective function of FCM yields a straightforward solution.

Firstly fix the number of the clusters "c" and then fix the value of "m", ($1 \leq m < \infty$).

Then, using the procedure below, set the iteration number i=1, initialize the probabilistic c-partition P^t, and estimate the value of Y_i.

$$P(T,V)=\sum_{i=1}^{c}\sum_{j}^{n}(t_{ik})^m (d_{ij})^2, \tag{6}$$

T is the set of prototypes (cluster centers) for each "c" class. V is a fuzzy c-partition that consists of the membership values of each point in each class, where a row represents one class and consists of the membership values in the class denoted by "i". In this case, "n" indicates the total number of clusters, while "j" represents the clusters, which will range from 1 to n. Furthermore, Possibilistic C-objective Mean's function is as follows;

$$min_{T,v}\left\{P(T,V;X,Y)=\sum_{k=1}^{n}\sum_{i=1}^{c}(t_{ix})^m x_k - v_{i\ A}^{2}+\sum_{i=1}^{c}Y_i\sum_{k=1}^{n}(1-t_{ik})^m\right\}, \tag{7}$$

$$P_m^{(i,j)}(T,V)=t_{ij}^m D_{ijA}^2 + Y_i(1-t_{ij})^m, \tag{8}$$

Where,

$Y_i>0$, $1\leq i\leq c$, $u_i \in R$, $m>1$

Where Y_i is the "bandwidth, scale, or resolution" parameter that is calculated from data. The distance is determined by the parameter. It is calculated as;

$$Y_i = k\frac{\sum_{k=1}^{n} t_{ik}^m D_{ikA}^2}{\sum_{k=1}^{n} t_{ik}^m}, \tag{9}$$

Where, $1\leq i\leq c$; $1\leq k\leq n$ and $k>0$ (the most common choice for k is 1).

The following formula may be used to compute the membership value t_{ik}, which is continually adjusted to calculate the objective function,

$$t_{ik} = \frac{1}{1 + \left(\frac{D_{ikA}^2}{Y_i} \right)^{\frac{1}{m-1}}}, \tag{10}$$

Where, $1 \le i \le c$; $1 \le k \le n$.

Here, v_i mentioned in the above minimization formula can be calculated by following formula;

$$v_i = \frac{\sum_{k=1}^{n} t_{ik}^m x_k}{\sum_{k=1}^{n} t_{ik}^m}, \tag{11}$$

Where, $1 \le i \le c$; $1 \le k \le n$

The objective function and membership value given above satisfy the maximizing requirements as well as the following fuzzy criterion (also applicable for FCM) mentioned below;

$t_{ik} \in [0,1]$; $\forall$i,j and $0 < \sum_{j=1}^{n} t_{ik} \le 1, \forall \mathrm{i}$

Update the prototype using P^t, as indicated and then compute the value of P^{t+1} using the algorithm and hence increment in the "i" until the terminating condition satisfies i.e. $P^t - P^{t+1} < \varepsilon$, where ε is a very small positive number.

If the terminating condition is satisfied then the partition has been done else get back to the step where we define the membership function and amend it accordingly to the given algorithm and iterate it until the termination condition fulfilled. The outcomes of the possibilistic algorithms, like any other clustering approach, are dependent on initialization. Clusters in possibilistic algorithms have limited mobility because each data point sees only one cluster at a time rather than all clusters simultaneously. As a result, for the algorithms to converge to the global minimum, a sufficiently good initialization is necessary. To obtain the initial partition, any acceptable (hard or fuzzy) clustering technique might be employed. The FCM technique, or one of its modifications, is a suitable candidate for initializing the relevant probabilistic algorithms, and Y_i estimates obtained using the resultant fuzzy partition are fairly acceptable. However, when there is too much noise, the fuzzy partition estimates of Y_i are not very good. This is due to the FCM's tendency to give relatively high memberships to noise points in excellent clusters. To address this issue, it appears that in very noisy scenarios, a reasonable method is to utilize the estimated Y_i just for a few iterations in the probabilistic process, re-estimate them, and then use them until convergence. This is all about the possibilistic C-mean algorithm.

Numerical Examples

Here, we'll look at a few examples of each method and analyze the images we'll take.

a) FCM Algorithm
   i) Example Image 1

Figure 1. image of human brain taken using the MRI (magnetic Resonance imaging)

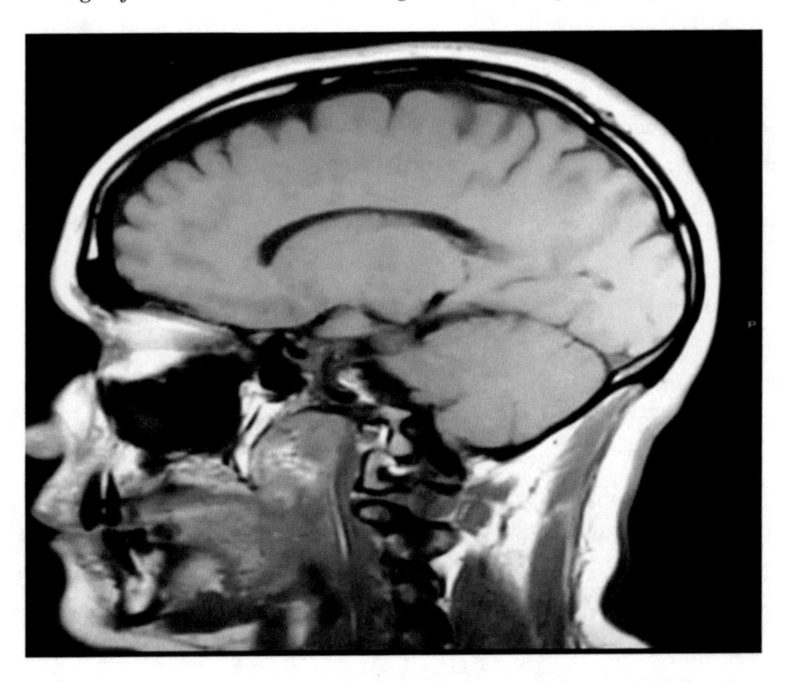

So we will take the data from the image and provide the results using FCM clustering method.

Table 1 below shows the data (co-ordinates) taken from the image.

Value of centers

$$V=\begin{bmatrix} 546.388 & 149.9860 \\ 718.6474 & 611.8613 \end{bmatrix}$$

Table 1.

X1	172	379	561	755	793	863	844	783	722	466
X2	184	99	98	115	209	317	453	628	769	769

Figure 2. Plot represents the data centers for the image coordinates using FCM of Figure 1

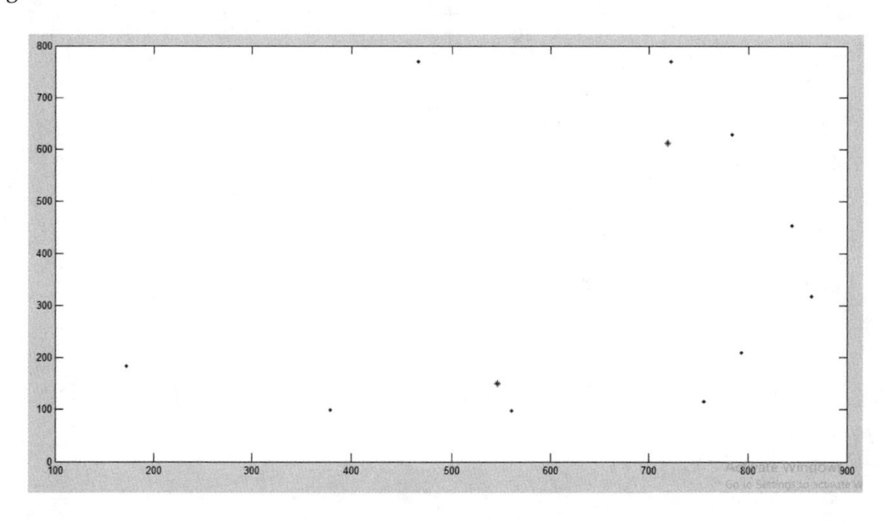

ii) Example Image 2

Figure 3. Image of human brain (top view) using MRI

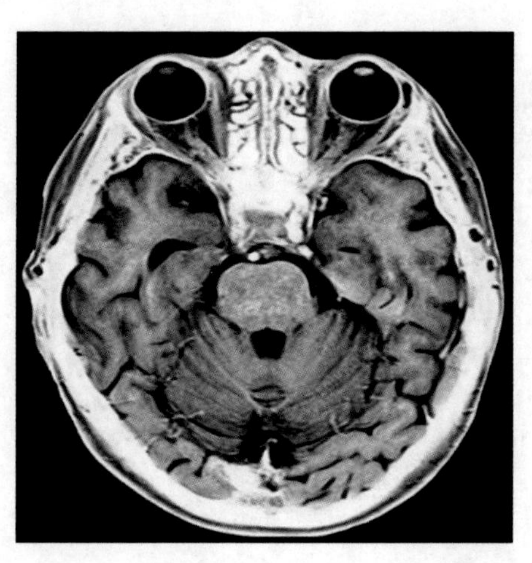

So, we will take the data from the image and provide the results using FCM clustering method.

Table 2 below shows the data (co-ordinates) taken from the image.

Table 2.

X_1	168	248	559	658	90	365	613	739	199
X_2	112	116	107	107	281	280	276	277	444

Value of center

$$V=\begin{bmatrix} 204.9784 & 237.9793 \\ 630.2012 & 240.3268 \end{bmatrix}$$

Figure 4. Plot Represents the data centers for the image coordinates using FCM of Figure 3

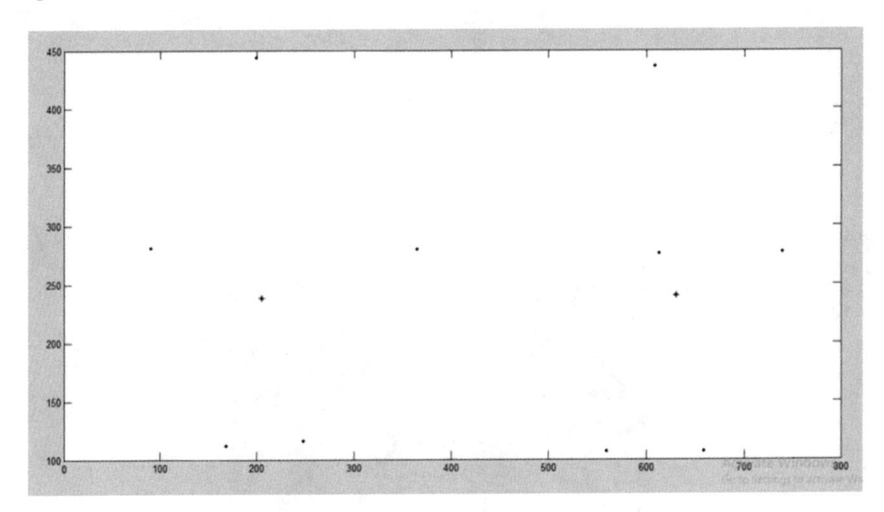

b) PCM Algorithm

i) Example Image 1

So, we will take the data from the image and provide the results using PCM clustering method.

Figure 5. Image of human brain taken using the MRI (magnetic Resonance imaging)

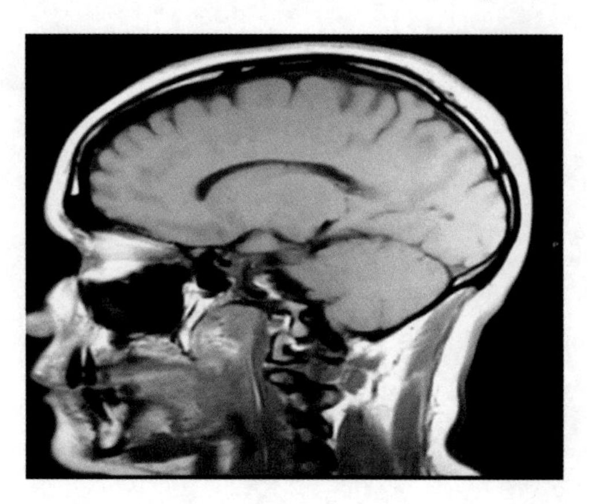

Table 3 below shows the data (co-ordinates) taken from the image.

Table 3.

X_1	172	379	561	755	793	863	844	783	722	466
X_2	184	99	98	115	209	317	453	628	769	769

Value of centers using previous algorithm i.e. FCM
Initially,

$$V_0 = \begin{bmatrix} 546.388 & 149.9860 \\ 718.6474 & 611.8613 \end{bmatrix}$$

We will now find out the value of new centers using the algorithm of PCM. Value of centers calculated using the PCM is,

$$V_{pcm} = \begin{bmatrix} 368.3888 & 180.4288 \\ 718.6474 & 611.8613 \end{bmatrix}$$

Figure 6. Plot represents the data centers for the image coordinates using PCM of Figure 5

ii) Example Image 2

Figure 7. Image of human Brain, skull (top view) using MRI

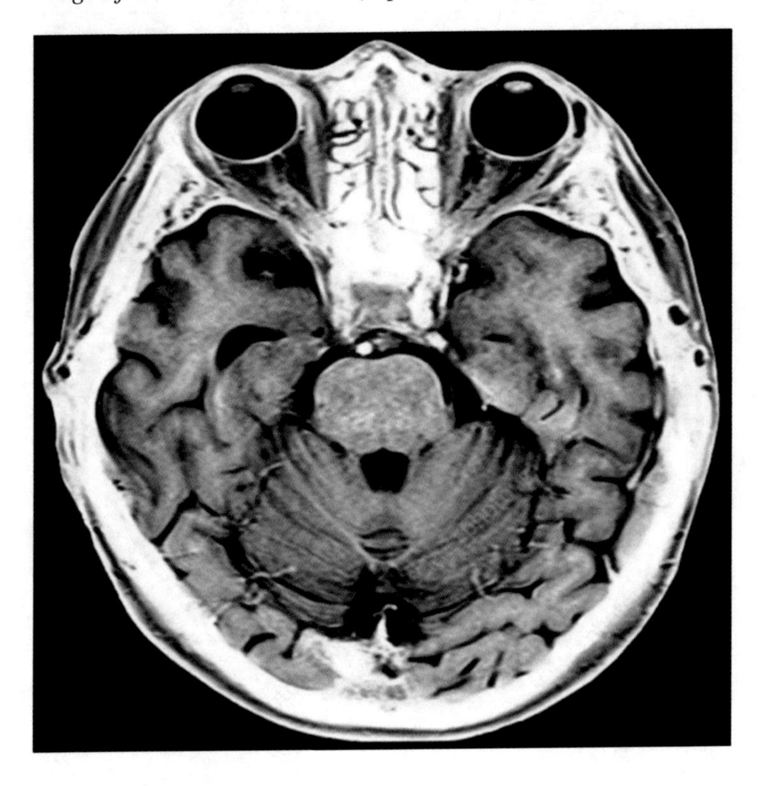

So, we will take the data from the image and provide the results using PCM clustering method.

Table 4 below shows the data (co-ordinates) taken from the image.

Table 4.

X_1	168	248	559	658	90	365	613	739	199
X_2	112	116	107	107	281	280	276	277	444

Value of centers using previous algorithm i.e. FCM

Initially,

$$V_0 = \begin{bmatrix} 204.9784 & 237.9793 \\ 630.2012 & 240.3268 \end{bmatrix}$$

We will now find out the value of new centers using the algorithm of PCM. Value of centers calculated using the PCM is,

$$V_{pcm} = \begin{bmatrix} 172.2530 & 273.9793 \\ 630.2012 & 240.3268 \end{bmatrix}$$

Figure 8. Plot represents the data centers for the image coordinates using PCM of Figure 7

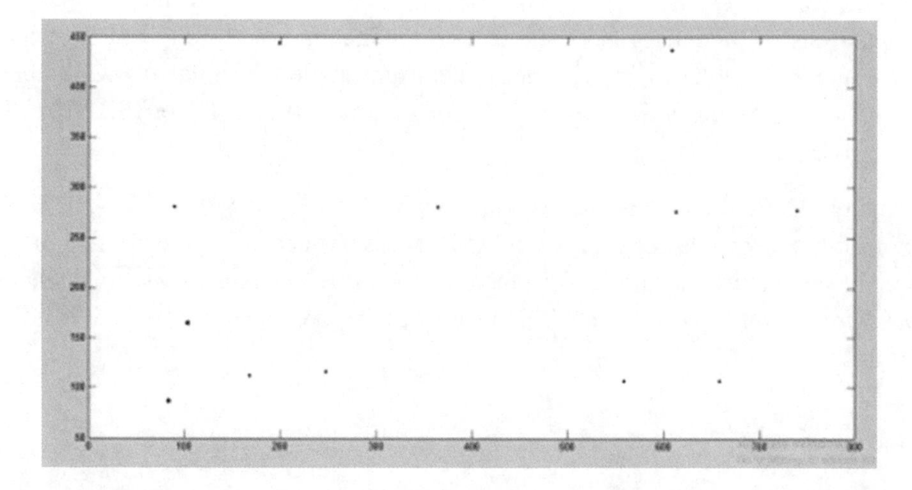

CONCLUSION

Applications today require many kinds of photographs as knowledge sources through elaboration and study. Degradation happens as a picture is converted from one type to another such as digitizing, processing, and transmitting, storage, etc. The resulting picture will then undergo a procedure called picture enhancement, which also involves a set of approaches that aim to improve an image's visual appearance. Image processing essentially enhances the interpretability or awareness of information for noises created in pictures and offers more input for numerous other completely automated image processing systems. Fuzzy image processing is a potent technique for expert knowledge edge preparation and the mixing of erroneous information from several sources. The desired fuzzy rules are an appealing result in order to increase the quality of edges as much as feasible. We demonstrated this by acquiring the coordinates of random images and then evaluating the photos with various methodologies such as FCM and PCM to show that we can process any image on a large scale in this way. These techniques are not limited to FCM and PCM. We have suggested that both membership and typicality values are required in clustering. There are more techniques, such as FPCM and PFCM, but for now, we have just discussed about FCM and PCM.

REFERENCES

Auephanwiriyakul, S., & Keller, J. M. (2002). Analysis and efficient implementation of a linguistic fuzzy C-means. *IEEE Transactions on Fuzzy Systems*, *10*(5), 563–582. doi:10.1109/TFUZZ.2002.803492

Chandrawat, R. K., Kumar, R., Garg, B. P., Dhiman, G., & Kumar, S. (2017). An analysis of modeling and optimization production cost through fuzzy linear programming problem with symmetric and right angle triangular fuzzy number. *Advances in Intelligent Systems and Computing*, *546*, 197–211. doi:10.1007/978-981-10-3322-3_18

Chandrawat, R. K., Kumar, R., Makkar, V., Yadav, M., & Kumari, P. (2019). A comparative fuzzy cluster analysis of the Binder's performance grades using fuzzy equivalence relation via different distance measures. In *Communications in Computer and Information Science* (Vol. 955). Springer Singapore. doi:10.1007/978-981-13-3140-4_11

Chankong, T., Theera-Umpon, N., & Auephanwiriyakul, S. (2014). Automatic cervical cell segmentation and classification in Pap smears. *Computer Methods and Programs in Biomedicine, 113*(2), 539–556. doi:10.1016/j.cmpb.2013.12.012 PMID:24433758

Cimino, M., & Frosini, G. (2007). On the noise distance in robust fuzzy c-means. *International Journal on Engineering, Computing and Technology,* 361–364. http://www2.ing.unipi.it/~r000099/publications/cimino_pub19.pdf

Del Moral, P. (2020). Theory and applications. *Mean Field Simulation for Monte Carlo Integration*, 85–124. doi:10.1201/b14924-7

Informa, F., Number, W. R., House, M., Street, M., & Dunn, J. C. (2008). *Well-Separated Clusters and Optimal Fuzzy Partitions Well-Separated Clusters and Optimal Fuzzy Partitions*. Academic Press.

Kumar, R. (2021). *A Comparative Study of Fuzzy Optimization through Fuzzy Number*. Academic Press.

Kumar, R., Chandrawat, R. K., Sarkar, B., Joshi, V., & Majumder, A. (2021). An Advanced Optimization Technique for Smart Production Using α-Cut Based Quadrilateral Fuzzy Number. *International Journal of Fuzzy Systems, 23*(1), 107–127. doi:10.100740815-020-01002-9

Pal, N. R., Pal, K., Keller, J. M., & Bezdek, J. C. (2005). A possibilistic fuzzy c-means clustering algorithm. *IEEE Transactions on Fuzzy Systems, 13*(4), 517–530. doi:10.1109/TFUZZ.2004.840099

Pedrycz, W., & Vulkovich, G. (2004). Fuzzy clustering with supervision. *Pattern Recognition, 37*(7), 1339–1349. doi:10.1016/j.patcog.2003.11.005

Rodríguez Ramos, A., Llanes-Santiago, O., Bernal de Lázaro, J. M., Cruz Corona, C., Silva Neto, A. J., & Verdegay Galdeano, J. L. (2017). A novel fault diagnosis scheme applying fuzzy clustering algorithms. *Applied Soft Computing, 58*, 605–619. doi:10.1016/j.asoc.2017.04.071

Senthilnath, J., Omkar, S. N., & Mani, V. (2011). Clustering using firefly algorithm: Performance study. *Swarm and Evolutionary Computation, 1*(3), 164–171. doi:10.1016/j.swevo.2011.06.003

Srinivasa, N., & Medasani, S. (2004). Active fuzzy clustering for collaborative filtering. *IEEE International Conference on Fuzzy Systems, 3*, 1697–1702. 10.1109/FUZZY.2004.1375436

Yang, M. S., Hwang, P. Y., & Chen, D. H. (2004). Fuzzy clustering algorithms for mixed feature variables. *Fuzzy Sets and Systems*, *141*(2), 301–317. doi:10.1016/S0165-0114(03)00072-1

ADDITIONAL READING

Askari, S. (2021). Fuzzy C-Means clustering algorithm for data with unequal cluster sizes and contaminated with noise and outliers: Review and development. *Expert Systems with Applications*, *165*, 113856. doi:10.1016/j.eswa.2020.113856

Atanassov, K. (2017). Type-1 Fuzzy Sets and Intuitionistic Fuzzy Sets. *Algorithms*, *10*(3), 106. doi:10.3390/a10030106

Bustince, H., Barrenechea, E., Pagola, M., Fernandez, J., Xu, Z., Bedregal, B., Montero, J., Hagras, H., Herrera, F., & De Baets, B. (2016). A historical account of types of fuzzy sets and their relationships. *IEEE Transactions on Fuzzy Systems*, *24*(1), 179–194. doi:10.1109/TFUZZ.2015.2451692

Chatzis, S. P. (2011). A fuzzy c-means-type algorithm for clustering of data with mixed numeric and categorical attributes employing a probabilistic dissimilarity functional. *Expert Systems with Applications*, *38*(7), 8684–8689. doi:10.1016/j.eswa.2011.01.074

Kannan, S. R., Devi, R., Ramathilagam, S., & Takezawa, K. (2013). Effective FCM noise clustering algorithms in medical images. *Computers in Biology and Medicine*, *43*(2), 73–83. doi:10.1016/j.compbiomed.2012.10.002 PMID:23219569

Kumar, R., & Gupta, S. (2013). Application of Fuzzy c- means clustering for Facility location and Transportation problems. *International Transactions in Applied Sciences*, *5*, 35–42.

Kumar, R., & Joshi, V. (2020). A New Approach to Optimize the Membership Grade in Fuzzy Linear Programming Problem. *European Journal of Molecular & Clinical Medicine*, *7*(7), 3774–3786.

Peng, X., & Selvachandran, G. (2019). Pythagorean fuzzy set: State of the art and future directions. *Artificial Intelligence Review*, *52*(3), 1873–1927. doi:10.100710462-017-9596-9

Ran, X., Zhou, X., Lei, M., Tepsan, W., & Deng, W. (2021). A novel K-means clustering algorithm with a noise algorithm for capturing urban hotspots. *Applied Sciences (Switzerland)*, *11*(23), 11202. Advance online publication. doi:10.3390/app112311202

Tsai, D. M., & Lin, C. C. (2011). Fuzzy C-means based clustering for linearly and nonlinearly separable data. *Pattern Recognition*, *44*(8), 1750–1760. doi:10.1016/j.patcog.2011.02.009

Xu, D., & Tian, Y. (2015). A Comprehensive Survey of Clustering Algorithms. *Annals of Data Science*, *2*(2), 165–193. doi:10.100740745-015-0040-1

KEY TERMS AND DEFINITIONS

Centroid: The location that represents the cluster's centre, whether it is real or imagined, is called a centroid. Each data point is then placed in a distinct cluster by reducing the in-cluster sum of squares.

Fuzzy Numbers: In contrast to a traditional real number, which can only ever refer to one specific value, a fuzzy number can refer to an infinitely large collection of related values, each of which is assigned a relative importance between zero and one. The concept of fuzzy numbers is a logical expansion of the classical number system.

Fuzzy Sets: In 1965, Lotfi A. Zadeh introduced fuzzy sets. Fuzzy sets are those sets whose elements have a degree of membership i.e., every fuzzy set is characterized by a membership function.

Image Processing: Image processing is a technique for altering or extracting information from an image by the application of various mathematical, statistical, and computational methods. It's a form of signal processing where the input is an image and the output could be the same image or some of the image's features.

Membership Function: Membership function shows the degrees of belongingness of elements of universe of discourse say X to set A where $A \subset X$. Simply put, it is a function that maps some set of real numbers to the interval [0, 1]. i.e. μA X®[0,1].

Noise: Data points that are anomalous or do not form a part of any significant cluster are referred to as noise.

Outliers: Since the majority of clustering methods require a minimum number of data points to construct a cluster, outliers are the ungrouped data points. Even if the outliers form a cluster, it is quite isolated from other clusters.

Unlabeled Data: Unlabeled data comprises of data extracted from nature or manufactured by humans in order to investigate the underlying scientific patterns. When it comes to unsupervised learning, clustering is by far the most critical challenge. Finding a pattern in an unlabeled data collection is at the heart of this challenge, as it is with others of its kind.

Unsupervised Learning: By applying machine learning algorithms to the analysis and classification of unlabeled datasets, unsupervised learning (also known as unsupervised machine learning) is able to shed light on previously opaque data. Without the help of a human, these algorithms can unearth previously unseen patterns or groups of related data.

Chapter 10
Survey or Review on the Deep Learning Techniques for Retinal Image Segmentation in Predicting/Diagnosing Diabetic Retinopathy

Sowmiya R.
Puducherry Technological University, India

Kalpana R.
Puducherry Technological University, India

ABSTRACT

Artificial intelligence (AI)-based image segmentation plays an important role in image processing and computer vision. AI can be used in the medical field (e.g., ophthalmology, disease prediction which involves direct visualization and imaging) as a frequent method for diagnosis. Deep learning comes under machine learning and as a part of AI. Deep learning algorithms have yielded considerable results in the medical field. Diabetic retinopathy is one of the most common causes of blindness, which is diagnosed by examining the appearance of the retina. The diabetic retinopathy stages are determined based on the changes seen in retina or retinal image. This chapter gives a detailed survey on different algorithms used for diagnosing diabetic retinopathy and different deep learning techniques used for medical image segmentation.

DOI: 10.4018/978-1-6684-4405-4.ch010

INTRODUCTION

Deep learning architecture has various kinds of layers such as convolutional, fully connected and recurrent layers. It also includes supervised and unsupervised learning of feature representation with various layers. The hidden layers of an Artificial Neural Network are also included in deep learning layers. To maximize the development of deep learning algorithms in different fields, distinct deep learning algorithms have different algorithms. Deep learning has a huge impact in healthcare. It has enabled the sector to improve patient monitoring and diagnostics (Alyoubi, 2020). Deep learning can interpret medical images like X-ray, MRI scan, CT scan etc. An image is made up of a number of distinct pixels. Image segmentation is used to group pixels with similar properties together. Image segmentation is the process of dividing an image into multiple segments. An object type is allocated to each pixel in the image throughout this process. As some area of the image contain no information, it is not necessary to process the entire image. Therefore, image segmentation is done to extract the key segments for processing. The Semantic segmentation and instance segmentation are the two types of image segmentation. All objects of the same type are identified by a single class label in semantic segmentation as in Figure 1. But in instance segmentation, related objects are identified by their own labels. Recognizing the pixels of organs or lesions from background medical pictures such as CT or MRI scans are the key challenges in medical image processing in order to offer important information on the shapes and sizes of these organs.

Figure 1. Types of Segmentation

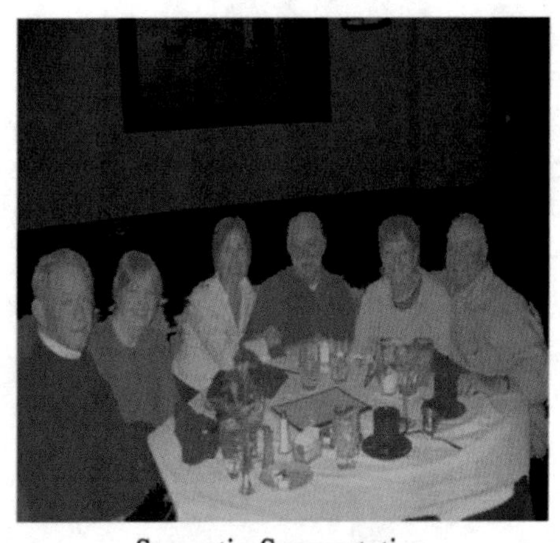

Semantic Segmentation

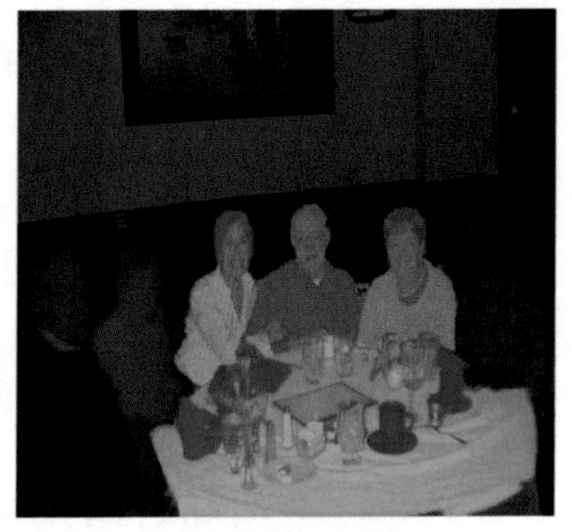

Instance Segmentation

For example, Cancer has long been seen as a fatal disease. Even in today's technologically advanced world, cancer can be lethal if it is not detected early enough. Early detection of malignant cells can save millions of lives. The morphology of the malignant cells are crucial in evaluating the aggressive stages of cancer. Object detection will not be useful here, even by putting the pieces together. Pin Wang (2016) has stated that only bounding boxes can be generated, which will not assist us in determining the form of the cells. In this case, Image segmentation techniques will have a significant impact. They enable us to take a more granular approach to the problem and produce more useful outcomes, as in Figure 2.

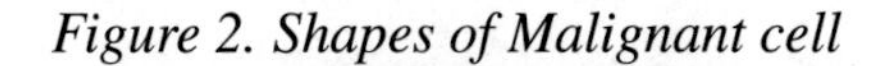

Figure 2. Shapes of Malignant cell

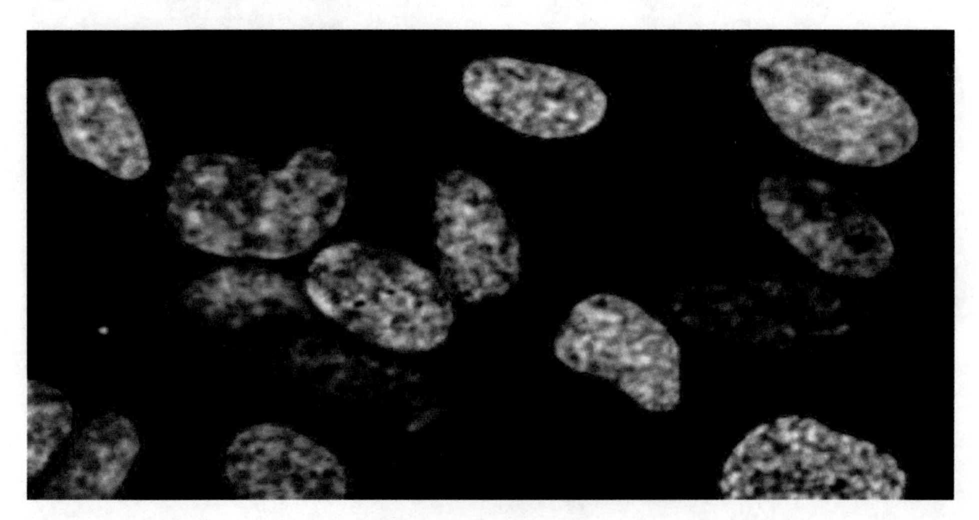

The remainder of the paper is organized as follows. In Section 2, the Diabetic Retinopathy is explained, Section 3, the related work is presented. In Section 4, datasets and its sources are given. Section 5 is composed of various techniques of diagnosing medical images. And finally, Section 6 presents the conclusion of the review.

DIABETIC RETINOPATHY (DR)

Diabetes mellitus (DM) is a collection of metabolic illnesses marked by hyperglycemia caused by insulin production, insulin action, or both. Diabetes-related chronic hyperglycemia is strongly associated to long-term damage, dysfunction, and failure of number of organs, as well as the eyes, kidneys, nerves, heart, and blood vessels (Priya, 2013). Diabetes is caused by a number of different pathogenic mechanisms.

Figure 3. Normal retina and Diabetic Retinopathy

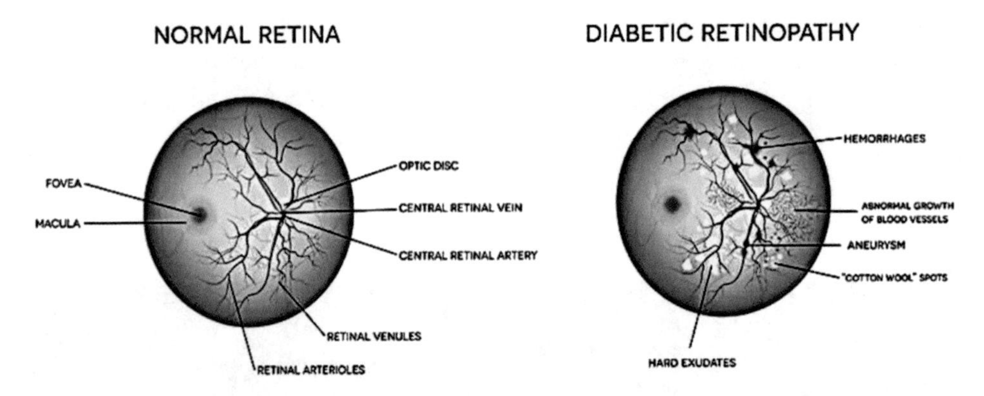

Signs of DR

The signs of DR as shown in Figure 3 are

- Microaneurysms(MA)
- Hemorrhages (HM)
- Exudates (EX)
- Neovascularization (NV)

Microaneurysm (MA)

Microaneurysms are small red dots in the retina that are often encircled by yellow rings, which are caused by vascular dilatations as in Figure 4. Microaneurysms have no other symptoms or indicators, and they have no effect on eyesight (Kou, 2020). The early signs of diabetic retinopathy are usually microaneurysms. This means that microaneurysms are extremely important symptoms since early identification of them in the eye can lead to earlier treatment of diabetic retinopathy, lowering the risk of vision loss.

Figure 4. Microaneurysm

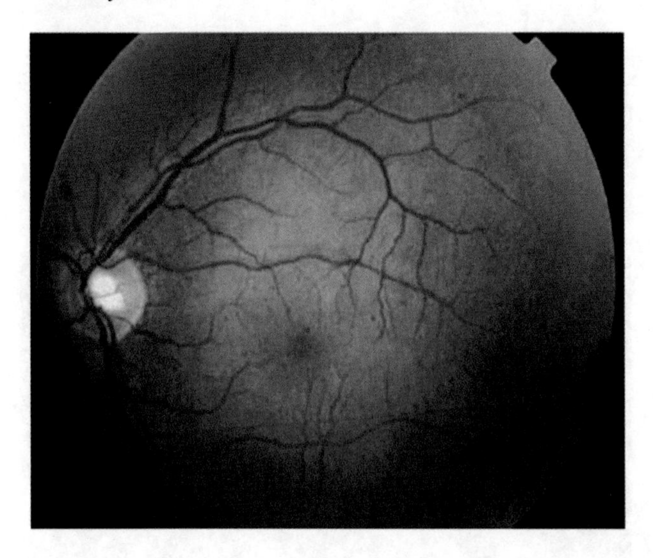

Hemorrhage (HM)

Retinal hemorrhage is an ophthalmic condition in which the retina, the light-sensitive tissue on the rear wall of the eye bleeds as in Figure 5. It may be present near optic disc or only in retinal periphery (Kiranyaz, 2015).

Figure 5. Hemorrhage

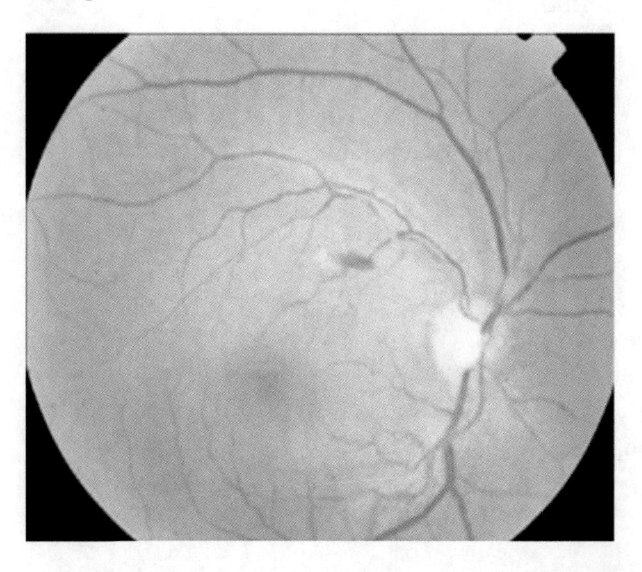

Exudates (EX)

The yellow flecks are called hard exudates. In Figure 6, the residual leakage of lipids from damaged capillaries is shown.

Figure 6. Exudates

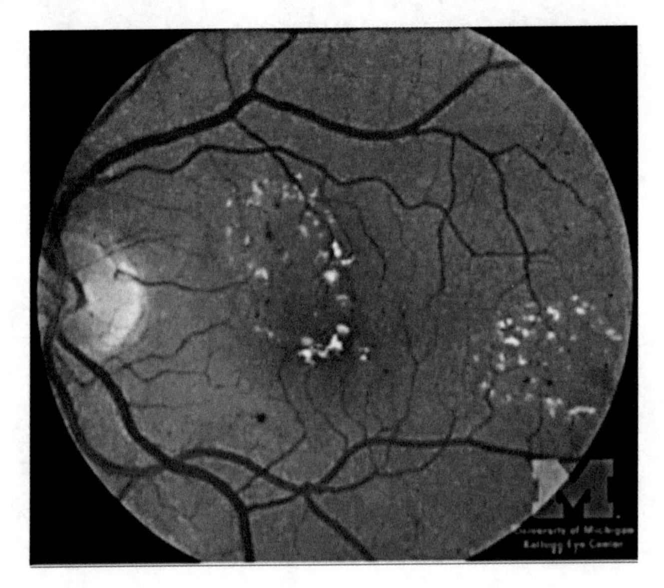

Neovascularization (NV)

The development of new tiny retinal blood vessels is known as neovascularization. When these new blood vessels grow to the surface of the retina, they are referred to as intraretinal micro vascular anomalies or retinal NV as shown in Figure 7.

Symptoms of DR

- Blurred vision
- Impaired color vision
- Poor night vision
- A blind spot in the center of the vision
- A sudden loss of vision

Figure 7.

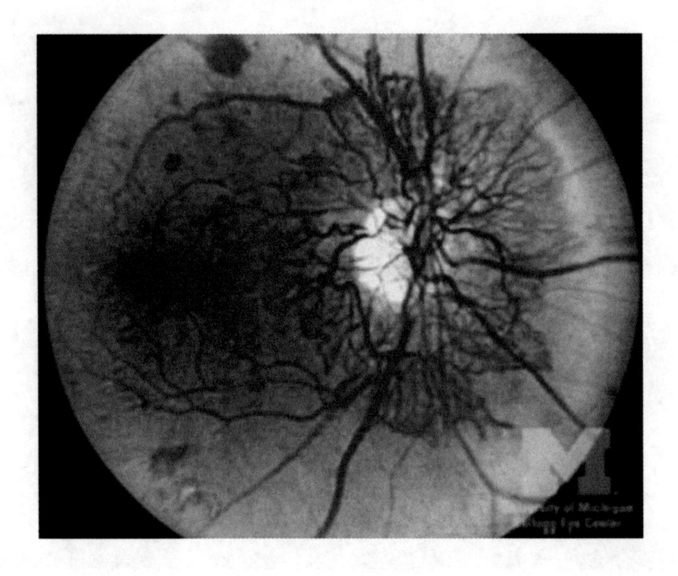

Grades of DR

The presence of one, two or all of these features in the retina determines the DR stages (Lim, 2014). Patients with early DR grades usually have no noticeable symptoms, while patients with advanced DR grades may experience symptoms such as distortion, blurred vision, and gradual visual severity loss. Therefore, DR grades can be classified into Non-Proliferative DR (NPDR) and Proliferative DR (PDR). NPDR is again subgraded into mild, moderate, and severe. Mild is indicated by appearance of Microaneurysm (MA), whereas moderate reflects appearance of Hemorrhage (HM) and/or Exudate (EX). The severe NPDR reflects increasing in retinal ischemia by appearing small, abnormal, and weak BV, which are called Neovascularization (NV). This severe grade is called PDR. Fig. 8 shows the various grades of DR by showing the pathological changes such as HM and EX etc.. Besides, NVs increase the area of BV and cause ischemia in the retina. The range of diminution of vision resulting from the gradual development of DR can vary. As in Table.1, the two major stages of DR: Non-Proliferative DR (NPDR) and Proliferative DR (PDR), which is characterized by neovascularization or vitreous/ preretinal hemorrhage (Roychowdhury, 2013).

Figure 8. DR Grades

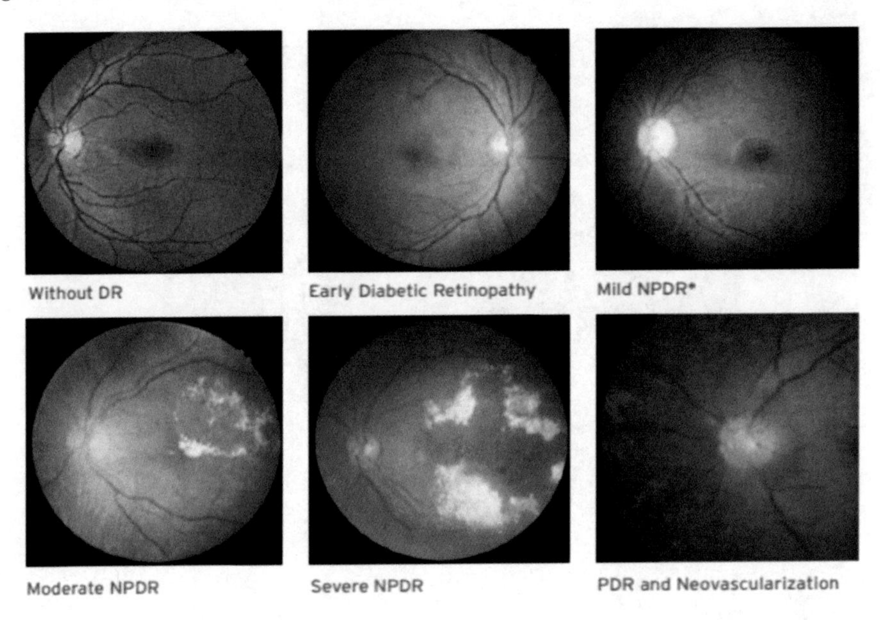

Annually up to 10% of diabetic patient without any signs of diabetic retinopathy develops NPDR. It is reported as there is 75% risk of development of PDR by a severe NPDR patient in one year. Commonly it takes many years for a patient to become PDR from normal status. The three sub-stages of NPDR are: mild, moderate, and severe NPDR. The different stages have to be treated with their own treatment options. Regular screening at a time interval is enough for patients with no DR or mild NPDR. For patients with moderate NPDR or worse, the treatment options vary.

Thus, the severity of the DR should be graded first for providing a proper treatment to the patients. The fundus pictures are used to diagnose the DR clinically. The fundus photographs are taken by the fundus camera directly. The hard or soft exudates, microaneurysms and hemorrhages are the common lesions that indicate DR. All of these lesions can be identified from fundus images.

RELATED WORKS

Worldwide 463 Million people (9%) of the global population, of which 72.96 million diabetic retinopathy case are from India. DR affects three out of four diabetic patients after 15 years of disease duration. In 1846, the French ophthalmologist and professor of Hygiene in Paris, Brouchardat reported the development of visual loss in the absence of cataract in diabetes. Abnormal retinal changes induced by diabetes was observed by Nettleship and Sir Steven Mackenzie.

Table 1. Severity Level with its findings

DR Severity Level	Lesions
No DR	Absent of lesions
Mild non-proliferative DR	MA only
Moderate non-proliferative DR	More than just MA but less than severe DR
Severe non-proliferative DR	Any of the following: • More than 20 intraretinal HM in each of 4 quadrants • Definite venous beading in 2+quadrants • Prominent intraretinalmicrovascular abnormalities in 1+ quadrant • No signs of proliferative DR
Proliferative DR	One or more of the following: • Vitreous/Pre-retinal HM • Neovascularization

A tree structured diagram which indicates the types of techniques available for DR is shown in Fig.9

Figure 9. Techniques used for DR

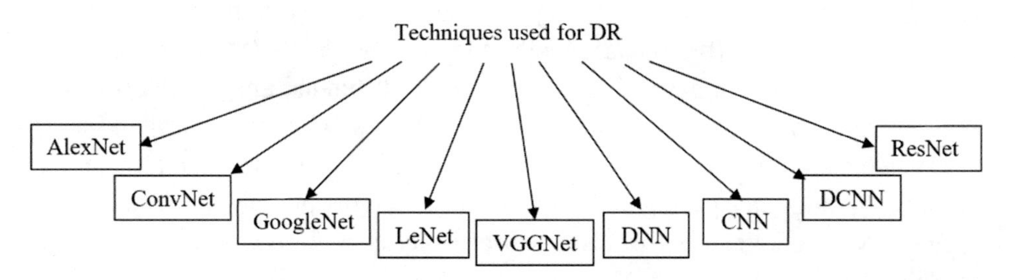

Biran (2016) has differentiated Hemorrhage (HM) from Exudate (EX) to detect DR. They first detected OD from the green channel. They used Contrast Limited Adaptive Histogram Equalization (CLAHE) to improve image contrasts. The combination of CLAHE and Gabor filters are used to partition the Exudate (EX)and then thresholding is done. Extraction of Hemorrhage (HM) is done using the Circular Hough Transform (CHT). Only EX and HM were segmented, not the DR grade.

Parasuraman (2018) extracted Gray Level Co-occurrence Matrix (GLCM), Gray Level Run Length Matrix (GLRLM), and Speeded Up Robust Features (SURF). The normal and DR images were classified. The Adaptive Neuro-Fuzzy Inference System (ANFIS) was utilized to extract the HM. The authors segmented HM as a symptom of DR, however HM alone cannot be used to determine the DR grade.

Orlando (2016) applied the Support Vector Machine (SVM) technique to extract BV. The pair wise interaction was weighed according to the related distance of pixels. The 2D Gabor filter and line detector unary potentials are used to standardize all of the images. The authors also overlooked the benefits of automated segmentation, which can have a detrimental impact on the outcomes.

Fadafen (2018) extracted EX by morphological after excluding OD. The authors used brightness, width, and direction to detect BV using edge and feature-based detection. Their findings were based on the visual system of humans, which is sensitive to intensity and direction. Despite the fact that EX is a significant indicator for DR detection, the authors were unable to classify the DR grades. They also didn't use any contrast enhancement techniques.

Safitri (2017) have diagnosed the fundus images into normal and DR. The authors enhanced the contrast by CLAHE. The blood vessel is segmented by thresholding and the matched filter. Finally, they used the box-counting technique to calculate fractal dimension and the K-Nearest Neighbor (KNN) classification method. The results, however, were influenced by the fractal dimension parameters. Their performance measures did not sufficient in ML imbalanced dataset.

Abdelmaksoud (2020) classified the healthy and the DR grades by extracting EX, MA, HM, and BV. They utilized matched filter with a first-order Gaussian derivative filter and some morphological operations. They extracted the GLCM, areas of lesions, and BP counts. Finally, they utilized MLSVM classifier. Using traditional approaches, extracting many signs from fundus images is difficult. It puts a strain on the developer, especially when dealing with enormous datasets.

Tymchenko (2020) made some augmentation processes such as horizontal and vertical flipping, transposing and rotation. Based on the pretrained ImageNet, the EfficientNet model is used. But the dataset is not enough to validate the real life model.

Hagos (2019) utilized the pre trained Inception-V3 model to differentiate the DR into normal and abnormal. The cropping and resizing the images are done during preprocessing. They used softmax classifier and stochastic GD optimizer. But the result shows the presence or absence of DR, not about the grades of DR.

Li (2019) used fractional MP in CNN to detect five classes of DR. The image is preprocessed by rescaling and clipping. The two CNN model was built with different layers to get different feature space and combined the best prediction by SVM classifier. But the prediction for class 3 and 4 is not accurate.

The following are the primary limitations of conventional methods and DL designs in diagnosing DR grades from color fundus images, as determined by the preceding review of the current literature:

- Most studies focused on detecting the presence or absence of DRs, while ignoring the DR grades. The research that primarily focused on segmenting DR indications were only able to segment one or two of the DR pathological abnormalities (EX, HM, BV, and MA).
- A lot of state-of-the-art systems diagnose DR grades without segmenting and showing the various DR variances for ophthalmologists.
- The majority of research skipped over preprocessing steps, despite the fact that noise and low contrast have an impact on segmentation and classification accuracy as in Table.2.

Table 2. Performance of different methodologies from various datasets

ANALYSIS TYPE	METHODOLOGY	DATASET	PERFORMANCE	DEMERITS
Segmenting EX and HM (Biran, 2016)	CLAHE, Gabor filter, CHT followed by thresholding	DRIVE,STARE	ACC 86.12%	Segmentation of EX and HM is only done without diagnosing the DR grades
Segmenting HM and DR detection (Parasuraman,2018)	GLCM,GLRLM and SURF for feature extraction and ANFIS for classification	MESSIDOR	ACC 92.56%	Segmentation of HM are only done, but the DR grade cannot be diagnosed using HM alone.
Blood Vessel Segmentation (Orlando, 2016)	2D Gabor filter and SVM	STARE	ACC 94.01%, SPE 95.5%, SEN 75.81%	Only blood vessels segmentation is done, whereas other lesions are not done
Segmenting EX (Fadafen, 2018)	Morphological Operations	DIARETDB1	AUC 90.12%	Only EX segmentation is done with poor quality of images.
Segmenting BV and DR detection (Safitri, 2017)	Box counting and KNN	MESSIDOR	ACC 89.17%	Results are dependent on fractal dimensional values. Not suitable for imbalanced datasets.
Lesion segmentation and DR grading (Abdel Maksoud,2020)	Matched filter with first order gaussian derivative, Morphological operations and MLSVM	DRIVE,STARE,MESSIDOR and IDRiD	ACC 89.2%, AUC 85.20%, SEN 85.1%, SPE 85.2%	Not easy to extract many signs from the fundus images using conventional methods. Not suitable for large datasets.
DR classification (Tymchenko, 2020)	EfficientNet	APTOS 2019	Kappa score 0.925	Not enough to validate the real life model.
DR detection (Hagos, 2019)	Inception-V3	KAGGLE	ACC 90.9%	Only the presence or absence of DR is done

DATASETS

There are various datasets that have been used in the literature either for the classification of DR or for grading of DR as in Table.3. These are depicted below

Table 3. Datasets

Dataset	Images	Resolution	Private/ PublicDataset	Link
DRIVE (Digital Retinal Images for vessel Extractor)	40 20 color fundus images	768*584	Public Dataset	https://drive.grand-challenge.org/
STARE (Structured Analysis of the Retina)	400 raw images	605 x &700 pixels	Public Dataset	https://cecas.clemson.edu/-ahoover/stare/
ImageRet (DIARETDBO DIARET DB1)	130 color fundus images	1500*1152	Public Dataset	https://www.it.lut.fi/project/imageret/
DR1	1077 fundus images	640x480	Public Dataset	https://figshare.com/articles/dataset/AdvancingBagofVisualWordsRepresentations_for_Lesion_Classification_in_RetinalImages/953671
DR2	435 fundus Images	640x480	Public Dataset	https://figshare.com/articles/dataset/AdvancingBagofVisualWordsRepresentations_for_Lesion_Classification_in_RetinalImages/953671
VICAVR	58 fundus images	768x584	Public Dataset	http://www.varpa.es/research/ophthalmology.html
AVR DB	100 Coloured fundus images	1504x1000 pixels	Private Dataset	http://biomisa.org/index.php/dataset-for-hypertensive-retinopathy
INSPIRE-AVR	40 retinal Images	-	Public Dataset	https://medicine.uiowa.edu/eye/inspire-datasets
CHASE DBI	28 fundus Images	1280x960	Public Dataset	https://blogs.kingston.ac.uk/retinal/chasedbl/
E-Ophtha	47 fundus images with exudates 35 fundus images without lesions 148 images with MAs and small HEM 233 fundus images with no lesions	1440x960 pixels to 2544 x 1696 pixels	Public Dataset	http://www.adets.net/en/third-party/e-ophtha/

Dataset Size

The size of target dataset is also a role-playing parameter to decide about the level of transfer learning technique. Full adaptation may result in over fitting if the target dataset is limited and the number of parameters is considerable (deeper networks). As a result, partial adaptation is a better option. On the other hand, if the target dataset is substantially larger, overfitting will not occur, and full adaptation will work perfectly (Kauppi, 2006 & 2007). Tajbakhsh (2016) has investigated the effect of dataset size on a full adaption approach. Lim (2014) demonstrated the results that extending the dataset from a quarter to the entire amount of the training dataset improves sensitivity by 10% (from 62 to 72%).

DIFFERENT TYPES OF ALGORITHMS

The different types of algorithms, their working and their applications in the medical field are as follows.

CNN

A CNN is a type of neural network that consists of a stack of layers, each of which performs a distinct task. e.g., convolution, pooling, loss calculation, etc. The output of the previous layer is sent into each intermediate layer. As shown in Figure 10 First is an input layer, in which the image is taken as an input, where the number of neurons are equal to the number of pixels. Second is the convolutional layer that has several filters to perform the convolution operations. Rectified Linear Unit (ReLU) is used to perform operations on elements. The output is a rectified feature map.

Figure 10. Conventional CNN

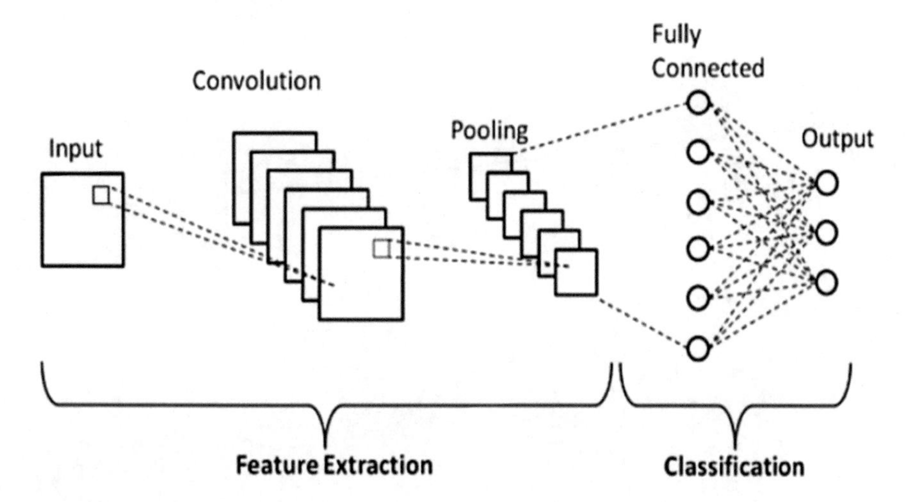

This rectified featured map next is fed into a Pooling layer. Pooling is a type of down sampling that minimizes the size of the featured map. By flattening the two-dimensional arrays from the pooled feature map, the pooling layer turns them into a single, long, continuous, linear vector (Zeiler, 2014). A fully connected layer is formed, when the flattened matrix from the pooling layer is fed as an input, which classifies and identifies the image. It is known as conventional CNN. The use of CNN in medical image interpretation of brain, breast, lung, and other organ diseases has been critically and completely examined. Researchers have successfully used

CNNs to detect tumors and classify them as benign or malignant (Arevalo, 2016), detect skin lesions (Nasr-Esfahani, 2016), interpret optical coherence tomography images (Kermany, 2018), detect colon cancer (Sirinukunwattana, 2016) and blood cancer, breast cancer (Kallenberg,, 2016),chest, eye and other medical image understanding applications.

FCN

A Fully Convolutional Network (FCN) has proved to be a powerful tool for semantic segmentation. The image pixels are transformed into pixel classes by FCN using CNN as shown in Fig.11. A fully connected network, unlike the CNNs for image classification and object recognition, turns the height and width of intermediate feature maps back to those of the input image. As a result, at the pixel level, the classification output and the input image have alone-to-one correspondence: the channel dimensions at any output pixel stores the classification results for the input pixel at the same spatial position.

Figure 11. FCN

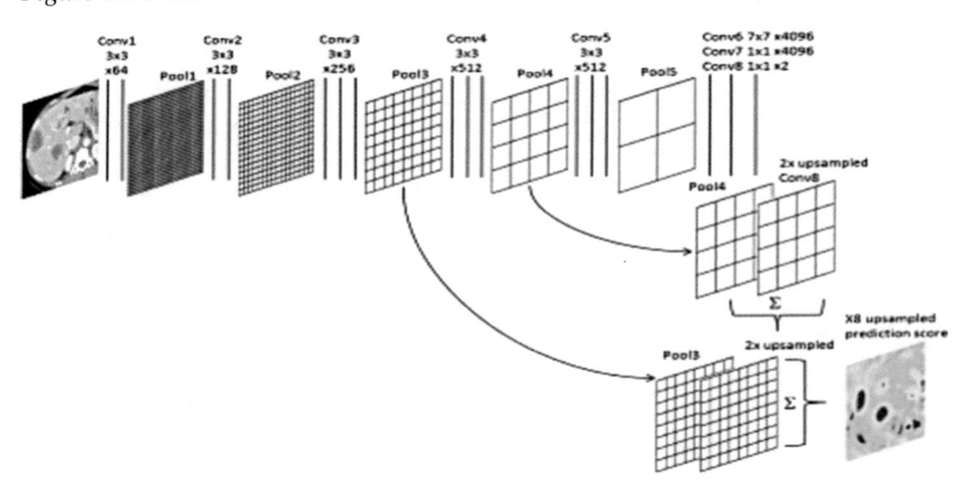

Shelhamer (2015) used a fully convolutional architecture for segmentation and detection of liver metastates in CT examinations. Fully Convolutional Networks (FCN) use efficient inference and learning to take input of any size and produce output of the same size. For the segmentation of 19 organs in3D CT images, Zhou (2017) used the FCN in a 2.5D approach. Hu (2017) used FCN to segment various organs from 3D images. Roth (2017) used a hierarchical coarse-to-fine technique that considerably improved tiny organ segmentation outcomes. Wu (2017) looked into cascaded FCN and saw whether it would improve FCN's ability to detect fetal boundaries in ultrasound images. Zeng (2018) used the multi-stream technique on 3D FCN to enhance the use of contextual information from multiple image resolutions while using a multimodality technique to improve the system robustness.

U-Net

U-Net, being one of the CNN's most essential semantic segmentation frameworks, which plays the major role in medical image analysis. As shown in Fig.12, the U- net network is made up of up sampling and down sampling. The primary notion is that a fixed-size image is dimensionally shrunk to fit the display area and thumbnails of the matching image are generated to extract deeper image features (Zeng, 2017). The image is then enlarged using up sampling and each layer features with down sampling and up sampling capabilities. Applications of U-Net based networks are Computed Tomography (CT), Magnetic Resonance Imaging (MRI), Ultrasound, X-ray, Optical Coherence Tomography (OCT), and Positron Emission Computed Tomography (PECT) are six imaging techniques and medical image analysis. G.D.Zeng (2018) used deeply supervised 3D U-net network for 3D MRI proximal femoral segmentation.

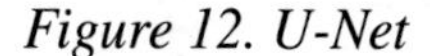

Figure 12. U-Net

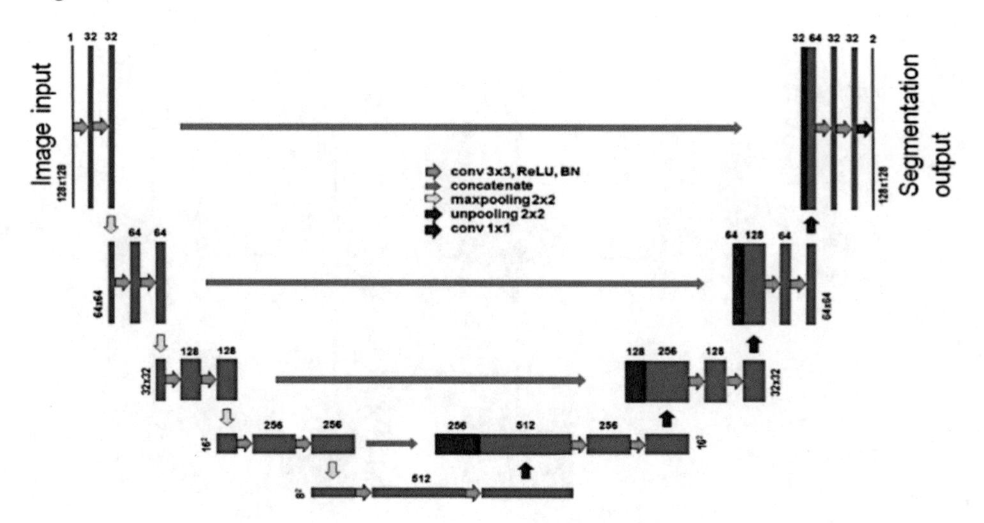

Multi-layer depth monitoring is aimed to reduce the problem of the gradient fading throughout the training process. Huang (2018) used the DCNN to suggest an automatic hepatic blood vessel extraction approach. In which, a 3D U-net network is chosen for accurate hepatic blood vessel extraction, and data augmentation technology is applied. Kim (2018) used a U-net-based DL approach for the automatic segmentation of mammary glands and fibrous glands. This solution not only eliminates the problem of MRI artefacts, but it also overcomes the problem of change in breast MRI. Dalmis (2017), a novel DL network is suggested that can successfully divide inter vertebral discs and their complicated borders from magnetic resonance scans of the spine. Using the cascade learning method which improves the convolutional layer and pooling layer of the classic U- net and solves the structural limitation of the maximum pooling layer in the traditional U-net.

RNN

A Recurrent Neural Network (RNN) is a type of artificial neural network in which nodes in a directed graph are connected in a temporal sequence. The two broad classes of RNN are finite impulse and infinite impulse. The RNN is equipped with recurrent connections, which allow it to remember patterns from previous inputs as shown in Fig.13.

Figure 13. RNN

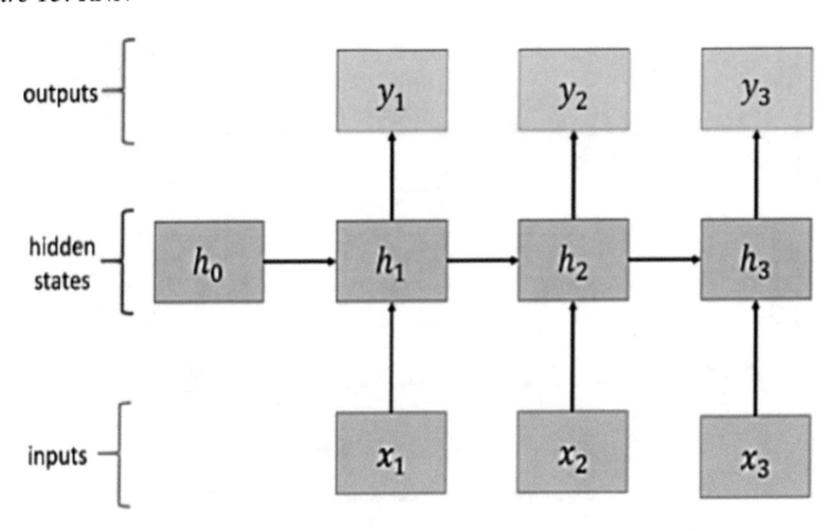

The inputs to a conventional LSTM network must be vectored, which is a drawback in medical image segmentation as the spatial information is lost (Zheng, 2015). Therefore, Srivastava (2015) and Xingjian (2015) used convolutional LSTM in which the convolutional operation has been used to replace vector multiplication. Cai (2017) used CLSTM to the deep CNN output layer in order to establish a more precise segmentation by gathering contextual information across. Cheng (2017) used GRU (Gated Recurrent Unit) which is an LSTM adjacent slices version that eliminates memory cells, resulting in a simpler structure with no performance loss. Xie (2016) used Clock Work RNN (CW-RNN) for muscle perimysium.

Transfer Learning

Transfer learning is defined as the capability of a system to recognize and employ the knowledge learned in a previous source domain to a novel task (Shie, 2015). Fine-tuning a network pre-trained on general images (Yosinski, 2014) and fine-tuning a network pre-trained on medical images for a different target organ or task are two techniques to transfer learning. When the tasks of the source and target networks are more comparable, transfer learning outperforms random initialization, and even transferring the weights of far-flung jobs outperforms random initialization. The weights are derived from a generic network (VGG16) and fine-tuned using ultrasound prenatal image segmentation (Zeiler, 2014). Similarly, the original weights were collected from a remote application and used to locate polyps (Tajbakhsh, 2016). As a result, the authors had to fine-tune all of the layers. By fine-tuning all layers instead of just the final, they were able to achieve a 25% increase in sensitivity. However, other trials showed that training from scratch produced better outcomes than fine-tuning a pre-trained network (Tran, 2016).

There are three major levels to transfer learning: (1) full network adaptation, which involves using a pre-trained network to initialize the weights (rather than a random initialization) and updating them all during training (Wang, 2016, Chen, 2015). (2) Partial network adaptation, which involves using a pre-trained network to establish the network parameters but freezing the weights for the first few layers and updating the last layers during training (Ren, 2016, Shin, 2016, Chen,2016). (3) Zero adaptation, in which the weights for the entire network are initialized from a pre-trained model and no changes are made. Alyoubi (2020) due to the wide range of organ (target) appearance, a zero-adaptation strategy from another medical network is often not recommended. It's especially risky if the sources have just been exposed to generic photos. Furthermore, because the objects in biomedical images might have a wide range of look and size, transfer learning from models with large differences in organ appearance may not improve segmentation results.

CONCLUSION

Deep learning methodologies have sparked a lot of interest in every field where traditional machine learning techniques were previously used. Finally, deep learning is the most powerful, supervised, and stimulating machine learning technique. It can give researchers a rapid assessment of the application's hidden and incredible difficulties in order to produce better and more accurate results. Application of these techniques will definitely help in screening patient for diabetic retinopathy and help them to get early treatment by consulting with their doctors. It is believed that deep learning will rapidly grow in more and more applications in the coming years, resulting in a big boom.

REFERENCES

Abdel Maksoud, E., Barakat, S., & Elmogy, M. (2020). A comprehensive diagnosis system for early signs and different diabetic retinopathy grades using fundus retinal images based on pathological changes detection. *Computers in Biology and Medicine*, *126*, 104039.

Alyoubi, W. L., Shalash, W. M., & Abulkhair, M. F. (2020). Diabetic retinopathy detection through deep learning techniques: A review. *Informatics in Medicine Unlocked*, *20*, 100377. doi:10.1016/j.imu.2020.100377

Alyoubi, W. L., Shalash, W. M., & Abulkhair, M. F. (2020). Diabetic retinopathy detection through deep learning techniques: A review. *Informatics in Medicine Unlocked*, *20*, 100377.

Arevalo, J., González, F. A., Ramos-Pollán, R., Oliveira, J. L., & Lopez, M. A. G. (2016). Representation learning for mammography mass lesion classification with convolutional neural networks. *Computer Methods and Programs in Biomedicine*, *127*, 248–257.

Biran, A., Bidari, P. S., & Raahemifar, K. (2016). Automatic method for exudates and hemorrhages detection from fundus retinal images. *International Journal of Computer and Information Engineering*, *10*(9), 1599–1602.

Cai, J., Lu, L., Xie, Y., Xing, F., & Yang, L. (2017). *Improving deep pancreas segmentation in CT and MRI images via recurrent neural contextual learning and direct loss function*. arXiv preprint arXiv:1707.04912.

Chen, H., Ni, D., Qin, J., Li, S., Yang, X., Wang, T., & Heng, P. A. (2015). Standard plane localization in fetal ultrasound via domain transferred deep neural networks. *IEEE Journal of Biomedical and Health Informatics*, *19*(5), 1627–1636.

Chen, H., Qi, X., Yu, L., & Heng, P. A. (2016). DCAN: deep contour-aware networks for accurate gland segmentation. In *Proceedings of the IEEE conference on Computer Vision and Pattern Recognition* (pp. 2487-2496). IEEE.

Cheng, D., & Liu, M. (2017, October). Combining convolutional and recurrent neural networks for Alzheimer's disease diagnosis using PET images. In *2017 IEEE International Conference on Imaging Systems and Techniques (IST)* (pp. 1-5). IEEE.

Dalmış, M. U., Litjens, G., Holland, K., Setio, A., Mann, R., Karssemeijer, N., & Gubern-Mérida, A. (2017). Using deep learning to segment breast and fibroglandular tissue in MRI volumes. *Medical Physics*, *44*(2), 533–546.

Fadafen, M. K., Mehrshad, N., &Razavi, S. M. (2018). Detection of diabetic retinopathy using computational model of human visual system. *Biomedical Research, 29*(9).

Hagos, T. (2019). Setup. In Android Studio IDE Quick Reference (pp. 1-9). Apress.

Hu, P., Wu, F., Peng, J., Bao, Y., Chen, F., & Kong, D. (2017). Automatic abdominal multi-organ segmentation using deep convolutional neural network and time-implicit level sets. *International Journal of Computer Assisted Radiology and Surgery*, *12*(3), 399–411.

Huang, Q., Sun, J., Ding, H., Wang, X., & Wang, G. (2018). Robust liver vessel extraction using 3D U-Net with variant dice loss function. *Computers in Biology and Medicine*, *101*, 153–162.

Kallenberg, M., Petersen, K., Nielsen, M., Ng, A. Y., Diao, P., Igel, C., ... Lillholm, M. (2016). Unsupervised deep learning applied to breast density segmentation and mammographic risk scoring. *IEEE Transactions on Medical Imaging*, *35*(5), 1322–1331.

Kauppi, T., Kalesnykiene, V., Kamarainen, J. K., Lensu, L., Sorri, I., Raninen, A., . . . Pietilä, J. (2007, September). The diaretdb1 diabetic retinopathy database and evaluation protocol. In BMVC (Vol. 1, pp. 1-10). Academic Press.

Kauppi, T., Kalesnykiene, V., Kamarainen, J. K., Lensu, L., Sorri, I., Uusitalo, H., . . . Pietilä, J. (2006). DIARETDB0: Evaluation database and methodology for diabetic retinopathy algorithms. Machine Vision and Pattern Recognition Research Group, Lappeenranta University of Technology.

Kermany, D. S., Goldbaum, M., Cai, W., Valentim, C. C., Liang, H., Baxter, S. L., ... Zhang, K. (2018). Identifying medical diagnoses and treatable diseases by image-based deep learning. *Cell, 172*(5), 1122–1131.

Kim, S., Bae, W. C., Masuda, K., Chung, C. B., & Hwang, D. (2018). Fine-grain segmentation of the intervertebral discs from MR spine images using deep convolutional neural networks: BSU-Net. *Applied Sciences (Basel, Switzerland), 8*(9), 1656.

Kiranyaz, S., Ince, T., & Gabbouj, M. (2015). Real-time patient-specific ECG classification by 1-D convolutional neural networks. *IEEE Transactions on Biomedical Engineering, 63*(3), 664–675. doi:10.1109/TBME.2015.2468589 PMID:26285054

Kou, C., Li, W., Yu, Z., & Yuan, L. (2020). An enhanced residual U-Net for microaneurysms and exudates segmentation in fundus images. *IEEE Access: Practical Innovations, Open Solutions, 8*, 185514–185525. doi:10.1109/ACCESS.2020.3029117

Li, Y. H., Yeh, N. N., Chen, S. J., & Chung, Y. C. (2019). Computer-assisted diagnosis for diabetic retinopathy based on fundus images using deep convolutional neural network. *Mobile Information Systems.*

Lim, G., Lee, M. L., Hsu, W., & Wong, T. Y. (2014, June). Transformed representations for convolutional neural networks in diabetic retinopathy screening. *Workshops at the Twenty-Eighth AAAI Conference on Artificial Intelligence.*

Lim, G., Lee, M. L., Hsu, W., & Wong, T. Y. (2014, June). Transformed representations for convolutional neural networks in diabetic retinopathy screening. *Workshops at the Twenty-Eighth AAAI Conference on Artificial Intelligence.*

Long, J., Shelhamer, E., & Darrell, T. (2015). Fully convolutional networks for semantic segmentation. In *Proceedings of the IEEE conference on computer vision and pattern recognition* (pp. 3431-3440). IEEE.

Nasr-Esfahani, E., Samavi, S., Karimi, N., Soroushmehr, S. M. R., Jafari, M. H., Ward, K., & Najarian, K. (2016, August). Melanoma detection by analysis of clinical images using convolutional neural network. In *2016 38th Annual International Conference of the IEEE Engineering in Medicine and Biology Society (EMBC)* (pp. 1373-1376). IEEE.

Orlando, J. I., Prokofyeva, E., & Blaschko, M. B. (2016). A discriminatively trained fully connected conditional random field model for blood vessel segmentation in fundus images. *IEEE Transactions on Biomedical Engineering, 64*(1), 16–27. doi:10.1109/TBME.2016.2535311 PMID:26930672

Parasuraman, K. (2018). Detection of retinal hemorrhage from fundus images using ANFIS classifier and MRG segmentation. *Biomedical Research, 29*(7).

Priya, R., & Aruna, P. (2013). Diagnosis of diabetic retinopathy using machine learning techniques. *ICTACT Journal on Soft Computing, 3*(4), 563-575.

Ren, S., He, K., Girshick, R., & Sun, J. (2016). Faster R-CNN: Towards real-time object detection with region proposal networks. *IEEE Transactions on Pattern Analysis and Machine Intelligence*, *39*(6), 1137–1149.

Roth, H. R., Oda, H., Hayashi, Y., Oda, M., Shimizu, N., Fujiwara, M., . . . Mori, K. (2017). *Hierarchical 3D fully convolutional networks for multi-organ segmentation*. arXiv preprint arXiv:1704.06382.

Roychowdhury, S., Koozekanani, D. D., & Parhi, K. K. (2013). DREAM: Diabetic retinopathy analysis using machine learning. *IEEE Journal of Biomedical and Health Informatics*, *18*(5), 1717–1728. doi:10.1109/JBHI.2013.2294635 PMID:25192577

Safitri, D. W., & Juniati, D. (2017, August). Classification of diabetic retinopathy using fractal dimension analysis of eye fundus image. In AIP conference proceedings (Vol. 1867, No. 1, p. 020011). AIP Publishing LLC.

Shie, C. K., Chuang, C. H., Chou, C. N., Wu, M. H., & Chang, E. Y. (2015, August). Transfer representation learning for medical image analysis. In *2015 37th annual international conference of the IEEE Engineering in Medicine and Biology Society (EMBC)* (pp. 711-714). IEEE.

Shin, H. C., Roth, H. R., Gao, M., Lu, L., Xu, Z., Nogues, I., ... Summers, R. M. (2016). Deep convolutional neural networks for computer-aided detection: CNN architectures, dataset characteristics and transfer learning. *IEEE Transactions on Medical Imaging*, *35*(5), 1285–1298.

Sirinukunwattana, K., Raza, S. E. A., Tsang, Y. W., Snead, D. R., Cree, I. A., & Rajpoot, N. M. (2016). Locality sensitive deep learning for detection and classification of nuclei in routine colon cancer histology images. *IEEE Transactions on Medical Imaging*, *35*(5), 1196–1206.

Srivastava, N., Mansimov, E., & Salakhudinov, R. (2015, June). Unsupervised learning of video representations using lstms. In *International conference on machine learning* (pp. 843-852). PMLR.

Tajbakhsh, N., Shin, J. Y., Gurudu, S. R., Hurst, R. T., Kendall, C. B., Gotway, M. B., & Liang, J. (2016). Convolutional neural networks for medical image analysis: Full training or fine tuning? *IEEE Transactions on Medical Imaging*, *35*(5), 1299–1312.

Tajbakhsh, N., Shin, J. Y., Gurudu, S. R., Hurst, R. T., Kendall, C. B., Gotway, M. B., & Liang, J. (2016). Convolutional neural networks for medical image analysis: Full training or fine tuning? *IEEE Transactions on Medical Imaging, 35*(5), 1299–1312.

Tran, D., Bourdev, L., Fergus, R., Torresani, L., & Paluri, M. (2016). Deep end2end voxel2voxel prediction. In *Proceedings of the IEEE conference on computer vision and pattern recognition workshops* (pp. 17-24). IEEE.

Tymchenko, B., Marchenko, P., & Spodarets, D. (2020). *Deep learning approach to diabetic retinopathy detection.* arXiv preprint arXiv:2003.02261.

Wang, J., MacKenzie, J. D., Ramachandran, R., & Chen, D. Z. (2016, October). A deep learning approach for semantic segmentation in histology tissue images. In *International Conference on Medical Image Computing and Computer-Assisted Intervention* (pp. 176-184). Springer.

Wang, P., Hu, X., Li, Y., Liu, Q., & Zhu, X. (2016). Automatic cell nuclei segmentation and classification of breast cancer histopathology images. *Signal Processing, 122*, 1–13. doi:10.1016/j.sigpro.2015.11.011

Wu, L., Xin, Y., Li, S., Wang, T., Heng, P. A., & Ni, D. (2017, April). Cascaded fully convolutional networks for automatic prenatal ultrasound image segmentation. In *2017 IEEE 14th international symposium on biomedical imaging (ISBI 2017)* (pp. 663-666). IEEE.

Xie, Y., Zhang, Z., Sapkota, M., & Yang, L. (2016, October). Spatial clockwork recurrent neural network for muscle perimysium segmentation. In *International Conference on Medical Image Computing and Computer-Assisted Intervention* (pp. 185-193). Springer.

Xingjian, S. H. I., Chen, Z., Wang, H., Yeung, D. Y., Wong, W. K., & Woo, W. C. (2015). Convolutional LSTM network: A machine learning approach for precipitation now casting. In Advances in neural information processing systems (pp. 802-810). Academic Press.

Yosinski, J., Clune, J., Bengio, Y., & Lipson, H. (2014). *How transferable are features in deep neural networks?* arXiv preprint arXiv:1411.1792.

Zeiler, M. D., & Fergus, R. (2014, September). Visualizing and understanding convolutional networks. In *European conference on computer vision* (pp. 818-833). Springer.

Zeiler, M. D., & Fergus, R. (2014, September). Visualizing and understanding convolutional networks. In *European conference on computer vision* (pp. 818-833). Springer.

Zeng, G., Yang, X., Li, J., Yu, L., Heng, P. A., & Zheng, G. (2017, September). 3D U-net with multi-level deep supervision: fully automatic segmentation of proximal femur in 3D MR images. In *International workshop on machine learning in medical imaging* (pp. 274-282). Springer.

Zeng, G., & Zheng, G. (2018, April). Multi-stream 3D FCN with multi-scale deep supervision for multi-modality isointense infant brain MR image segmentation. In *2018 IEEE 15th International Symposium on Biomedical Imaging (ISBI 2018)* (pp. 136-140). IEEE.

Zeng, G., & Zheng, G. (2018). Deep learning-based automatic segmentation of the proximal femur from MR images. In *Intelligent Orthopaedics* (pp. 73–79). Springer.

Zheng, S., Jayasumana, S., Romera-Paredes, B., Vineet, V., Su, Z., Du, D., ... Torr, P. H. (2015). Conditional random fields as recurrent neural networks. In *Proceedings of the IEEE international conference on computer vision* (pp. 1529-1537). IEEE.

Zhou, X., Takayama, R., Wang, S., Hara, T., & Fujita, H. (2017). Deep learning of the sectional appearances of 3D CT images for anatomical structure segmentation based on an FCN voting method. *Medical Physics*, *44*(10), 5221–5233.

Chapter 11
Adaptive Clinical Treatments and Reinforcement Learning for Automatic Disease diagnosis

Pawan Whig
Vivekananda Institute of Professional Studies, India

Ketan Gupta
https://orcid.org/0000-0002-2953-0385
University of the Cumberlands, USA

Nasmin Jiwani
https://orcid.org/0000-0002-7360-0264
University of the Cumberlands, USA

Shama Kouser
Jazan University, Saudi Arabia

Mayank Anand
BridgeLabz Solutions Pvt. Ltd., India

ABSTRACT

Machine learning models are taught how to make a series of decisions depending on a set of inputs in reinforcement learning. The agent learns how to accomplish a goal in an unexpected, maybe complex environment. Reinforcement learning places artificial intelligence in a game-like environment. It solves the problem by trial and error. Artificial intelligence is rewarded or punished based on its actions. Its purpose is to maximize the amount of money paid out in total. In addition to providing the game's rules, the designer does not give any feedback or recommendations on how to win the model. To maximize reward, the model must determine the optimum way to do a job, beginning with purely random trials and progressing to complex techniques and superhuman abilities. Reinforcement learning, with its power of

DOI: 10.4018/978-1-6684-4405-4.ch011

search and diversity of trials, is likely the most effective strategy for hinting at a system's originality. Unlike humans, AI can learn from thousands of concurrent gameplays if a reinforcement learning algorithm is run on sufficiently efficient computer infrastructure.

INTRODUCTION

Reinforcement learning is a type of machine learning. It is about acting appropriately in a given situation to maximize gain. Various apps and computers utilize it to evaluate the best potential behavior or course of action to take in a particular event (Jiwani et al., 2021).

Developers create a system for rewarding desired activities and penalizing undesirable Reinforcement learning. This strategy motivates the agent by assigning positive values to preferred activities and negative values to undesired behaviors. To arrive at an appropriate solution, the agent is trained to seek the highest long-term and total benefit (Whig, Velu, & Naddikatu, 2022).

These long-term goals are critical to preventing the agent from becoming stuck on smaller targets. Through time and experience, he or she learns to avoid the bad and focus on the good(Whig, Velu, & Sharma, 2022). This learning strategy has been used in artificial intelligence (AI) to drive unsupervised machine learning using incentives and penalties. Figure 1 depicts the fundamentals of reinforcement learning, while Figure 2 depicts how it works.

Reinforcement Learning

The primary elements necessary for Reinforcement Learning are defined as follows: Input might be regarded as a beginning state from which the model will begin. O/P: There are several possible outputs for a range of solutions to a given problem. Learning: Depending on the input, the model will return a state, and the user's feedback will determine whether to reward or penalize the model based on the outcome(Alkali et al., 2022a).

The model is still learning.

The optimal answer is determined by the highest possible payment.

Figure 1. Fundamentals of reinforcement learning

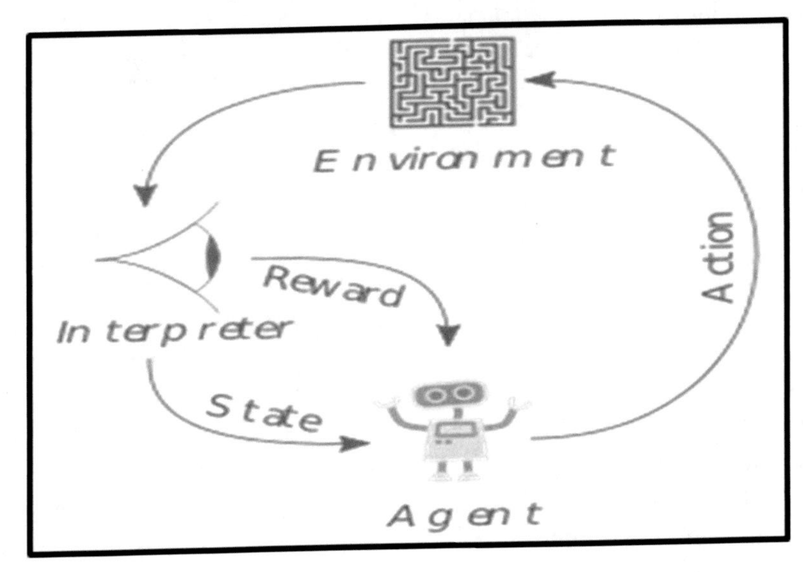

Figure 2. Working of RL

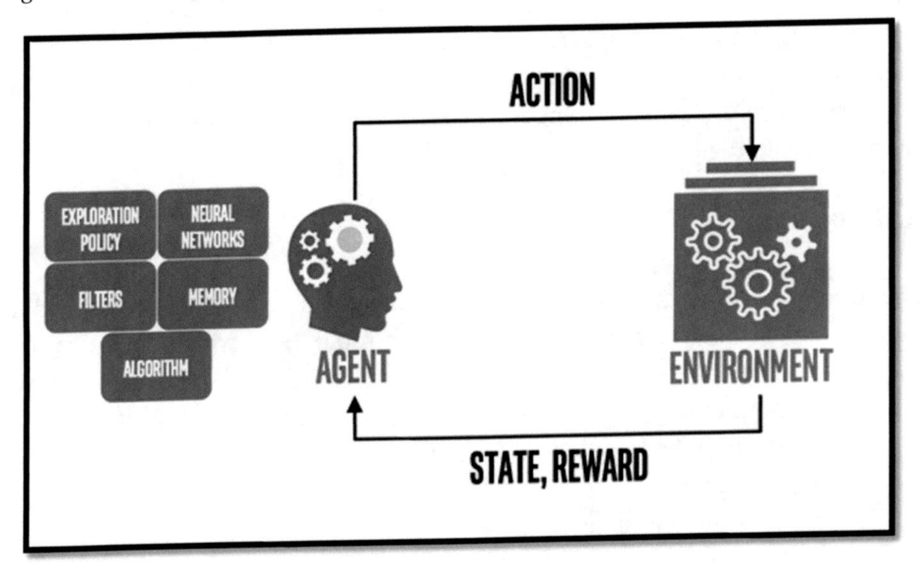

Types of Machine Learning

Different Types of Machine Learning are described below in Figure 3

- Supervised

- Unsupervised
- Reinforcement learning

Figure 3. Types of ML

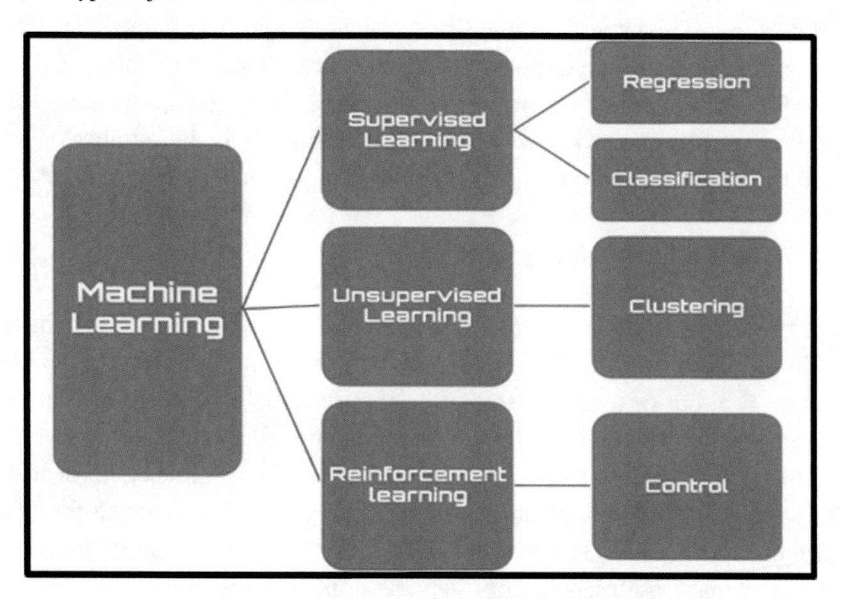

Supervised

The first type of shallow machine learning is supervised learning. And it is exactly what the term implies(Whig, Kouser, Velu, et al., 2022; Whig, Velu, & Ready, 2022). When the developer names the variables with which the machine will interact, this type of learning happens. In this domain, there are two forms of learning: regression and classification.

The system can recognize and organize numbers to make predictions. The total square footage of a property, the number of bathrooms, and the number of bedrooms, for example, can all be evaluated. By collecting diverse samples of houses and learning from their variables, it can anticipate the cost of a property using linear regression.

Unsupervised

The preceding example of playing flashcards with a machine will help you understand unsupervised learning (Jupalle et al., 2022; Whig, Velu, & Nadikattu, 2022). Except that this time, instead of other humans, the machine is playing a game of flashcards with itself. On one side of the picture, a cat or dog appears. There is a blank spot on the back of the card. As an example, the computer may recognize that cats have pointed ears and dogs have floppy ears, indicating a distinction between the two. Cats and dogs are separated into different heaps. The process of gathering items together is referred to as clustering(Whig, Velu, & Bhatia, 2022). The system can also detect many items at the same time, which is quite beneficial. The computer software may have observed the cats' four legs, green eyes, and pointy ears. There are also four-legged dogs with brown eyes and floppy ears. It employs fewer features and decreases factors associated with the images, such as the number of legs, to discern between cats and dogs. This is referred to as dimension reduction.

Reinforcement Learning

Reinforcement learning is the process of teaching a computer positive behavior by rewarding it. This one will be easier to understand if we imagine a mouse trying to find its way out of a maze. Before the mouse (machine) begins, he is given a thousand points. The aim is for him to maintain and enhance his points (M. Anand et al., 2022). It loses points if it runs into a dead wall or a mousetrap, or if it goes in the wrong direction. Points are granted for successfully traversing the maze or choosing the correct turn that leads to the cheese. As a consequence, the computer is obliged to make proper predictions and respond appropriately.

When a mouse can cognitively model a labyrinth and plan out a set of paths and steps to take, it is said to be learning by reinforcement. Model-free learning happens when the mouse establishes a habit of repeatedly traversing the labyrinth.

They each have their own set of benefits and drawbacks. Supervised learning via regression and classification is the most successful method for predicting speech and visual data. Unsupervised learning has a variety of uses, including the development of advertising concepts (Alkali et al., 2022b). Reinforcement learning, which involves learning through rewards, is used by physical robots. Figure 4 depicts the distinction between various ML.

Types of Reinforcement

There are two forms of reinforcement: Positive-positive reinforcement happens as a result of an event that occurs as a result of a given behavior, and it increases the strength as well as the frequency of the behavior. In other words, it has a positive effect on individual behavior (Chopra & WHIG, 2022a).

"Negative Reinforcement" refers to behavior that is encouraged as a result of preventing or avoiding an unpleasant situation. Figures 5 and 6 highlight the differences and features between the two kinds.

Figure 4. Difference between different ML Blogs

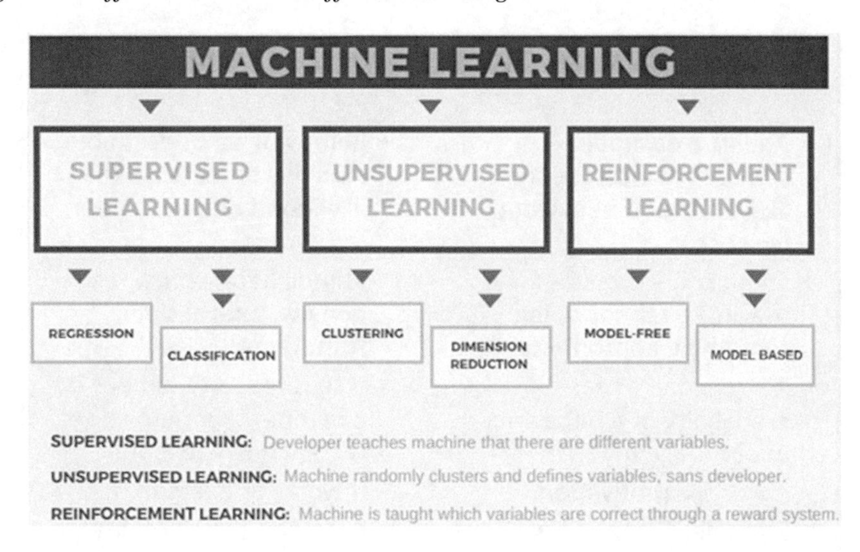

Figure 5. Characteristics of different RL

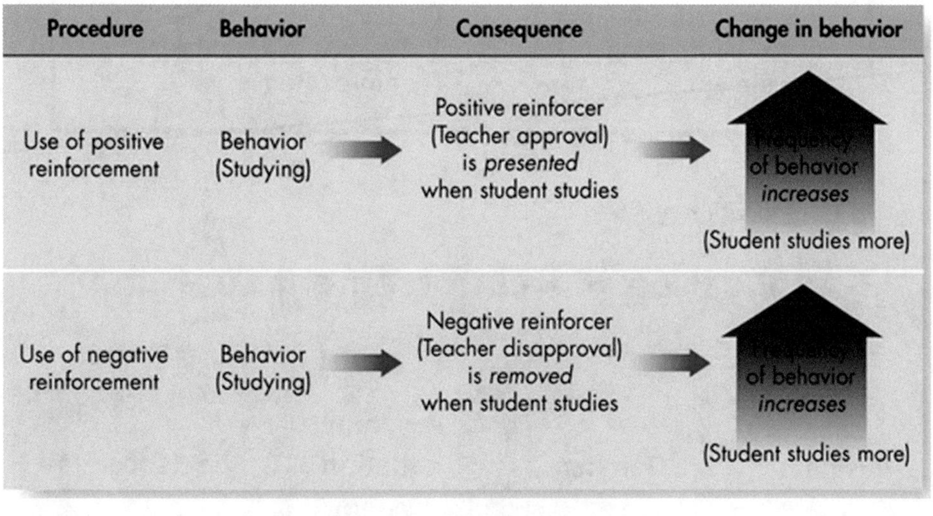

Procedure	Behavior	Consequence	Change in behavior
Use of positive reinforcement	Behavior (Studying)	Positive reinforcer (Teacher approval) is *presented* when student studies	Frequency of behavior *increases* (Student studies more)
Use of negative reinforcement	Behavior (Studying)	Negative reinforcer (Teacher disapproval) is *removed* when student studies	Frequency of behavior *increases* (Student studies more)

Various Practical Applications of Reinforcement Learning

The various RL applications are shown in Figure 7

- RL may be used in industrial robotics to automate processes.
- Machine learning and data processing can benefit from RL.
- Students' needs can be met using RL-based training methods.

Figure 6. Difference between PRL and NRL

Positive Reinforcement	Negative Reinforcement
• Adding a desirable stimulus to increase the likelihood of a behaviour to reoccur	• Removing an undesirable stimulus to increase the likelihood of a behaviour to reoccur
• Stimuli here work as a reward, given for doing something appropriate	• Stimuli here work as a penalty, for not doing something
• It strenghtens the probability of a behaviour to occur again.	• It teaches us to behave in a manner that help us get rid of a nasty respones.
• It works a motivation.	• It works as a lesson.
• Example: Going out with friends to watch a movie if you finish your assignment. Thus, increasing the likelihood of you completing assignment.	• Example: Taking umbrella with you even and using it when it starts to rain. Thus, preventing you from getting wet and teaching you to carry umbrella more often.

Figure 7. Application of RL

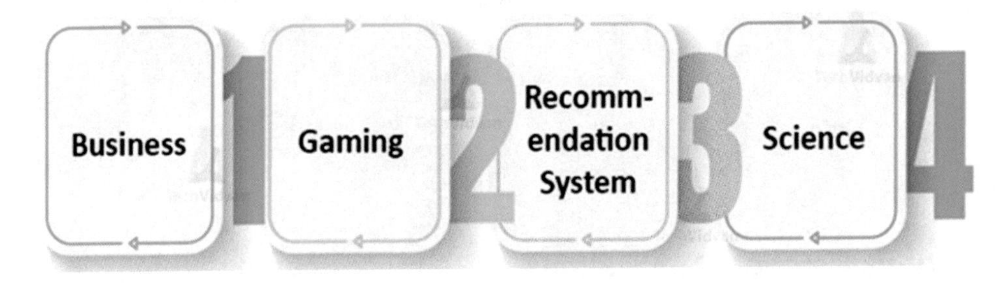

RL can be used in large environments in the following situations

- The environment has a model, but there is no analytical solution; There is only a simulation model of the environment provided (the subject of simulation-based optimization)

- The only way to collect information about the environment is to interact with it

Common RL Algorithms

Reinforcement learning is not a single method, but rather a set of algorithms that use a variety of methodologies (Chopra & WHIG, 2022b; Whig, Nadikattu, & Velu, 2022). The majority of the differences may be linked to how they investigate their environment. Although there are various RL algorithms, as seen in Fig. 8, some of the most essential methods are covered here.

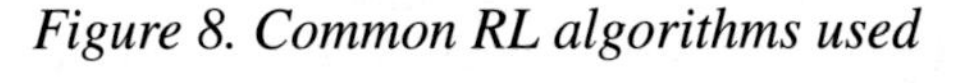

Figure 8. Common RL algorithms used

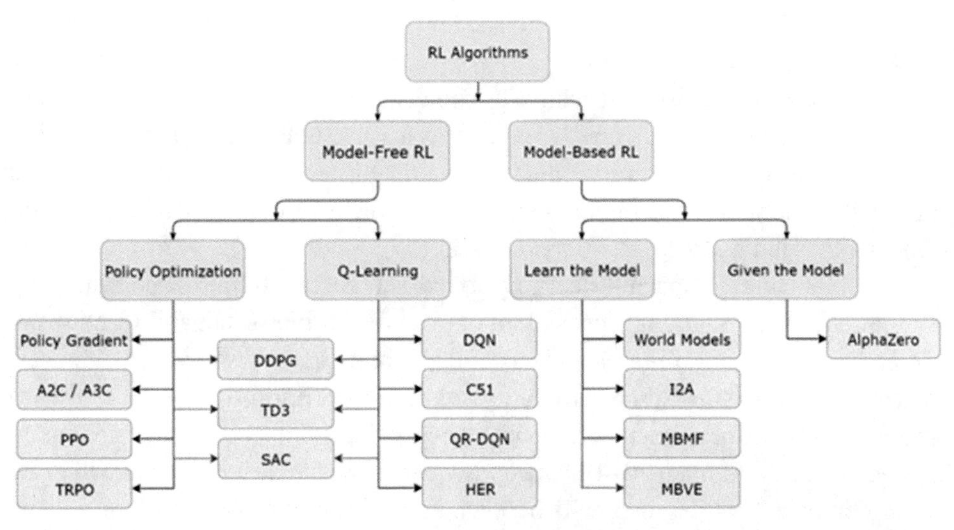

State-action-reward-state-action. The agent is provided a policy as a first step. In essence, the policy is a probability that informs it of the likelihood that specific behaviors would result in rewards or favorable states for the policy.

Q-learning. This strategy approaches reinforcement learning in an entirely new way. As a result, the agent's exploration of the environment becomes increasingly self-directed.

An in-depth look at Q-Networks. These algorithms employ neural networks in addition to reinforcement learning methodologies (Velu & Whig, 2022). Self-directed world exploration underpins reinforcement learning. A random sample of helpful behaviors from the past is employed in the neural network to predict future actions.

RL in Healthcare

Healthcare has always been an early adopter and major beneficiary of technological improvements. Reinforcement learning has consistently resulted in improved outcomes in the healthcare system. Reinforcement learning, in addition to being a branch of machine learning, aims to increase an individual's capacity to make decisions based on their interactions with the world around them and deliver feedback (Chopra & WHIG, 2022c).

Traditionally, reward indications were utilized in supervised learning procedures, but the reinforcement learning approach incorporates a progressive decision-making process that is sampling, evaluative, and delayed at the same time. The distinct qualities of reinforcement learning make it a feasible alternative for developing cutting-edge solutions in a variety of healthcare disciplines. As a result, diagnostic decisions or treatment regimens are often distinguished by a lengthy and sequential procedure.

Machine learning (a subset of AI) is becoming essential in many healthcare organizations. As a result, machine learning has given birth to a slew of new applications in the healthcare system. It has also significantly assisted in the improvement of administrative operations in health facilities, the personalization of health treatments, and the mapping and treatment of communicable diseases, among other things (Whig & Ahmad, 2011).

The application of machine learning affects general practitioners and healthcare systems as well, because it is critical for clinical resolution sustainability, allowing for early diagnosis of diseases and customized treatment ways to achieve the best outcomes. Doctors and patients can use machine learning to observe and learn about potential illness courses and consequences, as well as dissimilar treatment options(Whig & Ahmad, 2014). As a consequence, healthcare structures will grow more competent while costs will be decreased. Generations of wisdom will be required to enhance the creation of new drugs and assure the delivery of old ones.

In healthcare systems, machine learning algorithms have been created to aid both patients and personnel, with the most common areas of application being:

THE SMART RECEIVER

Health Quotient

With this software, Quotient Health wants to lower the costs of sustaining electronic medical records by refining and standardizing the techniques used to construct these systems. A clear aim is to improve the healthcare system while lowering costs (Whig & Ahmad, 2016).

The Second is KenSci

KenSci uses reinforcement learning to forecast diseases and treatments, allowing doctors and patients to intervene earlier in the process. It also helps predict public health risks by recognizing patterns, raising warning signals, and anticipating sickness development, among other aspects.

Ciox Health

Ciox Health uses machine learning to regulate and manipulate health data. Furthermore, it aids in the expansion and improvement of patient access, as well as the accuracy of health data.

As a result, RL is great for systems with inherent delays, such as autonomous vehicles, robotics, video games, financial and business management, and, yes, healthcare. According to Yu et al., RL's distinct progressive decision-making model is suited for healthcare applications because it "addresses sequential decision-making challenges with sampling, evaluative, and delayed data concurrently." To make fairly well-informed decisions, RL is also adaptable enough to account for the delayed effects of medicines and does not require as much contextual knowledge.

As a result, RL is great for systems with inherent delays, such as autonomous vehicles, robotics, video games, financial and business management, and, yes, healthcare. According to Yu et al., RL's distinct progressive decision-making model is suited for healthcare applications because it "addresses sequential decision-making challenges with sampling, evaluative, and delayed data concurrently." RL is also flexible enough to accommodate for the delayed effects of treatments and does not require as much contextual information to make fairly well-informed judgments(S. Anand et al., 2016.).

The researchers claim that "RL can discover optimal policies using just previous experiences, without requiring any prior knowledge of the mathematical model of biological systems." RL is more appealing than many present medicines due to nonlinear, unpredictable, and delayed interactions between therapies and human bodies.

RL IN HEALTHCARE APPLICATIONS

RL is employed in several heal health caretings, but it has proven to be particularly effective in the implementation of dynamic treatment regimens (DTRs) for patients with chronic illnesses or disorders. It has also demonstrated some capacity in automated medical diagnosis, health resource scheduling and resource allocation, drug research and development, and health management.

DR

The creation and maintenance of DTRs for patients with chronic conditions are the most common real-world health care use of RL. DTRs grow increasingly detailed in terms of treatment alternatives, such as therapy type, drug dose, and appointment schedule, as a patient's medical history and circumstances evolve. The algorithm creates therapeutic options that will provide the patient with the best-desired environment state based on clinical observations and patient evaluations as input data. RL is used in these treatment regimes to automate decision-making. DTRs have previously been used to treat several chronic conditions, including cancer and HIV. Figure 9 depicts an example of DTR.

Figure 9. Example of DTR

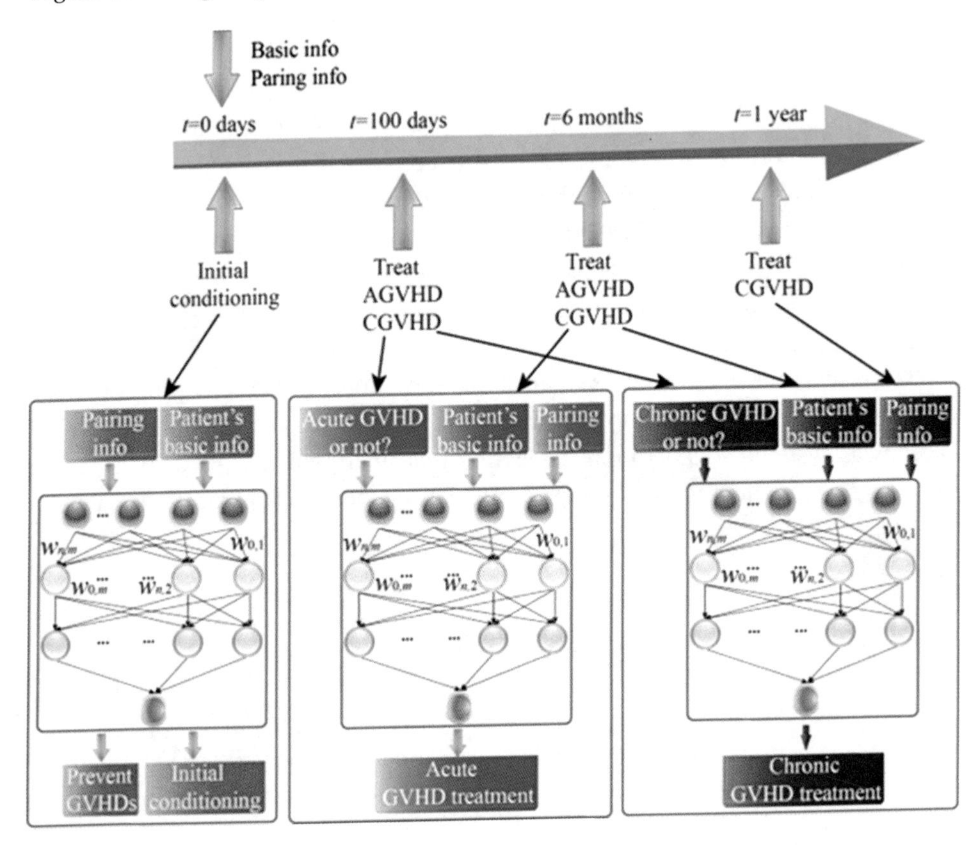

AMD ("Automated Medical Diagnosis")

To match the appropriate disease profile, patient information (such as history and current symptoms) is used. While it may appear to be a simple operation, it may be a time-consuming and cognitively demanding one for busy professionals.

Misdiagnosis costs were discussed in a recent blog post: Over the preceding 25 years, misdiagnosed patients were reimbursed for more than $40 billion. Machine learning algorithms are used by both doctors and patients to improve diagnosis. It's just that ML diagnostic solutions require massive amounts of labeled data to learn. In contrast, RL agents require less labeled data. Figure 10 is an example of AMD.

Figure 10. Example of AMD

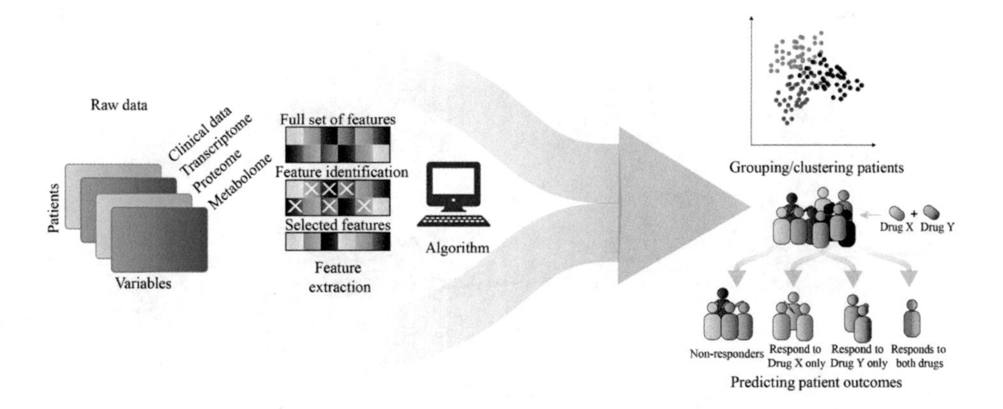

Scheduling and Distribution of Health Care Resources

In the healthcare market, patients are the consumers, while healthcare resources are the service providers. Because of its well-documented suitability, business process management (BPM) can benefit from RL. By analyzing seasonal trends, current inpatient and staffing levels, and other data sources, RL can help hospitals and clinics manage their daily operations.

Discovery, Design, and Development of Pharmaceuticals

Traditional drug development's human-driven, the trial-and-error technique has numerous flaws, the most serious of which is that it is time- and cost-prohibitive. This is still true today when studying the behavior of molecules and atoms using modern methodologies such as computer models and simulations (M&S). Despite all of this work and investment, success rates remain low, with less than 10% of compounds making it to the first phase of clinical trials. RL approaches are rapidly being used in de novo drug development to automate and improve drug design assumptions and molecule selection. Figure 11 depicts a flowchart of pharmaceutical design and development.

Figure 11. Flowchart of design and development of pharmaceuticals

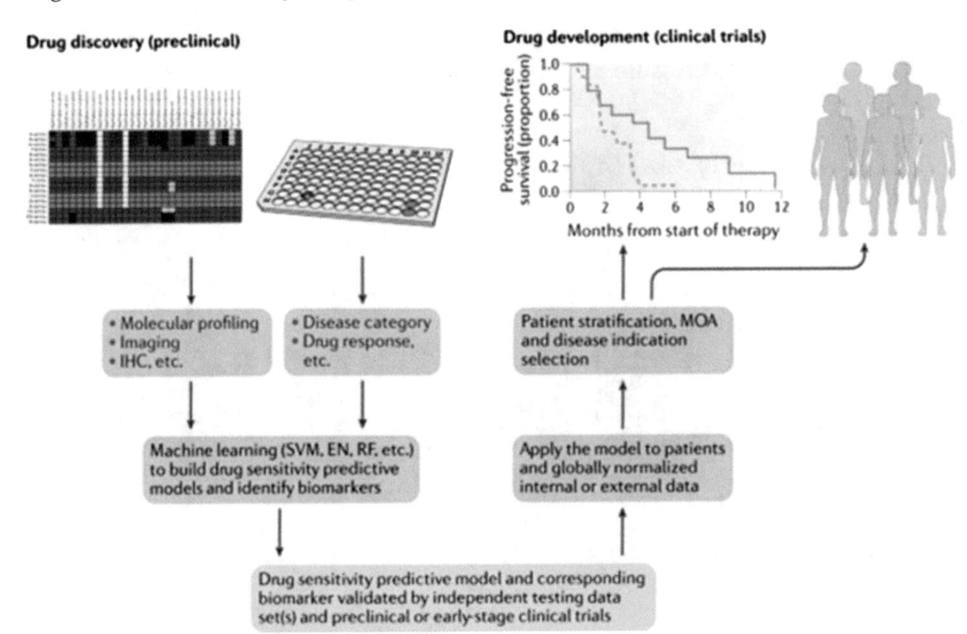

Management of the Health

Researchers have also used RL to create adaptive and personalized therapies for long-term health management, like as exercise and weight-control regimes for obese or diabetic patients. Artificial intelligence has already enhanced patient engagement and compliance with health management programs. Figure 12 depicts management in the healthcare sector.

Figure 12. Management in the health care sector

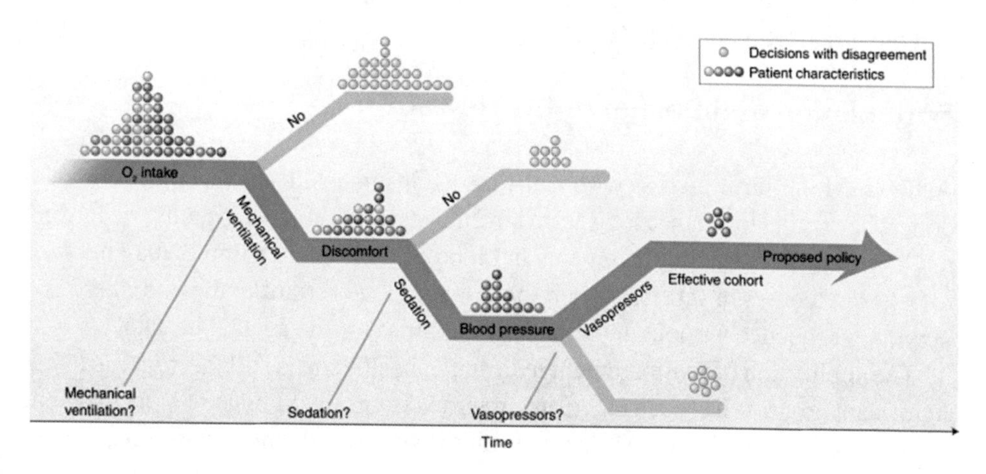

CHALLENGES OF RL

As promising as RL in health care is, there are numerous obstacles to overcome before it can be used on a wide basis in clinical practice. It can be difficult to transfer a real-time agent from a training or simulated environment to the actual world, and because the agent can only understand rewards and punishments, upgrading or adjusting the algorithm can be challenging(Verma et al., 2015).

This video from OpenAI shows an RL agent figuring out how to receive prizes without finishing the race.

Shortage of Data

Isaac Godfried, a deep learning researcher, points out that utilizing actual patients to train RL algorithms isn't always the most ethical method, even though RL agents learn best on the job. To do so, they must train in simulated environments using historical observational data on specific therapies, which is sometimes challenging for numerous reasons, including HIPPA compliance and personal health information (PHI)(Sharma et al., 2015).

Partial Observability

Even while real-time agents can frequently account for the complete state of simulated settings, the human body is considerably more complicated and dynamic than even the most thorough simulations or historical data sets can capture. It's fairly uncommon for RL agents in healthcare settings to have a partial awareness of their surroundings because of the partial observability of blood pressure, temperature, and other data(Rupani et al., 2017).

Formulation and Design of the Reward

Achieving long-term success with real-time agents in health care is easier said than done when trying to balance long-term advantages with short-term gains. According to Godfried, "periodic improvements in blood pressure, for example, may not lead to better outcomes in sepsis." When there is only one reward at the end, there is a very long sequence without any intermediate input for the agent," he said.

The application of reinforcement learning in healthcare is still far from ideal, but significant progress has been made on numerous fronts, including the more efficient and precise construction of DTRs for chronic diseases and other conditions, among other things (Asopa et al., 2021). It is certain that as reward policies are adjusted and more data is made available to construct settings for RL agents, we will witness additional gains – and, in the end, better health outcomes for patients and more efficient operations for health organizations.

RESULTS AND CONCLUSION

However, this strategy is not always applicable because machine learning bases promises of improvement on gains in performance over expected statistical procedures. The impact of a machine learning algorithm must be assessed.

With its ability to influence final actions within a particular environment, reinforcement learning is an intriguing promise in the field of healthcare. With its application, a more complete and exact therapy is delivered at a lesser cost.

Reinforcement learning, if well-implemented, is projected to have a considerable influence on the treatment and control of chronic diseases in the next years by connecting patient-centered health information with external variables such as weather and economic dynamics or pollution exposure. It will easily develop precise pharmacological treatments that are suited to each individual's unique traits by utilizing readily available genetic information.

CONCLUSION

Different sectors seem to be taking notice of Reinforcement learning and other machine learning techniques. This Book Chapter is very useful for the researchers working in the same field.

REFERENCES

Alkali, Y., Routray, I., & Whig, P. (2022a). Strategy for Reliable, Efficient and Secure IoT Using Artificial Intelligence. *IUP Journal of Computer Sciences, 16*(2).

AlkaliY.RoutrayI.WhigP. (2022b). Study of various methods for reliable, efficient and Secured IoT using Artificial Intelligence. *Available at* SSRN 4020364. doi:10.2139/ssrn.4020364

Anand, M., Velu, A., & Whig, P. (2022). Prediction of Loan Behaviour with Machine Learning Models for Secure Banking. *Journal of Computing Science and Engineering: JCSE, 3*(1), 1–13.

Anand, S., Whig, P., & Shrivastava, S. (n.d.). *FEM Analysis of Impact of Cylindrical Tool on Composite Laminated Plate*. Academic Press.

Asopa, P., Purohit, P., Nadikattu, R. R., & Whig, P. (2021). Reducing carbon footprint for sustainable development of smart cities using IoT. *2021 Third International Conference on Intelligent Communication Technologies and Virtual Mobile Networks (ICICV)*, 361–367. 10.1109/ICICV50876.2021.9388466

Chopra, G., & Whig, P. (2022a). A clustering approach based on support vectors. *International Journal of Machine Learning for Sustainable Development, 4*(1), 21–30.

Chopra, G., & Whig, P. (2022b). Using machine learning algorithms classified depressed patients and normal people. *International Journal of Machine Learning for Sustainable Development, 4*(1), 31–40.

Gupta, Jiwani, Afreen, & D. (2022). Liver Disease Prediction using Machine learning Classification Techniques. *2022 IEEE 11th International Conference on Communication Systems and Network Technologies (CSNT),* 221-226.

Gupta, K., Jiwani, N., & Afreen, N. (2022). Blood Pressure Detection Using CNN-LSTM Model. *2022 IEEE 11th International Conference on Communication Systems and Network Technologies (CSNT),* 262-366. 10.1109/CSNT54456.2022.9787648

Jiwani, N., Gupta, K., & Afreen, N. (2022). A Convolutional Neural Network Approach for Diabetic Retinopathy Classification. *2022 IEEE 11th International Conference on Communication Systems and Network Technologies (CSNT),* 357-361. 10.1109/CSNT54456.2022.9787577

Jiwani, N., Gupta, K., & Afreen, N. (2022). Automated Seizure Detection using Theta Band. *2022 International Conference on Emerging Smart Computing and Informatics (ESCI),* 1-4.

Jiwani, N., Gupta, K., & Whig, P. (2021). Novel HealthCare Framework for Cardiac Arrest With the Application of AI Using ANN. *2021 5th International Conference on Information Systems and Computer Networks (ISCON)*, 1–5.

Jupalle, H., Kouser, S., Bhatia, A. B., Alam, N., Nadikattu, R. R., & Whig, P. (2022). Automation of human behaviors and its prediction using machine learning. *Microsystem Technologies*, *28*(8), 1–9. doi:10.100700542-022-05326-4

Rupani, A., Whig, P., Sujediya, G., & Vyas, P. (2017). A robust technique for image processing based on interfacing of Raspberry-Pi and FPGA using IoT. *2017 International Conference on Computer, Communications and Electronics (Comptelix)*, 350–353. 10.1109/COMPTELIX.2017.8003992

Sharma, A., Kumar, A., & Whig, P. (2015). On the performance of CDTA based novel analog inverse low pass filter using 0.35 μm CMOS parameter. *International Journal of Science, Technology & Management*, *4*(1), 594–601.

Velu, A., & Whig, P. (2022). Studying the impact of the COVID vaccination on the world using data analytics. *Vivekananda J Res*, *10*(1), 147–160.

Verma, T., Gupta, P., & Whig, P. (2015). Sensor Controlled Sanitizer Door Knob with Scan Technique. *Emerging ICT for Bridging the Future-Proceedings of the 49th Annual Convention of the Computer Society of India CSI*, *2*, 261–266.

Whig, P., & Ahmad, S. N. (2011). On the performance of ISFET-based device for water quality monitoring. *International Journal of Communications, Network and Systems Sciences*, *4*(11), 709–719. doi:10.4236/ijcns.2011.411087

Whig, P., & Ahmad, S. N. (2014). Simulation of linear dynamic macro model of photo catalytic sensor in SPICE. *COMPEL: The International Journal for Computation and Mathematics in Electrical and Electronic Engineering*.

Whig, P., & Ahmad, S. N. (2016). Ultraviolet Photo Catalytic Oxidation (UVPCO) sensor for air and surface sanitizers using CS amplifier. *Global Journal of Research in Engineering*.

Whig, P., Kouser, S., Velu, A., & Nadikattu, R. R. (2022). Fog-IoT-Assisted-Based Smart Agriculture Application. In *Demystifying Federated Learning for Blockchain and Industrial Internet of Things* (pp. 74–93). IGI Global. doi:10.4018/978-1-6684-3733-9.ch005

Whig, P., Nadikattu, R. R., & Velu, A. (2022). COVID-19 pandemic analysis using application of AI. *Healthcare Monitoring and Data Analysis Using IoT: Technologies and Applications*, 1.

Whig, P., Velu, A., & Bhatia, A. B. (2022). Protect Nature and Reduce the Carbon Footprint With an Application of Blockchain for IIoT. In *Demystifying Federated Learning for Blockchain and Industrial Internet of Things* (pp. 123–142). IGI Global. doi:10.4018/978-1-6684-3733-9.ch007

Whig, P., Velu, A., & Naddikatu, R. R. (2022). The Economic Impact of AI-Enabled Blockchain in 6G-Based Industry. In *AI and Blockchain Technology in 6G Wireless Network* (pp. 205–224). Springer. doi:10.1007/978-981-19-2868-0_10

Whig, P., Velu, A., & Nadikattu, R. R. (2022). Blockchain Platform to Resolve Security Issues in IoT and Smart Networks. In *AI-Enabled Agile Internet of Things for Sustainable FinTech Ecosystems* (pp. 46–65). IGI Global. doi:10.4018/978-1-6684-4176-3.ch003

Whig, P., Velu, A., & Ready, R. (2022). Demystifying Federated Learning in Artificial Intelligence With Human-Computer Interaction. In *Demystifying Federated Learning for Blockchain and Industrial Internet of Things* (pp. 94–122). IGI Global. doi:10.4018/978-1-6684-3733-9.ch006

Whig, P., Velu, A., & Sharma, P. (2022). Demystifying Federated Learning for Blockchain: A Case Study. In Demystifying Federated Learning for Blockchain and Industrial Internet of Things (pp. 143–165). IGI Global. doi:10.4018/978-1-6684-3733-9.ch008

KEY TERMS AND DEFINITIONS

Diagnosis: The identification of the nature of an illness or other problem by examination of the symptoms.

Healthcare: Health care or healthcare is the improvement of health via the prevention, diagnosis, treatment, amelioration, or cure of disease, illness, injury.

Machine Learning: Machine learning (ML) is a type of artificial intelligence (AI) that allows software applications to become more accurate at predicting outcomes without being explicitly programmed to do so.

Medical: Medical means relating to illness and injuries and to their treatment or prevention.

Reinforcement Learning: Reinforcement learning is a machine learning training method based on rewarding desired behaviors and/or punishing undesired ones.

Chapter 12
AI-Enabled Internet of Nano Things Methodology for Healthcare Information Management

Anand Singh Rajawat
School of Computer Sciences and Engineering, Sandip University, Nashik, India

S. B. Goyal
https://orcid.org/0000-0002-8411-7630
Faculty of Information Technology, City University, Malaysia

Piyush Pant
Sandip University, Nashik, India

Pradeep Bedi
https://orcid.org/0000-0003-1708-6237
Department of Computer Science and Engineering, Galgotias University, India

ABSTRACT

Internet of nano things (IoNT) is growing at an exponential rate due to a growing population, more communication between devices in networks, sensors, actuators, and so on. This rise shows up in many ways, such as volume, speed, diversity, honesty, and value. Getting important information and insights is hard work and a very important issue. One of the most important ways to solve a problem is to come to a conclusion based on a number of different criteria. This can help you choose the best solution from a number of options. AI-enabled algorithms and decision making that takes into account multiple factors can be useful in big data sets. During the deduction process, AI-enabled algorithms and evaluations based on multiple criteria are used. Because it works well and has a lot of potential, it is used in many different areas, such as computer science and information technology, agriculture, and business.

DOI: 10.4018/978-1-6684-4405-4.ch012

INTRODUCTION

Before the recent changes in wireless communication and networking paradigms, it was hard to think of ways to improve the way healthcare services ((Nwosu A.U. et al, 2021), (Rajawat A.S., Bei P. et al 2022), (D. S. Bin Abdul Hamid et al 2021), (Pradeep Bedi et al, 2021), (Goyal, S B. et al 2021)) were designed. According to the information in (P, K., & P, A. S., 2018) body area networks (BANs) can make it possible for patients' vital signs and health problems to be sensed and reported in a way that is very close to real time. With the help of mobile health (mHealth) and wearable health systems, medical care can be given on a number of mobile platforms, such as smartphones and other wearable devices. Sensor networks can send out warnings about things in the environment that are important to health. It is expected that the Internet of Things (IoT) will be able to provide health services that are more advanced and integrated. This is because the many different smart devices and sensor networks will be able to connect and work together. A wide range of medical applications can be made possible and supported by the networking paradigms listed above. However, at the moment, these paradigms are only useful for basic health monitoring and reporting, assisted and ambient living, and offline diagnostics. The health risks and precautions that must be taken make it hard to use these networking models. To create health and medical services and deliver sophisticated and fine-grained applications, networking paradigms with design primitives that allow smooth and noninvasive deployment in different contexts, such as a person's environment, on the body, and inside the body, are needed. Nanonetworks are a new way to connect computers that is made possible by recent discoveries in nanotechnology. They have a lot of potential to help medical applications go beyond just monitoring. It's very exciting to think about. Nanonetworks could be used for a lot of different things, such as stopping epidemics, doing surgery on a nanoscale level, and making drug delivery more effective. Nanomachines (M. N. M. Samsuddin et al. 2021), which are also called "nano-devices," are the building blocks of a nanonetwork. From one to a few hundred nanometers is how big they are. Nanomachines could be able to sense their surroundings and react to them. The information they gather could be sent to nano-devices called nano-routers. The data can then be sent by these nano-routers to bigger devices like micro-devices, cellphones, and access points. The human body has enough room for many different nanonetworks, each of which may have a different purpose. The nano-devices should be able to talk to each other mostly through chemical communication and Terahertz electromagnetic communication, which are two different technologies. The release of certain molecules and the reactions to those molecules can be thought of as a form of molecular communication, similar to how information signals are sent and received. This way of talking is easy to set up because nano-devices are so small and only work in a small area. For sending data at the nanoscale, radio waves with electromagnetic fields that work in the terahertz range are used. The nanomaterials that will be used to make the antenna determine both the bandwidth and the power for a given amount of input energy (S. Bandyopadhyay et al., 2022), Nanomachines can be used in biological systems like the human body and in a wide range of environmental settings without harming them. This is possible because of their small size, which is measured in nanometers. Nanomachines, on the other hand, are very limited at the nanoscale. They have very little energy, memory, and communication range, so they can only do the most basic calculations (Himanshi Babbar; et al.,2022). Nanonetworks can connect nanomachines so they can work together and share information, even though they are very small and have a limited range of communication. To make it easier for nanomachines to connect to the Internet, which is becoming known as the Internet of Nano-Things, the design of communication technologies that allow this kind of cooperation and give access to situations that would be hard for standard sensing devices needs to be rethought to take into account the different situations and sizes. This will help make what is being called the "Internet of Nano-Things" possible (IoNT). Researchers have recently proposed that molecular communication is the only way for nanonetworks to work. They called this possible future development the "Internet of BioNano-Things". This article talks at length about the architectural requirements and networking needs for Internet of Things-based health care applications. Instead of focusing on specific use cases, we give a broad classification of needs that can be traced back to the IoNT's generic application functionality. Instead of focusing on each use case, this is done. We also put a lot of attention on the possible benefits of using IoNT in the healthcare industry. We talk about the problems that come up when setting up and evaluating IoNT, such as deployment, communication, and compatibility with already-established networking paradigms. In the end, we'll talk more about the many problems that need to be solved in order to bring healthcare applications down to the nanoscale, with a focus on the networking stack's many layers. To be more specific, the structure of this document is described further down. In the second part of this paper, we will talk about the big picture of ubiquitous healthcare and the architectural requirements that will make the use of nanonetworks necessary. In the section 3, we'll talk about the IoNT's possible uses and benefits in the healthcare field. In Section 4, we talk about how the performance evaluation and the analysis are going right now. In Section 5, we talk about the IoNT networking requirements and problems that need to be solved for creative healthcare applications to be made possible. The conclusion is the last thing you will read in the paper.

PROBLEM FORMULATION

The problems we'll talk about below are not unique to the Internet of Nano Things, but they can make it harder. The biggest problem with using this technology more widely in medicine is that these nanosensors don't work well with each other. The people who make these nanosensors have a responsibility to make sure that their products don't hurt a patient's body and that they can stay in touch with other wearable devices. It's possible that, in order for designers to reach this goal, they will have to find and study a wide range of corporealities that can work with the human body. But to get these kinds of materials, you have to do a lot of research first, which slows down the process and makes it more likely that people will get the wrong idea. It won't be long before scientists figure out how to fix the problems that are holding back the Internet of Nano Things. Soon, the Internet of Nano Things will be accepted along with other new technologies like virtual reality. This will help make devices that are both smaller and more useful than their traditional counterparts. By putting these cutting-edge technologies together, business leaders will be able to find new ways to improve efficiency, make customers happier, and make more money.

Related Work

(A. Ali et al., 2015) Explore some of the ways the Internet of Things (IoT) could be used in healthcare, what the IoT needs to do to support these uses, and the possible healthcare service opportunities that lie behind these uses. In order to get a sense of how things are going with implementation right now, we take a quick look at the key actions that are being taken to analyse and assess IoNT performance.

(Y. A. Qadri et al.,2020) This study looks at how these technologies affect H-IoT systems and how they might change in the near or far future to improve service quality (QoS).

(J. Iannacci et al., 2022) In this paper, we look at the expected gap between current approaches to designing Hardware-Software (HW-SW) systems and the needs of AI-driven 6G when it comes to adaptability, flexibility, and evolution. We pay special attention to how these three things will play a role. Micro and nanotechnologies, devices, and systems are expected to play a big role in providing 6G functions, especially at the network edge. Also, it is expected that this will change the way people usually think about homework, making it more abstract.

(Fouad, H., et al., 2021) I In this study, we show a new IoBNT-based model and an improved Bio-Cyber communication interface for analysing and predicting blood clots in the vasculature. This study looks at both of these things. The model uses a bio-interface to get information about the circulatory system. This information is then turned into an electrical representation by the model. Also, the sensitivity to light or heat sets off a trigger that makes certain nano-carrier molecules, like liposomes, come out of hiding. These nano-carrier molecules can be made to travel through the bloodstream and passively enter the targeted area, where they then activate the right nano-devices to predict clots.

(El-Fatyany, et al., 2021) compartmental models in both the forward and backward biocyber interfaces of the IoBNT paradigm so you can see how well the suggested approach works. The results of the simulations that were run on the newly built model show that the IoBNT-based privacy method presented has the potential to improve the delivery of therapeutic drugs to the target cells and solve privacy problems at the same time.

(Mohamed, S., et al., 2022) The goal of this work is to combine the strengths of artificial neural networks (ANNs) and mathematical modelling. The suggested method takes a two-pronged approach, first employing non-linear least square to fit electro-bio and bio-electro interface model parameters, and then utilising ANN to learn the design underlying the model parameters (to acquire the parameter estimator).

(Al-Turjman et al., 2021) Two of the things that our data distribution system looks at are the number of hops and the amount of energy that is available. The suggested method for sending data has been shown to work through a lot of simulations, which have been confirmed by testbed results. Earlier energy-aware baseline approaches, which were written about in published research, were different from this. Table 1 shows the research gaps between several AI-enabled techniques for the Internet of Nano Things.

INTERNET OF NANO THINGS

With the help of the Internet of Nano Things and in-body nanosensors that can easily monitor a patient's health and physiological activity, a Body Sensor Network can be set up (i.e. BSN). Nanosensors(Al-Turjman, F.et al., 2020) on a wearable device will give both patients and medical professionals access to this information. By using IoNT, both patients and medical professionals will have instant access to health records that could save their lives. This kind of data can help a lot with both making medical reports and figuring out how successful a surgery was. Nanosensors can help find infectious diseases, even the ones that are known for being hard to find. Once pathogens like viruses or bacteria have been found, nanosensors will be able to send this information to both doctors and patients(Akkaş, M.A., et al.,2022). This will help them make better decisions about how to treat the disease. In figure 1, the basic working is described, how the sensors will be set up on the individual and the phone will act as a gateway to pass the changes and sensor readings. Later the data will be uploaded to internet, from where the healthcare service will be activated.

Table 1. Research Gaps between the different AI enabled Internet of nano things technique

Author	Year	Methodology/ Domain	Remark and research gap
A. Ali et al.	2015	Internet of Things (IoT) in healthcare	Examined prospective Internet of Things (IoT) uses in healthcare, the prerequisites for supporting these applications, and IoT's prospects for supporting healthcare services. We examine the major steps taken to analyse and assess IoNT performance to gauge implementation progress.
J. Iannacci et al.	2022	AI-driven 6G	This paper examines how current techniques to designing HW-SW systems may not meet the adaptability, flexibility, and evolution required of AI-driven 6G. We carefully analyse these three variables. Micro and nanotechnologies are likely to play a big role in 6G, especially at the network edge. This could make homework more abstract.
Fouad, H., et al.	2021	IoBNT-based model	This article describes an IoBNT-based methodology for analysing and forecasting blood clots. Both topics are covered. Bio-interface model gets circulatory data. The model electricalizes data. Heat or light sensitivity triggers liposome release. Nano-carrier molecules can enter the bloodstream passively and trigger clot-detecting nano-devices.
El-Fatyany, et al.	2020	IoBNT-based privacy	The outcomes of the simulations performed on the newly constructed model demonstrate that the IoBNT-based privacy strategy is capable of improving the delivery of therapeutic medications to the target cells while also resolving privacy issues.
Mohamed, S., et al.	2022	ANN and mathematical modelling	Our data distribution method considers energy and hops. Numerous calculations and testbed results prove the data transfer method's viability. Earlier work considered energy-aware baseline approaches.

Figure 1. The Internet of Nano things application in Healthcare

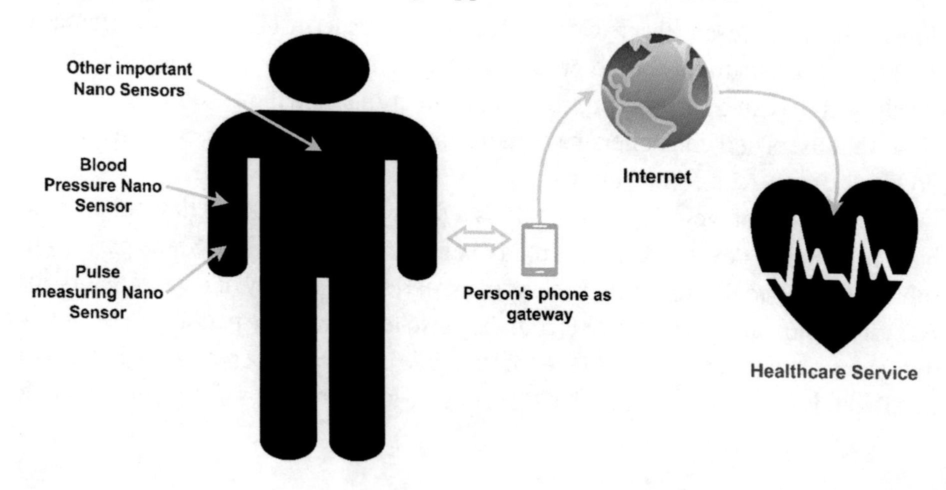

With the help of nanosensors, doctors may soon be able to find out what viruses like the Nipah virus are. Nanosensors could also be used to keep track of the temperatures of living cells in the body.

AI ENABLED IoNT

The integration of AI with networked technologies is rapidly becoming a standard practice as both AI and IoNT continue to get increasing amounts of attention.

Because it is something that pertains to all of us, it is imperative that everyone be able to successfully navigate the healthcare system. However, it is not easy to retain everything in one's thoughts at once. There is a limit to what the human intellect and body can accomplish. For this reason, the task of pushing limitations should be left to developing technologies such as the internet of things and artificial intelligence. The application of Iont and AI is welcomed in every sector of the economy, including the healthcare sector, which is not an exception to this rule (Farahzadi, A., et al., 2022). It is now possible to construct the whole digital ecosystem, which is an Internet of Things ecosystem consisting of connected gadgets. This encompasses municipal infrastructure, intelligent homes, retail, manufacturing, supply chain, education, healthcare, and life sciences, among other fields. Because it incorporates both AI and ML, the Internet of Things (IoNT) is increasingly being utilised to give customers with access to intelligent assistance. It is gradually taking the place of workers who perform manual labour across a wide range of businesses. The discipline of medicine is not an exception to this rule.

Combine IoNT and Artificial Intelligence

IoNT and AI need each other to work well. For the Internet of Things to work (Iannacci, J., 2021), it needs to be able to process and use a huge amount of information. So, AI algorithms can be used to improve IoNT functions, and they should be used to do so so that users and consumers have more satisfying experiences. So, what exactly do we get from AI's contributions to IoNT?

The Internet of New Things (IoNT) is a fairly new technology that connects the billions of smart devices that are already in use around the world. Some parts of the IoNT still need to be improved, such as the speed and accuracy of data transmission. AI systems not only act like people, but they also learn from the patterns of behaviour they show on their own. AI has to go through this process to get better at what it does. IoNT stands (El-Fatyany, A. et al., 2021) to gain a lot from AI's many abilities in the broadest sense. In its most narrow sense, the term refers to the artificial intelligence (AI) software that is built into Internet of Things (IoNT) devices, as well as the additional fog or edge computing solutions that give IoNT its intelligence. So, the large amounts of quickly processed sensor data from smart devices can only help machine learning, making physical objects smarter overall.

Artificial Intelligence and IoNT in Healthcare

When applied to the healthcare industry, the combination of AI and IoNT has the potential to significantly increase the efficiency of healthcare operations. AI algorithms embedded in Internet of Things devices make it possible to intelligently and effectively track (gather), monitor (analyse), control (plan), optimise (train), and automate (model, forecast) data. They are able to decrease the administrative burden that is placed on clinical staff when they cooperate with one another. Better clinical processes will directly result in more time being spent by doctors with patients, which in turn will lead to a more patient-centered approach to the delivery of healthcare. As a consequence of this, the following are the applications that make the most frequent use of IoNT's capabilities in AI(Akkaş, M.A., 2021) Management of supplies and patients, as well as the scheduling and rotation of medical personnel. We have shown Figure 2 use of IoNTs capabilities in AI. Medication and Therapeutics for the Care of Patients with Chronic Illness. The reduction of the amount of time that patients have to wait in order to be seen in Disease Management from a Distance.

Figure 2. Use of IoNT's Capabilities in AI

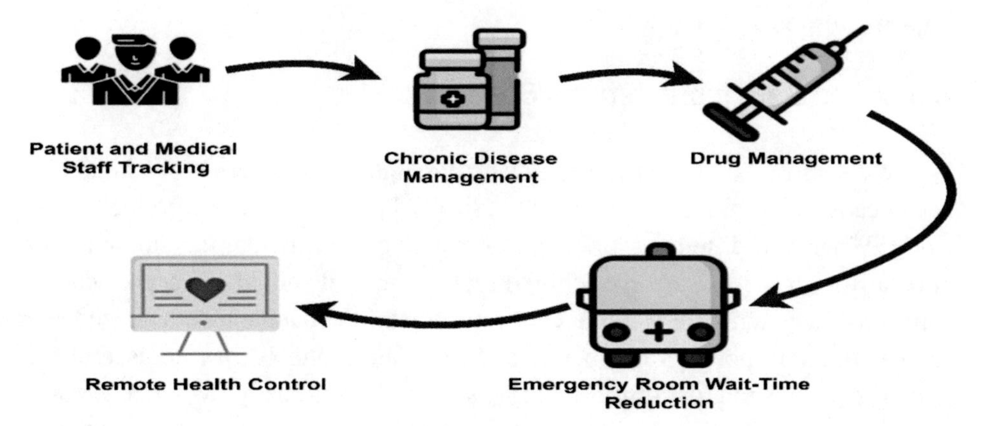

IoNT Operational Principles in the Medical Field

Even though it makes sense to be interested in the results of such an innovative process, it is not really important to know what happened. The easiest way to explain why AI-enabled IoNT needs to be used in healthcare is to give a deeper understanding of how the Internet of Things (IoNT) works. This gives a more nuanced understanding(Rajawat, A.S.,et al., 2021) of where IoNT could be used in the healthcare system.

Devices with Physical Interfaces to/from the Real World

Every service a customer could ask for in the field of healthcare has some kind of material basis. Also, both caregivers and patients, as well as the technology itself, need to be in the same room with each other for services to be delivered. These networks of devices, like those used in medical robotics, can connect to the outside world in many different ways. Because of this, it is inevitable that the development of user-friendly physical interfaces with different communication technologies (like Bluetooth, NFC, WiFi, and USB) will improve the quality of this interaction. This will make the flow of data between IoNT robots more efficient and give people a more accurate picture of and way to track services. When an IoNT-based solution is put into place, the physical connections can be used to make wireless networks. There seems to be a concerted effort to group the Internet of Things nodes that support different sensor devices. This will make it easier for devices to connect to the Internet's larger infrastructure and for established exchange procedures to work. This is being done to make it easier for devices to connect to the Internet's infrastructure as a whole.

Structured Data Input through Sensors

Wireless sensor networks have been made possible by the Internet of Things. As has already been said, these networks basically link the real world to the virtual world. When two different worlds are exchanging information, the smooth flow of data is what makes sure everything keeps going as it should. After the sensors collect the data and send it to the data control hub, the data is then analyzed and processed. Even though a number of different data channels may be used at the same time, collecting data from multiple sensors is done with low latency. Also, edge analytics keeps data records short and well-structured even as the number of data sources grows exponentially, and the high dynamism of IoNT devices makes it possible (A.S.R. et al., 2021) to get missing information from nearby devices to fill in the gaps. This way, missing information can be filled in.

Tiny Input/Output Devices

The shape and size of IO devices must meet certain requirements. Also, when changing the device's specs, the conditions under which it works should be taken into account. In this way, the wired or wireless interfaces of IoNT devices receive data from sensors, which are small because they use micro-electromechanical systems (MEMS) technology and send data back to mobile or cloud computers. In contrast, human interfaces need input and output devices that are pretty big. So, not only is there a need for in, but there is also a chance that the size of the sensors and IO devices could be cut down. This is because there is a need for. Think about technologies like heart-rhythm monitors that are implanted and measure and track biochemical data all the time. More and more people are using these kinds of devices. We have shown multiple integration of input and output devices in Figure 3.

Figure 3. Integration of I/O devices

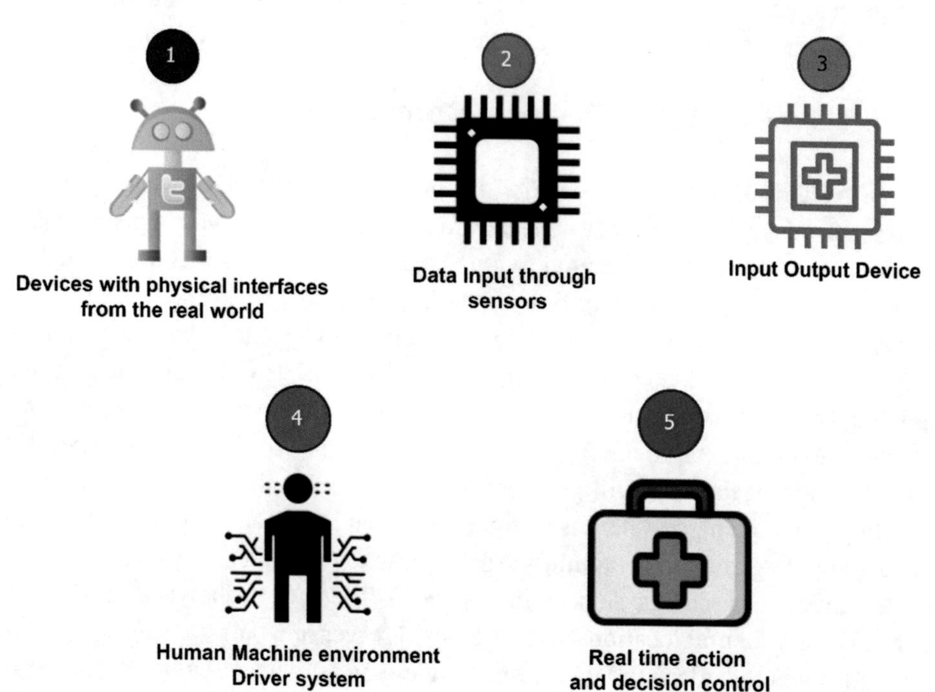

Human-Machine-Environment System Drivers

HMI, which stands for “human-machine interaction,” is a term that describes how people and machines share information and ideas. On the other hand, the Internet of Things is built on how people, machines, and the natural world are all linked to each other. The word “environment” refers to all of the physical and social factors that affect a patient’s care. Both of these factors are important. Since IoNT technology will make it even more important for the healthcare industry to be able to track this factor in real time, the term “environment” refers to all physical and social factors.

Most Internet of Things sensors are wireless, which means they can connect local networks of devices. This pairing makes no sense unless all three of these things are taken into account. So, it’s important to remember that Internet of Things (IoNT) technologies are made by people and made to be used by people(Rajawat AS, et al., 2022). They can also be used in a variety of situations. IoNT data should be used as inferrable information and made sense of with the help of AI to learn about a person’s mental and physical states, emotions, behaviours, and intentions. This can be done by using the IoNT data that can be generated by multi-modal sensors.

Real-Time Action and Decision Control

When AI and IoNT are used together, it’s easier to keep track of what’s going on and react quickly. This shows a shift toward a more intelligent way to manage data, active patient participation, and individualized treatment plans that are carried out in real time. In order to do real-time analysis, you need a steady stream of data. It is very unlikely that advanced processing systems will be able to handle the almost constant stream of data coming from different sensors. It is a real-time artificial intelligence system that could make smart data management easier by cutting down on the amount of data. In the future, Internet of Things (IoNT) systems, especially those used in healthcare, will put a lot of value on AI technologies that are built in. One of the main goals here is to figure out what localized data means by using edge computing and fog computing. Again, close to real-time analysis can be done on the Internet of Things devices themselves if the data is analyzed at the edge instead of in a central location (such as a cloud server or a data center). The use of AI algorithms to understand data from a wide range of smart sensors on the edge of the Internet of Things is a good sign for the future of condition monitoring and preventive maintenance in general.

Healthcare Cybersecurity Challenges with IoNT

Even though the Internet of Things is bringing many clear benefits, the technology also poses risks to the privacy of data, which is a key part of the healthcare system. This is because traditional algorithms have a hard time organizing and protecting unstructured data that doesn't live in databases (such as electronic documents and reports). There is a good chance that the problem can be fixed by analyzing the data, and the powerful learning algorithms will be a big part of this. Data organization is a step in the right direction, but even though it is a step in the right direction, it does not guarantee safety against cyber-attacks (P. Pant et al., 2022). Because of this, the best thing to do is to push for the standardization of IoNT ecosystems. Most of the time, the devices and apps that make up the IoNT store private and confidential information. As a result, the Health Insurance Portability and Accountability Act's (HIPAA) privacy rule will protect such sensitive health information, and laws like the General Data Protection Regulation (GDPR) of the European Union will punish financially those who misuse data. When used together to manage a number of complex systems, the Internet of Things (IoNT) and artificial intelligence (AI) will, without a doubt, give the healthcare industry as a whole cutting-edge results. Still, health care services need to be given in a way that doesn't put people at risk.

RESULT AND DISCUSSION

The Internet of Nano Things (IoNT), the Internet of Things, sensors, actuators, and other factors are all contributing to the exponential growth of IoNT. Numerous indicators of this increase include volume, speed, diversity, honesty, and worth. Obtaining crucial knowledge and insights requires a lot of effort and is a crucial concern. Using a variety of diverse criteria to get a conclusion is one of the most crucial approaches to solve a problem. This might assist you in selecting the finest alternative out of several available ones. Big data sets can benefit from AI-enabled algorithms that take into account a variety of aspects. Deduction is carried out using AI-enabled algorithms and assessments based on a variety of factors. The proliferation of Internet-connected gadgets has increased the amount of sensor data available regarding various facets of human health. It will be critical to have a better method for storing and finding knowledge at some time in the future. There is no escape from creating more intelligent surroundings where humans and machines may collaborate more effectively and safely. Better prediction algorithms and a variety of artificial intelligence systems will be used to accomplish this. The Internet of Things (IoT) is playing a bigger and bigger role in how healthcare organizations run their daily business. Delivering individualized, customer-centered services is one of the long-term objectives. This is made feasible by the Internet of Things (IoT), artificial intelligence (AI), the edge, and fog.

The nano-sensors on the individual's body will monitor him and the changes and rating will be updated on the cloud with the help of the person's device like a smartphone, which would act as a gateway from the nano-sensors to the cloud. From there the medical service on the other side can track the individual's record and rating to provide him with the best possible support. This model is enhanced by Artificial Intelligence algorithms that allows the model to make decision and take actions as per it as the changes occur in the body of the individual. This would certainly allow the model to be energy efficient, smarter and better in terms of basic working.

CONCLUSION

The exponential rise of the Internet of Nano Things (IoNT), the Internet of Things, sensors, actuators, and other elements are all influencing this development. Volume, speed, diversity, honesty, and worth are only a few examples of the numerous signs of this growth. It takes a lot of work to acquire essential knowledge and insights, which is a vital worry. One of the most important methods to solve a problem is to use a range of different criteria to arrive at a conclusion. This might help you pick the best option from the several that are offered. With the rise of Internet-connected devices, there is now a lot of sensor data about different parts of human health. At some point in the future, it will be important to have a better way to store and find information. There is no way around building smarter environments where people and machines can work together better and safer. This will be done by using a lot of different kinds of artificial intelligence and better prediction algorithms. The Internet of Things (IoNT) is becoming more and more important to the day-to-day operations of healthcare organizations. Long-term goals include delivering services that are customer-centered and customized. The Internet of Things (IoNT), artificial intelligence (AI), the edge, and fog make this possible.

REFERENCES

Akkaş, M. A. (2021). Nano-Sensor Modelling for Intra-Body Nano-Networks. *Wireless Personal Communications*, *118*(4), 3129–3143. doi:10.100711277-021-08171-2

Akkaş, M. A., & Sokullu, R. (2022). Wıreless Communıcatıons Beyond 5 g: Teraherzwaves, Nano-Communıcatıons and the Internet of Bıo-Nano-Thıngs. *Wireless Personal Communications*. Advance online publication. doi:10.100711277-022-09878-6

Al-Turjman, F. (2019). A rational data delivery framework for disaster-inspired internet of nano-things (IoNT) in practice. *Cluster Computing*, *22*(S1), 1751–1763. doi:10.100710586-017-1357-7

Al-Turjman, F. (2020). A Cognitive Routing Protocol for Bio-Inspired Networking in the Internet of Nano-Things (IoNT). *Mobile Networks and Applications*, *25*(5), 1929–1943. doi:10.100711036-017-0940-8

Ali, N. A., & Abu-Elkheir, M. (2015). Internet of nano-things healthcare applications: Requirements, opportunities, and challenges. *2015 IEEE 11th International Conference on Wireless and Mobile Computing, Networking and Communications (WiMob),* 9-14. 10.1109/WiMOB.2015.7347934

Babbar, H., Rani, S., & Kumar, N. (2022). *Internet of Things (IoT) Enabled Software Defined Networking (SDN) for Load Balancing, Edge, Cloud Computing in Healthcare. In IoT-enabled Smart Healthcare Systems, Services and Applications*. Wiley. doi:10.1002/9781119816829.ch3

Bandyopadhyay, S. (2022). *MediFi: An IoT based Wireless and Portable System for Patient's Healthcare Monitoring. In 2022 Interdisciplinary Research in Technology and Management*. IRTM. doi:10.1109/IRTM54583.2022.9791747

Bedi, Goyal, Kumar, & Patnaik. (2021). Machine Learning Aspects for Trustworthy Internet of Healthcare Things. In Internet of Healthcare Things: Machine Learning for Security and Privacy. doi:10.1002/9781119792468.ch4

Bin Abdul Hamid, D. S., Goyal, S. B., & Ghosh, A. (2021). Application of Deep Learning with Wearable IoT in Healthcare Sector. *2021 IEEE 6th International Conference on Computing, Communication and Automation (ICCCA)*, 697-701. 10.1109/ICCCA52192.2021.9666240

El-Fatyany, A., Wang, H., & Abd El-atty, S. M. (2021). Efficient Framework Analysis for Targeted Drug Delivery Based on Internet of Bio-NanoThings. *Arabian Journal for Science and Engineering*, *46*(10), 9965–9980. doi:10.100713369-021-05651-2 PMID:33907662

El-Fatyany, A., Wang, H., Abd El-atty, S. M., & Khan, M. (2020). Biocyber Interface-Based Privacy for Internet of Bio-nano Things. *Wireless Personal Communications*, *114*(2), 1465–1483. doi:10.100711277-020-07433-9

Farahzadi, A., Farahsary, P. S., & Rezazadeh, J. (2022). A survey on IoT fog nano datacenters. *Wireless Networks*, *28*(1), 173–207. doi:10.100711276-021-02829-2

Fouad, H., Hashem, M., & Youssef, A. E. (2021). Retraction Note: A Nano-biosensors model with optimized bio-cyber communication system based on Internet of Bio-Nano Things for thrombosis prediction. *Journal of Nanoparticle Research*, *23*(8), 182. doi:10.100711051-021-05263-9

Goyal, S. B., Bedi, P., Kumar, J., & Varadarajan, V. (2021). Deep learning application for sensing available spectrum for cognitive radio: An ECRNN approach. *Peer-to-Peer Networking and Applications*, *14*(5), 3235–3249. doi:10.100712083-021-01169-4

Iannacci, J. (2021). The WEAF Mnecosystem (water, earth, air, fire micro/nano ecosystem): A perspective of micro/nanotechnologies as pillars of future 6G and tactile internet (with focus on MEMS). *Microsystem Technologies*, *27*(10), 3943–3951. doi:10.100700542-020-05202-z

Iannacci, J., & Poor, H. V. (2022). Review and Perspectives of Micro/Nano Technologies as Key-Enablers of 6G. *IEEE Access: Practical Innovations, Open Solutions*, *10*, 55428–55458. doi:10.1109/ACCESS.2022.3176348

Mohamed, S., Dong, J., El-Atty, S. M. A., & Eissa, M. A. (2022). Bio-Cyber Interface Parameter Estimation with Neural Network for the Internet of Bio-Nano Things. *Wireless Personal Communications*, *123*(2), 1245–1263. doi:10.100711277-021-09177-6

Nwosu, A. U., Goyal, S. B., & Bedi, P. (2021). Blockchain Transforming Cyber-Attacks: Healthcare Industry. In A. Abraham, H. Sasaki, R. Rios, N. Gandhi, U. Singh, & K. Ma (Eds.), *Innovations in Bio-Inspired Computing and Applications. IBICA 2020. Advances in Intelligent Systems and Computing* (Vol. 1372). Springer. doi:10.1007/978-3-030-73603-3_24

P, K., & P, A. S. (2018). Intelligent Healthcare Monitoring in IoT. *International Journal of Advanced Engineering, Management and Science,* 441–445. doi:10.22161/ijaems.4.6.2

Pant, P. (2022). Blockchain for AI-Enabled Industrial IoT with 5G Network. *2022 14th International Conference on Electronics, Computers and Artificial Intelligence (ECAI),* 1-4. 10.1109/ECAI54874.2022.9847428

Qadri, Y. A., Nauman, A., Zikria, Y. B., Vasilakos, A. V., & Kim, S. W. (2020). The Future of Healthcare Internet of Things: A Survey of Emerging Technologies. IEEE Communications Surveys & Tutorials, 22(2), 1121-1167. doi:10.1109/COMST.2020.2973314

Rajawat, A. S., Barhanpurkar, K., Shaw, R. N., & Ghosh, A. (2021). Risk Detection in Wireless Body Sensor Networks for Health Monitoring Using Hybrid Deep Learning. In S. Mekhilef, M. Favorskaya, R. K. Pandey, & R. N. Shaw (Eds.), *Innovations in Electrical and Electronic Engineering. Lecture Notes in Electrical Engineering* (Vol. 756). Springer. doi:10.1007/978-981-16-0749-3_54

Rajawat, A. S., Bedi, P., Goyal, S. B., Shaw, R. N., Ghosh, A., & Aggarwal, S. (2022). AI and Blockchain for Healthcare Data Security in Smart Cities. In V. Piuri, R. N. Shaw, A. Ghosh, & R. Islam (Eds.), *AI and IoT for Smart City Applications. Studies in Computational Intelligence* (Vol. 1002). Springer. doi:10.1007/978-981-16-7498-3_12

Rajawat, A.S., Goyal, S.B., Bedi, P., Verma, C., Safirescu, C.O., & Mihaltan, T.C. (2022). Sensors Energy Optimization for Renewable Energy-Based WBANs on Sporadic Elder Movements. *Sensors, 22*(15), 5654. doi:10.3390/s22155654

Rajawat, A. S., Rawat, R., Barhanpurkar, K., Shaw, R. N., & Ghosh, A. (2021). Depression detection for elderly people using AI robotic systems leveraging the Nelder–Mead Method. *Artificial Intelligence for Future Generation Robotics, 2021*, 55–70. doi:10.1016/B978-0-323-85498-6.00006-X

Samsuddin, M. N. M., Raffei, A. F. M., & Rahman, N. S. A. (2021). IoT Based Sport Healthcare Monitoring System. *2021 International Conference on Software Engineering & Computer Systems and 4th International Conference on Computational Science and Information Management (ICSECS-ICOCSIM),* 316-319. 10.1109/ICSECS52883.2021.00064

ADDITIONAL READING

Babbar, H., Rani, S., & Alqahtani, S. A. (2022). Intelligent Edge Load Migration in SDN-IIoT for Smart Healthcare. *IEEE Transactions on Industrial Informatics, 1*, 1. Advance online publication. doi:10.1109/TII.2022.3172489

KEY TERMS AND DEFINITIONS

AI-Driven 6G: With the introduction of the 6G communication network, also called the sixth-sense next-generation communication network, the Internet of Things (IoT) will become more valuable. 6G will usher in a new era of artificial intelligence, which will open up huge opportunities in a wide range of fields, such as improving how humans think, the Internet of Things, experience quality, life expectancy, and many more. Thanks to improvements in artificial intelligence and 6G networking technology, the internet of things will soon be replaced by the internet of intelligence.

Artificial Intelligence: The term "artificial intelligence" (AI) refers to the attempt made by machines (often computers) to simulate the capabilities of human intelligence. Expert systems, natural language processing, machine learning, and machine vision are some specialized applications of AI.

Bio-Cyber Communication: All over the world, thrombosis is always near the top of the list of the main causes of death. Even though people often don't take the situation seriously, thrombosis is still one of the leading causes of death, killing one out of every four people. Scientists have been baffled by it for a long time, especially when it comes to figuring out how to predict and stop it in its early stages.

Body Sensor Network: The wireless body area network (WBAN) is another innovative piece of technology. It uses wearable sensors to let a remote system keep an eye on a patient and gather information for his or her medical record.

Deep Learning: Deep learning is a type of machine learning and artificial intelligence (AI) that imitates the way humans gain certain types of knowledge. Deep learning is an important element of data science, which includes statistics and predictive modeling.

Decision Making: In order to make decisions, one must first acknowledge the existence of a problem, then gather all of the pertinent evidence, and finally consider the relative merits of the various prospective solutions. You are able to make choices that are more deliberate and well thought out when you use decision-making processes that involve a series of steps. These processes can help you organise relevant information and establish alternatives.

Healthcare Cybersecurity: The main goal of cybersecurity in healthcare is to stop attacks from happening. This goal includes protecting networks from things like the wrong use of sensitive patient information, its theft, or its being made public. It is of the utmost importance to make sure that accurate and private patient information that could save their lives can be accessed.

Healthcare Information Management: Managers of patient health information are responsible for the organization, monitoring, and protection of the data related to the patient's health, which may include the patient's symptoms, diagnoses, medical histories, test results, and procedures.

Internet of Nano Things: The Internet of Nano-Things is a network of tiny sensors that can send data wirelessly over a local area network (LAN) or a cellular data network (cellular network) to a remote server in the cloud (IoNT). These sensors can be put inside of both everyday things and living things. Data transfer, data caching, and the use of energy are all big problems in the IoNT right now.

Internet of Things (IoT): The "Internet of Things" is a network of computers, appliances, and other physical things that are all connected to each other and can collect and send data using built-in sensors, processors, software, and other technologies. People often call this kind of network the "Internet of Things."

Machine Learning: Machine learning (ML) lets programs make better predictions over time, even if they haven't been trained. Machine learning algorithms produce predictions from historical data.

Mobile Health: The term "mobile health," or "mHealth" for short, refers to the delivery of medical and public health services using wireless mobile devices.

Nanomachines: The term "mobile health," or "mHealth" for short, refers to the delivery of medical and public health services using wireless mobile devices.

Nanonetworks: By interconnecting nanomachines and forming nanonetworks, the capacities of single nanomachines are expected to be enhanced, as the ensuing information exchange will allow them to cooperate towards a common goal.

Nanosensors: Nanosensors are chemical or mechanical nanoscale sensors that can detect chemical species and nanoparticles and monitor physical factors such as temperature.

Compilation of References

Abdel Maksoud, E., Barakat, S., & Elmogy, M. (2020). A comprehensive diagnosis system for early signs and different diabetic retinopathy grades using fundus retinal images based on pathological changes detection. *Computers in Biology and Medicine*, *126*, 104039.

Abdel-Zaher, A. M., & Eldeib, A. M. (2016). Breast cancer classification using deep belief networks. *Expert Systems with Applications*, *46*, 139–144. doi:10.1016/j.eswa.2015.10.015

Abie, H. (2019, May). Cognitive cybersecurity for CPS-IoT enabled healthcare ecosystems. In *2019 13th International Symposium on Medical Information and Communication Technology (ISMICT)* (pp. 1-6). IEEE.

Ahamed, F., & Farid, F. (2018, December). Applying internet of things and machine-learning for personalized healthcare: Issues and challenges. In *2018 International Conference on Machine Learning and Data Engineering (iCMLDE)* (pp. 19-21). IEEE.

Akçayır, M., & Akçayır, G. (2017). Advantages and challenges associated with augmented reality for education: A systematic review of the literature. *Educational Research Review*, *20*, 1–11. doi:10.1016/j.edurev.2016.11.002

Akkaş, M. A. (2021). Nano-Sensor Modelling for Intra-Body Nano-Networks. *Wireless Personal Communications*, *118*(4), 3129–3143. doi:10.100711277-021-08171-2

Akkaş, M. A., & Sokullu, R. (2022). Wıreless Communıcatıons Beyond 5 g: Teraherzwaves, Nano-Communıcatıons and the Internet of Bıo-Nano-Thıngs. *Wireless Personal Communications*. Advance online publication. doi:10.100711277-022-09878-6

Al Omar, A., Bhuiyan, M. Z. A., Basu, A., Kiyomoto, S., & Rahman, M. S. (2019). Privacy-friendly platform for healthcare data in cloud based on blockchain environment. *Future Generation Computer Systems*, *95*, 511–521. doi:10.1016/j.future.2018.12.044

Alexander, T., Westhoven, M., & Conradi, J. (2017). Virtual environments for competency-oriented education and training. In *Advances in Human Factors, Business Management, Training and Education* (pp. 23–29). Springer International Publishing. doi:10.1007/978-3-319-42070-7_3

Alferaidi, A., Yadav, K., Alharbi, Y., Razmjooy, N., Viriyasitavat, W., Gulati, K., ... Dhiman, G. (2022a). Distributed Deep CNN-LSTM Model for Intrusion Detection Method in IoT-Based Vehicles. *Mathematical Problems in Engineering.*

Alferaidi, A., Yadav, K., Alharbi, Y., Viriyasitavat, W., Kautish, S., & Dhiman, G. (2022b). Federated Learning Algorithms to Optimize the Client and Cost Selections. *Mathematical Problems in Engineering.*

Alharbi, Y., Alferaidi, A., Yadav, K., Dhiman, G., & Kautish, S. (2021). Denial-of-Service Attack Detection over IPv6 Network Based on KNN Algorithm. *Wireless Communications and Mobile Computing.*

Ali, A., Glackin, C., Cannings, N., Wall, J., Sharif, S., & Moniri, M. (2019). *A Framework for Augmented Reality Based Shared Experiences.* doi:10.1007/978-3-030-23089-0#about

Ali, N. A., & Abu-Elkheir, M. (2015). Internet of nano-things healthcare applications: Requirements, opportunities, and challenges. *2015 IEEE 11th International Conference on Wireless and Mobile Computing, Networking and Communications (WiMob),* 9-14. 10.1109/WiMOB.2015.7347934

Alkali, Y., Routray, I., & Whig, P. (2022a). Strategy for Reliable, Efficient and Secure IoT Using Artificial Intelligence. *IUP Journal of Computer Sciences, 16*(2).

AlkaliY.RoutrayI.WhigP. (2022). Study of various methods for reliable, efficient, and Secured IoT using Artificial Intelligence. *Available at* SSRN 4020364. doi:10.2139/ssrn.4020364

Al-Turjman, F. (2019). A rational data delivery framework for disaster-inspired internet of nano-things (IoNT) in practice. *Cluster Computing, 22*(S1), 1751–1763. doi:10.100710586-017-1357-7

Al-Turjman, F. (2020). A Cognitive Routing Protocol for Bio-Inspired Networking in the Internet of Nano-Things (IoNT). *Mobile Networks and Applications, 25*(5), 1929–1943. doi:10.100711036-017-0940-8

Alyoubi, W. L., Shalash, W. M., & Abulkhair, M. F. (2020). Diabetic retinopathy detection through deep learning techniques: A review. *Informatics in Medicine Unlocked, 20*, 100377. doi:10.1016/j.imu.2020.100377

Anand, S., Whig, P., & Shrivastava, S. (n.d.). *FEM Analysis of Impact of Cylindrical Tool on Composite Laminated Plate.* Academic Press.

Anand, M., Velu, A., & Whig, P. (2022). Prediction of Loan Behaviour with Machine Learning Models for Secure Banking. *Journal of Computing Science and Engineering: JCSE, 3*(1), 1–13.

Araújo, T., Aresta, G., Castro, E., Rouco, J., Aguiar, P., Eloy, C., Polónia, A., & Campilho, A. (2017). Classification of breast cancer histology images using convolutional neural networks. *PLoS One, 12*(6), e0177544. doi:10.1371/journal.pone.0177544 PMID:28570557

Arevalo, J., González, F. A., Ramos-Pollán, R., Oliveira, J. L., & Lopez, M. A. G. (2016). Representation learning for mammography mass lesion classification with convolutional neural networks. *Computer Methods and Programs in Biomedicine, 127*, 248–257.

Asopa, P., Purohit, P., Nadikattu, R. R., & Whig, P. (2021). Reducing carbon footprint for sustainable development of smart cities using IoT. *2021 Third International Conference on Intelligent Communication Technologies and Virtual Mobile Networks (ICICV)*, 361–367. 10.1109/ICICV50876.2021.9388466

Auephanwiriyakul, S., & Keller, J. M. (2002). Analysis and efficient implementation of a linguistic fuzzy C-means. *IEEE Transactions on Fuzzy Systems*, *10*(5), 563–582. doi:10.1109/TFUZZ.2002.803492

Azuma, Baillot, Behringer, Feiner, Julier, & MacIntyre. (2001). *Recent Advances in Augmented Reality*. Academic Press.

Babbar, H., Rani, S., & Kumar, N. (2022). *Internet of Things (IoT) Enabled Software Defined Networking (SDN) for Load Balancing, Edge, Cloud Computing in Healthcare. In IoT-enabled Smart Healthcare Systems, Services and Applications*. Wiley. doi:10.1002/9781119816829.ch3

Badrinarayanan, V., Handa, A., & Cipolla, R. (2015). *SegNet: A deep convolutional encoder-decoder architecture for robust semantic pixel-wise labelling*. https://arxiv.org/abs/1505.07293

Bandyopadhyay, S. (2022). *MediFi: An IoT based Wireless and Portable System for Patient's Healthcare Monitoring. In 2022 Interdisciplinary Research in Technology and Management*. IRTM. doi:10.1109/IRTM54583.2022.9791747

Banerjee, A., Chakraborty, C., Kumar, A., & Biswas, D. (2020). Emerging trends in IoT and big data analytics for biomedical and health care technologies. In *Handbook of data science approaches for biomedical engineering* (pp. 121–152). Academic Press.

Basavanhally, A., Feldman, M. D., Shih, N., Mies, C., Tomaszewski, J.E., Ganesan, S., Madabhushi, A. (2011). Multi-field of view strategy for image-based outcome prediction of multiparametricestrogen receptor-positive breast cancer histopathology: Comparison to oncotype dx. *J Pathol Inform*, *2*(1).

Bedi, Goyal, Kumar, & Patnaik. (2021). Machine Learning Aspects for Trustworthy Internet of Healthcare Things. In Internet of Healthcare Things: Machine Learning for Security and Privacy. doi:10.1002/9781119792468.ch4

Bejnordi, E. (2017). Diagnostic Assessment of Deep Learning Algorithms for Detection of Lymph Node Metastases in Women With Breast Cancer. *Journal of the American Medical Association*, *318*(22), 2199–2210. doi:10.1001/jama.2017.14585 PMID:29234806

Bellman, R. E., & Zadeh, L. A. (1970). Decision-Making in a Fuzzy Environment. *Management Science*, *17*(4), B-141–B-164. doi:10.1287/mnsc.17.4.B141

Ben Fekih, R., & Lahami, M. (2020). Application of Blockchain Technology in Healthcare: A Comprehensive Study. Lecture Notes in Computer Science, 12157, 268–276. doi:10.1007/978-3-030-51517-1_23

Benayoun, R., Tergny, J., & Laritchev, O. (n.d.). *Mathematical Programming*. North-Holland Publishing Company.

Bhatia, V., & Whig, P. (2013a). A secured dual-tune multi-frequency-based smart elevator control system. *International Journal of Research in Engineering and Advanced Technology, 4*(1), 1163–2319.

Bhatia, V., & Whig, P. (2014). Performance analysis of multi-functional bot system design using microcontroller. *International Journal of Intelligent Systems and Applications, 6*(2), 69–75. doi:10.5815/ijisa.2014.02.09

Bhoi, A., Balabantaray, R. C., Sahoo, D., Dhiman, G., Khare, M., Narducci, F., & Kaur, A. (2022). Mining social media text for disaster resource management using a feature selection based on forest optimization. *Computers & Industrial Engineering*, 108280.

Bin Abdul Hamid, D. S., Goyal, S. B., & Ghosh, A. (2021). Application of Deep Learning with Wearable IoT in Healthcare Sector. *2021 IEEE 6th International Conference on Computing, Communication and Automation (ICCCA)*, 697-701. 10.1109/ICCCA52192.2021.9666240

Biran, A., Bidari, P. S., & Raahemifar, K. (2016). Automatic method for exudates and hemorrhages detection from fundus retinal images. *International Journal of Computer and Information Engineering, 10*(9), 1599–1602.

Cai, J., Lu, L., Xie, Y., Xing, F., & Yang, L. (2017). *Improving deep pancreas segmentation in CT and MRI images via recurrent neural contextual learning and direct loss function*. arXiv preprint arXiv:1707.04912.

Caicedo, J. C., Goodman, A., Karhohs, K. W., Cimini, B. A., Ackerman, J., Haghighi, M., Heng, C. K., Becker, T., Doan, M., McQuin, C., Rohban, M., Singh, S., & Carpenter, A. E. (2019). Nucleus segmentation across imaging experiments: The 2018 Data Science Bowl. *Nature Methods, 16*(12), 1247–1253. doi:10.103841592-019-0612-7 PMID:31636459

Cameron, C. (2014). *Spanish students create AR science posters with Layar*. Available: https://www.layar.com/news/blog/2014/12/22/spanishstudents-create-AR-science-posters-with-layar/

Carmigniani, J., & Furht, B. (2011). Augmented Reality: An Overview. In B. Furht (Ed.), *Handbook of Augmented Reality*. Springer. doi:10.1007/978-1-4614-0064-6_1

Casino, F., Dasaklis, T. K., & Patsakis, C. (2019). A systematic literature review of blockchain-based applications: Current status, classification and open issues. *Telematics and Informatics, 36*, 55–81. doi:10.1016/j.tele.2018.11.006

Cerqueira, C. S., & Kirner, C. (2012). Developing Educational Applications with a Non-Programming Augmented Reality Authoring Tool. *Proceedings of World Conference on Educational Multimedia, Hypermedia and Telecommunications*, 2816-2825.

Chakravarty, S., Demirhan, H., & Baser, F. (2020). Fuzzy regression functions with a noise cluster and the impact of outliers on mainstream machine learning methods in the regression setting. *Applied Soft Computing, 96*, 106535.

Chandrawat, R. K., Kumar, R., Garg, B. P., Dhiman, G., & Kumar, S. (2017). An analysis of modeling and optimization production cost through fuzzy linear programming problem with symmetric and right angle triangular fuzzy number. *Advances in Intelligent Systems and Computing*, *546*, 197–211. doi:10.1007/978-981-10-3322-3_18

Chandrawat, R. K., Kumar, R., Makkar, V., Yadav, M., & Kumari, P. (2019). A comparative fuzzy cluster analysis of the Binder's performance grades using fuzzy equivalence relation via different distance measures. *Communications in Computer and Information Science*, *955*, 108–118. doi:10.1007/978-981-13-3140-4_11

Chang, G., Morreale, P., & Medicherla, P. (2011). Applications of Augmented Reality Systems in Education. *Proceedings of Society for Information Technology & Teacher Education International Conference*, *2010*, 1380–1385.

Chankong, T., Theera-Umpon, N., & Auephanwiriyakul, S. (2014). Automatic cervical cell segmentation and classification in Pap smears. *Computer Methods and Programs in Biomedicine*, *113*(2), 539–556. doi:10.1016/j.cmpb.2013.12.012 PMID:24433758

Channumsin, O., Pimpol, J., Thongsopa, C., & Tangsrirat, W. (2015). VDBA-based floating inductance simulator with a grounded capacitor. *2015 7th International Conference on Information Technology and Electrical Engineering (ICEE)*, 114–117.

Chatterjee, I. (2021). Artificial intelligence and patentability: Review and discussions. *International Journal of Modern Research*, *1*(1), 15–21.

Cheng, D., & Liu, M. (2017, October). Combining convolutional and recurrent neural networks for Alzheimer's disease diagnosis using PET images. In *2017 IEEE International Conference on Imaging Systems and Techniques (IST)* (pp. 1-5). IEEE.

Cheng, X., Chen, F., Xie, D., Sun, H., & Huang, C. (2020). Design of a Secure Medical Data Sharing Scheme Based on Blockchain. *Journal of Medical Systems*, *44*(2), 52. Advance online publication. doi:10.100710916-019-1468-1 PMID:31915982

Cheng, X., Chen, F., Xie, D., Sun, H., Huang, C., & Qi, Z. (2019). Blockchain-Based Secure Authentication Scheme for Medical Data Sharing. *Communications in Computer and Information Science*, *1058*, 396–411. doi:10.1007/978-981-15-0118-0_31

Chen, H., Ni, D., Qin, J., Li, S., Yang, X., Wang, T., & Heng, P. A. (2015). Standard plane localization in fetal ultrasound via domain transferred deep neural networks. *IEEE Journal of Biomedical and Health Informatics*, *19*(5), 1627–1636.

Chen, H., Qi, X., Yu, L., & Heng, P. A. (2016). DCAN: deep contour-aware networks for accurate gland segmentation. In *Proceedings of the IEEE conference on Computer Vision and Pattern Recognition* (pp. 2487-2496). IEEE.

Chenthara, S., Ahmed, K., Wang, H., Whittaker, F., & Chen, Z. (2020). Healthchain: A novel framework on privacy preservation of electronic health records using blockchain technology. *PLoS ONE*, *15*(12). doi:10.1371/journal.pone.0243043

Chopra, G., & Whig, P. (2022a). A clustering approach based on support vectors. *International Journal of Machine Learning for Sustainable Development, 4*(1), 21–30.

Chopra, G., & Whig, P. (2022b). Using machine learning algorithms classified depressed patients and normal people. *International Journal of Machine Learning for Sustainable Development, 4*(1), 31–40.

Cimino, M., & Frosini, G. (2007). On the noise distance in robust fuzzy c-means. *International Journal on Engineering, Computing and Technology,* 361–364. http://www2.ing.unipi.it/~r000099/publications/cimino_pub19.pdf

Clemente-Suárez. (2020). Dynamics of population immunity due to the herd effect in the COVID-19 pandemic. *Vaccines, 8*(2), 236.

Coffin, C., Bostandjiev, S., Ford, J., & Hollerer, T. (2008). *Enhancing Classroom and Distance Learning Through Augmented Reality*. Academic Press.

Cui, Y., Zhang, G., Liu, Z., Xiong, Z., & Hu, J. (2019). A deep learning algorithm for one-step contour aware nuclei segmentation of histopathology images. *Medical & Biological Engineering & Computing, 57*(9), 2027–2043. doi:10.100711517-019-02008-8 PMID:31346949

Dai, H., Han, J., & Lichtfouse, E. (2020). Who is running faster, the virus or the vaccine? *Environmental Chemistry Letters, 18*(6), 1761–1766. doi:10.100710311-020-01110-w PMID:33082737

Dakhel, M., & Hassan, S. (2020). A Secure Wireless Body Area Network for E-Health Application Using Blockchain. *Communications in Computer and Information Science, 1174*, 395–408. doi:10.1007/978-3-030-38752-5_31

Dalmış, M. U., Litjens, G., Holland, K., Setio, A., Mann, R., Karssemeijer, N., & Gubern-Mérida, A. (2017). Using deep learning to segment breast and fibroglandular tissue in MRI volumes. *Medical Physics, 44*(2), 533–546.

Davenport, T., & Kalakota, R. (2019). The potential for artificial intelligence in healthcare. *Future Healthcare Journal, 6*(2), 94–98. doi:10.7861/futurehosp.6-2-94 PMID:31363513

De Aguiar, E. J., Faiçal, B. S., Krishnamachari, B., & Ueyama, J. (2020). A Survey of Blockchain-Based Strategies for Healthcare. *ACM Computing Surveys, 53*(2), 1–27. Advance online publication. doi:10.1145/3376915

de Andres Sanchez, J., & Gómez, A. T. (2003b). Estimating a term structure of interest rates for fuzzy financial pricing by using fuzzy regression methods. *Fuzzy Sets and Systems, 139*(2), 313–331.

de Andrés Sánchez, J., & Gómez, A. T. (2004). Estimating a fuzzy term structure of interest rates using fuzzy regression techniques. *European Journal of Operational Research, 154*(3), 804–818.

de Andres Sanchez, J., & Terceño Gómez, A. (2003a). Applications of fuzzy regression in actuarial analysis. *The Journal of Risk and Insurance, 70*(4), 665–699.

Deep, K., Bansal, J. C., Das, K. N., Lal, A. K., Garg, H., Nagar, A. K., & Pant, M. (Eds.). (2017). *Proceedings of Sixth International Conference on Soft Computing for Problem Solving* (*Vol. 546*). Springer Singapore. 10.1007/978-981-10-3322-3

Del Moral, P. (2020). Theory and applications. *Mean Field Simulation for Monte Carlo Integration*, 85–124. doi:10.1201/b14924-7

Dhiman, G., Juneja, S., Mohafez, H., El-Bayoumy, I., Sharma, L. K., Hadizadeh, M., ... Khandaker, M. U. (2022a). Federated learning approach to protect healthcare data over big data scenario. *Sustainability*, *14*(5), 2500.

Dhiman, G., Juneja, S., Viriyasitavat, W., Mohafez, H., Hadizadeh, M., Islam, M. A., ... Gulati, K. (2022c). A novel machine-learning-based hybrid CNN model for tumor identification in medical image processing. *Sustainability*, *14*(3), 1447.

Dhiman, G., Rashid, J., Kim, J., Juneja, S., Viriyasitavat, W., & Gulati, K. (2022b). Privacy for healthcare data using the byzantine consensus method. *Journal of the Institution of Electronics and Telecommunication Engineers*, 1–12.

Dinesh Kumar, R., Golden Julie, E., Harold Robinson, Y., Vimal, S., Dhiman, G., & Veerasamy, M. (2022). Deep convolutional nets learning classification for artistic style transfer. *Scientific Programming*.

Dinesh Kumar, R., Golden Julie, E., Harold Robinson, Y., Vimal, S., Dhiman, G., & Veerasamy, M. (2022). Deep Convolutional Nets Learning Classification for Artistic Style Transfer. *Scientific Programming*.

Ding, H., Cao, X., Wang, Z., Dhiman, G., Hou, P., Wang, J., ... Hu, X. (2022). Velocity clamping-assisted adaptive salp swarm algorithm: Balance analysis and case studies. *Mathematical Biosciences and Engineering*, *19*(8), 7756–7804.

El-Elimat. (2021). Acceptance and attitudes toward COVID-19 vaccines: a cross-sectional study from Jordan. *Plos one*, *16*(4), e0250555.

El-Fatyany, A., Wang, H., & Abd El-atty, S. M. (2021). Efficient Framework Analysis for Targeted Drug Delivery Based on Internet of Bio-NanoThings. *Arabian Journal for Science and Engineering*, *46*(10), 9965–9980. doi:10.100713369-021-05651-2 PMID:33907662

El-Fatyany, A., Wang, H., Abd El-atty, S. M., & Khan, M. (2020). Biocyber Interface-Based Privacy for Internet of Bio-nano Things. *Wireless Personal Communications*, *114*(2), 1465–1483. doi:10.100711277-020-07433-9

Fadafen, M. K., Mehrshad, N., &Razavi, S. M. (2018). Detection of diabetic retinopathy using computational model of human visual system. *Biomedical Research, 29*(9).

Farahzadi, A., Farahsary, P. S., & Rezazadeh, J. (2022). A survey on IoT fog nano datacenters. *Wireless Networks*, *28*(1), 173–207. doi:10.100711276-021-02829-2

Fleck, S., & Simon, G. (2013). *An Augmented Reality Environment for Astronomy Learning in Elementary Grades. An Exploratory Study*. doi:10.1145/2534903.2534907

Forni, G., & Mantovani, A. (2021). COVID-19 vaccines: Where we stand and challenges ahead. *Cell Death and Differentiation*, *28*(2), 626–639. doi:10.103841418-020-00720-9 PMID:33479399

Fouad, H., Hashem, M., & Youssef, A. E. (2021). Retraction Note: A Nano-biosensors model with optimized bio-cyber communication system based on Internet of Bio-Nano Things for thrombosis prediction. *Journal of Nanoparticle Research*, *23*(8), 182. doi:10.100711051-021-05263-9

Froese, T., & Ziemke, T. (2009). Enactive artificial intelligence: Investigating the systemic organization of life and mind. *Artificial Intelligence*, *173*(3-4), 466–500. doi:10.1016/j.artint.2008.12.001

Gaggioli, A. (2018). Blockchain Technology: Living in a Decentralized Everything. *Cyberpsychology, Behavior, and Social Networking*, *21*(1), 65–66. doi:10.1089/cyber.2017.29097.csi

Gandomkar, Z., Brennan, P. C., & Mello-Thoms, C. (2018). MuDeRN: Multicategory classification of breast histopathological image using deep residual networks. *Artificial Intelligence in Medicine*, *88*, 14–24. doi:10.1016/j.artmed.2018.04.005 PMID:29705552

George, N., Muiz, K., Whig, P., & Velu, A. (2021, July). The framework of Perceptive Artificial Intelligence using Natural Language Processing (PAIN). *Artificial & Computational Intelligence*.

Ghanbari, R., Ghorbani-Moghadam, K., Mahdavi-Amiri, N., & de Baets, B. (2020). Fuzzy linear programming problems: Models and solutions. *Soft Computing*, *24*(13), 10043–10073. doi:10.100700500-019-04519-w

Girardi, F., De Gennaro, G., Colizzi, L., & Convertini, N. (2020). Improving the Healthcare Effectiveness: The Possible Role of EHR, IoMT and Blockchain. *Electronics, 9*(6), 884. doi:10.3390/electronics9060884

Gordon, W. J., & Catalini, C. (2018). Blockchain Technology for Healthcare: Facilitating the Transition to Patient-Driven Interoperability. *Computational and Structural Biotechnology Journal*, *16*, 224–230. doi:10.1016/j.csbj.2018.06.003 PMID:30069284

Goyal, S. B., Bedi, P., Kumar, J., & Varadarajan, V. (2021). Deep learning application for sensing available spectrum for cognitive radio: An ECRNN approach. *Peer-to-Peer Networking and Applications*, *14*(5), 3235–3249. doi:10.100712083-021-01169-4

Gregori, D., Petrinco, M., Bo, S., Desideri, A., Merletti, F., & Pagano, E. (2011). Regression models for analyzing costs and their determinants in health care: An introductory review. *International Journal for Quality in Health Care*, *23*(3), 331–341.

Griggs, K. N., Ossipova, O., Kohlios, C. P., Baccarini, A. N., Howson, E. A., & Hayajneh, T. (2018). Healthcare Blockchain System Using Smart Contracts for Secure Automated Remote Patient Monitoring. *Journal of Medical Systems*, *42*(7), 130. Advance online publication. doi:10.100710916-018-0982-x PMID:29876661

Gupta, Jiwani, Afreen, & D. (2022). Liver Disease Prediction using Machine learning Classification Techniques. *2022 IEEE 11th International Conference on Communication Systems and Network Technologies (CSNT),* 221-226.

Gupta, K., Jiwani, N., & Afreen, N. (2022). Blood Pressure Detection Using CNN-LSTM Model. *2022 IEEE 11th International Conference on Communication Systems and Network Technologies (CSNT),* 262-366. 10.1109/CSNT54456.2022.9787648

Gupta, N., Gupta, K., Gupta, D., Juneja, S., Turabieh, H., Dhiman, G., ... Viriyasitavat, W. (2022). Enhanced virtualization-based dynamic bin-packing optimized energy management solution for heterogeneous clouds. *Mathematical Problems in Engineering*.

Gupta, V. K., Shukla, S. K., & Rawat, R. S. (2022). Crime tracking system and people's safety in India using machine learning approaches. *International Journal of Modern Research, 2*(1), 1–7.

Gurcan, M. N., Boucheron, L. E., Can, A., Madabhushi, A., Rajpoot, N. M., & Yener, B. (2009). Histopathological image analysis: A review. *IEEE Reviews in Biomedical Engineering, 2*, 147–171. doi:10.1109/RBME.2009.2034865 PMID:20671804

Gutierrez, M., Guinters, E., & Perez-Lopez, D. (2012). *Improving Strategy of Self-Learning in Engineering: Laboratories with Augmented Reality*. Academic Press.

Hagos, T. (2019). Setup. In Android Studio IDE Quick Reference (pp. 1-9). Apress.

Hassan, L., Saleh, A., Abdel-Nasser, M., Omer, O. A., & Puig, D. (2021). Promising Deep Semantic Nuclei Segmentation Models for Multi-Institutional Histopathology Images of Different Organs. *International Journal of Interactive Multimedia and Artificial Intelligence, 6*(6), 35–45. doi:10.9781/ijimai.2020.10.004

He, K., Zhang, X., Ren, S., & Sun, J. (2016). Deep residual learning for image recognition. *Proc. IEEE Conf. Comput. Vis. Pattern Recognit. (CVPR)*, 770-778.

Hipp, J., Fernandez, A., Compton, C., & Balis, U. (2011). Why a pathology image should not be considered as a radiology image. *Journal of Pathology Informatics, 2*(1), 26. doi:10.4103/2153-3539.82051 PMID:21773057

Hose, D., & Hanss, M. (2019). Fuzzy linear least squares for the identification of possibilistic regression models. *Fuzzy Sets and Systems, 367*, 82–95.

Howard, A. G., Zhu, M., & Chen, B. (2017). *Mobilenets: Efficient convolutional neural networks for mobile vision applications*. Academic Press.

Hsu, J.-L., & Huang, Y.-H. (2011). *The Advent of Augmented-Learning: A Combination of Augmented Reality and Cloud Computing*. Academic Press.

Huang, G., Liu, Z., Van Der Maaten, L., & Weinberger, K. Q. (2017). Densely connected convolutional networks. *Proc. IEEE Conf. Comput. Vis. Pattern Recognit. (CVPR)*, 4700-4708.

Huang, Q., Sun, J., Ding, H., Wang, X., & Wang, G. (2018). Robust liver vessel extraction using 3D U-Net with variant dice loss function. *Computers in Biology and Medicine, 101*, 153–162.

Huang, X. (2019). Blockchain in Healthcare: A Patient-Centered Model. *Biomedical Journal of Scientific & Technical Research, 20*(3). Advance online publication. doi:10.26717/BJSTR.2019.20.003448 PMID:31565696

Hu, P., Wu, F., Peng, J., Bao, Y., Chen, F., & Kong, D. (2017). Automatic abdominal multi-organ segmentation using deep convolutional neural network and time-implicit level sets. *International Journal of Computer Assisted Radiology and Surgery, 12*(3), 399–411.

Iannacci, J. (2021). The WEAF Mnecosystem (water, earth, air, fire micro/nano ecosystem): A perspective of micro/nanotechnologies as pillars of future 6G and tactile internet (with focus on MEMS). *Microsystem Technologies, 27*(10), 3943–3951. doi:10.100700542-020-05202-z

Iannacci, J., & Poor, H. V. (2022). Review and Perspectives of Micro/Nano Technologies as Key-Enablers of 6G. *IEEE Access: Practical Innovations, Open Solutions, 10*, 55428–55458. doi:10.1109/ACCESS.2022.3176348

Informa, F., Number, W. R., House, M., Street, M., & Dunn, J. C. (2008). *Well-Separated Clusters and Optimal Fuzzy Partitions Well-Separated Clusters and Optimal Fuzzy Partitions*. Academic Press.

Irshad, H., Veillard, A., Roux, L., & Racoceanu, D. (2013). Methods for nuclei detection, segmentation, and classication in digital histopathology: A review Current status and future potential. *IEEE Reviews in Biomedical Engineering, 7*, 97–114. doi:10.1109/RBME.2013.2295804 PMID:24802905

Jiang, X., Coffee, M., Bari, A., Wang, J., Jiang, X., Huang, J., Shi, J., Dai, J., Cai, J., Zhang, T., Wu, Z., He, G., & Huang, Y. (2020). *Towards an Artificial Intelligence Framework for Data-Driven Prediction of Coronavirus Clinical Severity*. Academic Press.

Jiang, F., Jiang, Y., Zhi, H., Dong, Y., Li, H., Ma, S., ... Wang, Y. (2017). Artificial intelligence in healthcare: Past, present and future. *Stroke and Vascular Neurology, 2*(4).

Jiwani, N., Gupta, K., & Afreen, N. (2022). A Convolutional Neural Network Approach for Diabetic Retinopathy Classification. *2022 IEEE 11th International Conference on Communication Systems and Network Technologies (CSNT)*, 357-361. 10.1109/CSNT54456.2022.9787577

Jiwani, N., Gupta, K., & Whig, P. (2021). Novel HealthCare Framework for Cardiac Arrest With the Application of AI Using ANN. *2021 5th International Conference on Information Systems and Computer Networks (ISCON)*, 1–5.

Jiwani, N., Gupta, K., & Afreen, N. (2022). Automated Seizure Detection using Theta Band. *2022 International Conference on Emerging Smart Computing and Informatics (ESCI)*, 1-4.

Joshi, V., & Chandrawat, R. K. (2019). Comparative Analysis of Different Structure of the Crisp and Fuzzy Regression Equations Using Realistic Data. *Think India Journal, 22*(37), 1288–1303.

Juneja, S., Juneja, A., Dhiman, G., Jain, S., Dhankhar, A., & Kautish, S. (2021). computer Vision-Enabled character recognition of hand Gestures for patients with hearing and speaking disability. *Mobile Information Systems.*

Jupalle, H., Kouser, S., Bhatia, A. B., Alam, N., Nadikattu, R. R., & Whig, P. (2022). Automation of human behaviors and its prediction using machine learning. *Microsystem Technologies, 28*(8), 1–9. doi:10.100700542-022-05326-4

Kaggle. (n.d.). *2018 Data Science Bowl.* https://www.kaggle.com/c/data-science-bowl-2018

Kallenberg, M., Petersen, K., Nielsen, M., Ng, A. Y., Diao, P., Igel, C., ... Lillholm, M. (2016). Unsupervised deep learning applied to breast density segmentation and mammographic risk scoring. *IEEE Transactions on Medical Imaging, 35*(5), 1322–1331.

Kamal, M., Jalil, S. A., Muneeb, S. M., & Ali, I. (2018). A Distance Based Method for Solving Multi-Objective Optimization Problems. *Journal of Modern Applied Statistical Methods; JMASM, 17*(1), 2–23. doi:10.22237/jmasm/1532525455

Kanwal, S., Rashid, J., Kim, J., Juneja, S., Dhiman, G., & Hussain, A. (2022). Mitigating the coexistence technique in wireless body area networks by using superframe interleaving. *Journal of the Institution of Electronics and Telecommunication Engineers*, 1–15.

Kaplan, R. M., & Milstein, A. (2021). Influence of a COVID-19 vaccine's effectiveness and safety profile on vaccination acceptance. *Proceedings of the National Academy of Sciences.* 10.1073/pnas.2021726118

Katare, G., Padihar, G., & Qureshi, Z. (2018). Challenges in the integration of artificial intelligence and internet of things. *International Journal of System and Software Engineering, 6*(2), 10–15.

Kauppi, T., Kalesnykiene, V., Kamarainen, J. K., Lensu, L., Sorri, I., Raninen, A., . . . Pietilä, J. (2007, September). The diaretdb1 diabetic retinopathy database and evaluation protocol. In BMVC (Vol. 1, pp. 1-10). Academic Press.

Kauppi, T., Kalesnykiene, V., Kamarainen, J. K., Lensu, L., Sorri, I., Uusitalo, H., . . . Pietilä, J. (2006). DIARETDB0: Evaluation database and methodology for diabetic retinopathy algorithms. Machine Vision and Pattern Recognition Research Group, Lappeenranta University of Technology.

Kaur, P., Kumar, R., & Kumar, M. (2019). A healthcare monitoring system using random forest and internet of things (IoT). *Multimedia Tools and Applications, 78*(14), 19905–19916.

Kautish, S., Reyana, A., & Vidyarthi, A. (2022). SDMTA: Attack Detection and Mitigation Mechanism for DDoS Vulnerabilities in Hybrid Cloud Environment. *IEEE Transactions on Industrial Informatics.*

Kerawalla, Luckin, Seljeflot, & Woolard. (2006). "Making it real": Exploring the potential of augmented reality for teaching primary school science. *Virtual Reality, 10*(3), 163-174.

Kermany, D. S., Goldbaum, M., Cai, W., Valentim, C. C., Liang, H., Baxter, S. L., ... Zhang, K. (2018). Identifying medical diagnoses and treatable diseases by image-based deep learning. *Cell, 172*(5), 1122–1131.

Khera, Y., Whig, P., & Velu, A. (2021). efficient effective and secured electronic billing system using AI. *Vivekananda Journal of Research, 10*, 53–60.

Khezr, S., Moniruzzaman, M., Yassine, A., & Benlamri, R. (2019). Blockchain Technology in Healthcare: A Comprehensive Review and Directions for Future Research. *Applied Sciences, 9*(9), 1736. doi:10.3390/app9091736

Kim, S., Bae, W. C., Masuda, K., Chung, C. B., & Hwang, D. (2018). Fine-grain segmentation of the intervertebral discs from MR spine images using deep convolutional neural networks: BSU-Net. *Applied Sciences (Basel, Switzerland), 8*(9), 1656.

Kiranyaz, S., Ince, T., & Gabbouj, M. (2015). Real-time patient-specific ECG classification by 1-D convolutional neural networks. *IEEE Transactions on Biomedical Engineering, 63*(3), 664–675. doi:10.1109/TBME.2015.2468589 PMID:26285054

Kou, C., Li, W., Yu, Z., & Yuan, L. (2020). An enhanced residual U-Net for microaneurysms and exudates segmentation in fundus images. *IEEE Access: Practical Innovations, Open Solutions, 8*, 185514–185525. doi:10.1109/ACCESS.2020.3029117

Kour, K., Gupta, D., Gupta, K., Dhiman, G., Juneja, S., Viriyasitavat, W., ... Islam, M. A. (2022). Smart-hydroponic-based framework for saffron cultivation: A precision smart agriculture perspective. *Sustainability, 14*(3), 1120.

Krizhevsky, A., Sutskever, I., & Hinton, G. E. (2017). ImageNet classification with deep convolutional neural networks. *Communications of the ACM, 60*(6), 84–90. doi:10.1145/3065386

Kumar, R. (2021). *A Comparative Study of Fuzzy Optimization through Fuzzy Number*. Academic Press.

Kumar, A., Kaur, J., & Singh, P. (2011). A new method for solving fully fuzzy linear programming problems. *Applied Mathematical Modelling, 35*(2), 817–823. doi:10.1016/j.apm.2010.07.037

Kumari, A., Tanwar, S., Tyagi, S., & Kumar, N. (2018). Fog computing for Healthcare 4.0 environment: Opportunities and challenges. *Computers & Electrical Engineering, 72*, 1.

Kumar, R., Chandrawat, R. K., Garg, B. P., & Joshi, V. (2017). Comparison of optimized algorithms in facility location allocation problems with different distance measures. *AIP Conference Proceedings, 1860*, 020041. Advance online publication. doi:10.1063/1.4990340

Kumar, R., Chandrawat, R. K., & Joshi, V. (2020). Profit Optimization of products at different selling prices with fuzzy linear programming problem using situational based fuzzy triangular numbers. *Journal of Physics: Conference Series, 1531*(1), 012085. Advance online publication. doi:10.1088/1742-6596/1531/1/012085

Kumar, R., Chandrawat, R. K., Sarkar, B., Joshi, V., & Majumder, A. (2021). An advanced optimization technique for smart production using α-cut based quadrilateral fuzzy number. *International Journal of Fuzzy Systems*, *23*(1), 107–127.

Kumar, R., Chandrawat, R. K., Sarkar, B., Joshi, V., & Majumder, A. (2021). An Advanced Optimization Technique for Smart Production Using α-Cut Based Quadrilateral Fuzzy Number. *International Journal of Fuzzy Systems*, *23*(1), 107–127. doi:10.100740815-020-01002-9

Kumar, R., & Dhiman, G. (2021). A comparative study of fuzzy optimization through fuzzy number. *International Journal of Modern Research*, *1*(1), 1–14.

Kumar, R., Dhiman, G., Kumar, N., Chandrawat, R. K., Joshi, V., & Kaur, A. (2021). A novel approach to optimize the production cost of railway coaches of India using situational-based composite triangular and trapezoidal fuzzy LPP models. *Complex & Intelligent Systems*, *7*(4), 2053–2068. doi:10.100740747-021-00313-0

Kumar, R., Joshi, V., Dhiman, G., & Viriyasitavat, W. (2021). An improved exponential metric space approach for C-mean clustering analysing. *Expert Systems: International Journal of Knowledge Engineering and Neural Networks*, e12896. doi:10.1111/exsy.12896

Kumar, S., Raut, R. D., & Narkhede, B. E. (2020). A proposed collaborative framework by using artificial intelligence-internet of things (AI-IoT) in COVID-19 pandemic situation for healthcare workers. *International Journal of Healthcare Management*, *13*(4), 337–345. doi:10.1080/2047 9700.2020.1810453

Kumar, V. M. (2021). Strategy for COVID-19 vaccination in India: The country with the second highest population and number of cases. *NPJ Vaccines*, *6*(1), 1–7. PMID:33398010

Kuschel, N., & Rackwitz, R. (1997). Two Basic Problems in Reliability-Based Structural Optimization. In Mathematical Methods of Operations Research (Vol. 46). doi:10.1007/ BF01194859

Lal, S., Das, D., Alabhya, K., Kanfade, A., Kumar, A., & Kini, J. (2021). NucleiSegNet: Robust Deep Learning Architecture for the Nuclei Segmentation of Liver Cancer Histopathology Images. *Computers in Biology and Medicine*, *128*, 128. doi:10.1016/j.compbiomed.2020.104075 PMID:33190012

Lee, J. (2017). Lee-deep learning in medical imaging_gen. *Medical*, *18*, 570–584. PMID:28670152

Lee, T. F., Li, H. Z., & Hsieh, Y. P. (2021). A blockchain-based medical data preservation scheme for telecare medical information systems. *International Journal of Information Security*, *20*(4), 589–601. doi:10.100710207-020-00521-8

Li, Y. H., Yeh, N. N., Chen, S. J., & Chung, Y. C. (2019). Computer-assisted diagnosis for diabetic retinopathy based on fundus images using deep convolutional neural network. *Mobile Information Systems*.

Li, H., Xiao, F., Yin, L., & Wu, F. (2021). Application of Blockchain Technology in Energy Trading: A Review. *Frontiers in Energy Research*, *9*, 671133. Advance online publication. doi:10.3389/fenrg.2021.671133

Lim, G., Lee, M. L., Hsu, W., & Wong, T. Y. (2014, June). Transformed representations for convolutional neural networks in diabetic retinopathy screening. *Workshops at the Twenty-Eighth AAAI Conference on Artificial Intelligence.*

Liu, H., Crespo, R. G., & Martínez, O. S. (2020). Enhancing Privacy and Data Security across Healthcare Applications Using Blockchain and Distributed Ledger Concepts. *Healthcare, 8*(3), 243. doi:10.3390/healthcare8030243

Li, Y., Wu, J., & Wu, Q. (2019). Classification of Breast Cancer Histology Images Using Multi-Size and Discriminative Patches Based on Deep Learning. *IEEE Access: Practical Innovations, Open Solutions*, *7*, 21400–21408. doi:10.1109/ACCESS.2019.2898044

Long, J., Shelhamer, E., & Darrell, T. (2015). Fully convolutional networks for semantic segmentation. In *Proceedings of the IEEE conference on computer vision and pattern recognition* (pp. 3431-3440). IEEE.

Long, J., Shelhamer, E., & Darrell, T. (2015). Fully convolutional networks for semantic segmentation. *Proc. IEEE Conf. Comput. Vis. Pattern Recognit. (CVPR)*, 3431-3440.

Mackey, T. K., Kuo, T. T., Gummadi, B., Clauson, K. A., Church, G., Grishin, D., Obbad, K., Barkovich, R., & Palombini, M. (2019). "Fit-for-purpose?" - Challenges and opportunities for applications of blockchain technology in the future of healthcare. *BMC Medicine*, *17*(1), 68. Advance online publication. doi:10.118612916-019-1296-7 PMID:30914045

Macrinici, D., Cartofeanu, C., & Gao, S. (2018). Smart contract applications within blockchain technology: A systematic mapping study. *Telematics and Informatics*, *35*(8), 2337–2354. doi:10.1016/j.tele.2018.10.004

Madhu, G., Govardhan, A., & Ravi, V. (2022). *DSCN-net: a deep Siamese capsule neural network model for automatic diagnosis of malaria parasites detection. Multimed Tools Appl.* doi:10.100711042-022-13008-6

Marler, R. T., & Arora, J. S. (2010). The weighted sum method for multi-objective optimization: New insights. *Structural and Multidisciplinary Optimization*, *41*(6), 853–862. doi:10.100700158-009-0460-7

Martin, S., Diaz, G., Sancristobal, E., Gil, R., Castro, M., & Peire, J. (2011). New technology trends in education: Seven years of forecasts and convergence. *Computer Education*, *57*(3), 1893–1906. doi:10.1016/j.compedu.2011.04.003

McCauley-Bell, P. R., Crumpton-Young, L. L., & Badiru, A. B. (1999). Techniques and applications of fuzzy theory in quantifying risk levels in occupational injuries and illnesses. In *Fuzzy Theory Systems* (pp. 223–265). Academic Press.

McGhin, T., Choo, K. K. R., Liu, C. Z., & He, D. (2019). Blockchain in healthcare applications: Research challenges and opportunities. *Journal of Network and Computer Applications*, *135*, 62–75. doi:10.1016/j.jnca.2019.02.027

Mekala, M. S., Dhiman, G., Srivastava, G., Nain, Z., Zhang, H., Viriyasitavat, W., & Varma, G. P. S. (2022). A DRL-Based Service Offloading Approach Using DAG for Edge Computational Orchestration. *IEEE Transactions on Computational Social Systems*.

Mekala, M. S., Dhiman, G., Srivastava, G., Nain, Z., Zhang, H., Viriyasitavat, W., & Varma, G. P. S. (2022a). *A DRL-Based Service Offloading Approach Using DAG for Edge Computational Orchestration. IEEE Transactions on Computational Social Systems.*

Mekala, M. S., Srivastava, G., Lin, J. C. W., Dhiman, G., Park, J. H., & Jung, H. Y. (2022b). An efficient quantum based D2D computation and communication approach for the Internet of Things. *Optical and Quantum Electronics*, *54*(6), 1–19.

Mohamed, S., Dong, J., El-Atty, S. M. A., & Eissa, M. A. (2022). Bio-Cyber Interface Parameter Estimation with Neural Network for the Internet of Bio-Nano Things. *Wireless Personal Communications*, *123*(2), 1245–1263. doi:10.100711277-021-09177-6

Moorthy, T. V. K., Budati, A. K., Kautish, S., Goyal, S. B., & Prasad, K. L. (2022). Reduction of satellite images size in 5G networks using Machinelearning algorithms. *IET Communications*, *16*(5), 584–591. doi:10.1049/cmu2.12354

Morgan, J. A. (2018). *Yesterday's tomorrow today: Turing, Searle and the contested significance of artificial intelligence*. Academic Press.

Nadikattu, R. R., Mohammad, S. M., & Whig, P. (2020a). *Novel economical social distancing smart device for covid-19. International Journal of Electrical Engineering and Technology.*

Nair, R., Soni, M., Bajpai, B., Dhiman, G., & Sagayam, K. M. (2022). Predicting the Death Rate Around the World Due to COVID-19 Using Regression Analysis. *International Journal of Swarm Intelligence Research*, *13*(2), 1–13. doi:10.4018/IJSIR.287545

Nasr-Esfahani, E., Samavi, S., Karimi, N., Soroushmehr, S. M. R., Jafari, M. H., Ward, K., & Najarian, K. (2016, August). Melanoma detection by analysis of clinical images using convolutional neural network. In *2016 38th Annual International Conference of the IEEE Engineering in Medicine and Biology Society (EMBC)* (pp. 1373-1376). IEEE.

Naylor, P., Laé, M., Reyal, F., & Walter, T. (2019). Segmentation of nuclei in histopathology images by deep regression of the distance map. *IEEE Transactions on Medical Imaging*, *38*(2), 448–559. doi:10.1109/TMI.2018.2865709 PMID:30716022

Ng, E. Y. K. (2009). A review of thermography as promising non-invasive detection modality for breast tumor. *International Journal of Thermal Sciences*, *48*(5), 849–859. doi:10.1016/j.ijthermalsci.2008.06.015

Nwosu, A. U., Goyal, S. B., & Bedi, P. (2021). Blockchain Transforming Cyber-Attacks: Healthcare Industry. In A. Abraham, H. Sasaki, R. Rios, N. Gandhi, U. Singh, & K. Ma (Eds.), *Innovations in Bio-Inspired Computing and Applications. IBICA 2020. Advances in Intelligent Systems and Computing* (Vol. 1372). Springer. doi:10.1007/978-3-030-73603-3_24

OECD. (2021). *Coronavirus (COVID-19) vaccines for developing countries: An equal shot at recovery, OECD policy responses to coronavirus (COVID-19).* OECD.

Oliva, D., Esquivel-Torres, S., Hinojosa, S., Pérez-Cisneros, M., Osuna-Enciso, V., Ortega-Sánchez, N., Dhiman, G., & Heidari, A. A. (2021). Opposition-based moth swarm algorithm. *Expert Systems with Applications*, *184*, 115481.

Omala, A. A., Mbandu, A. S., Mutiria, K. D., Jin, C., & Li, F. (2018). Provably Secure Heterogeneous Access Control Scheme for Wireless Body Area Network. *Journal of Medical Systems*, *42*(6), 108. Advance online publication. doi:10.100710916-018-0964-z PMID:29705947

On the Performance of ISFET-based Device for Water Quality Monitoring. (n.d.). doi:10.4236/ijcns.2011.411087

Orlando, J. I., Prokofyeva, E., & Blaschko, M. B. (2016). A discriminatively trained fully connected conditional random field model for blood vessel segmentation in fundus images. *IEEE Transactions on Biomedical Engineering*, *64*(1), 16–27. doi:10.1109/TBME.2016.2535311 PMID:26930672

P, K., & P, A. S. (2018). Intelligent Healthcare Monitoring in IoT. *International Journal of Advanced Engineering, Management and Science,* 441–445. doi:10.22161/ijaems.4.6.2

Pal, N. R., Pal, K., Keller, J. M., & Bezdek, J. C. (2005). A possibilistic fuzzy c-means clustering algorithm. *IEEE Transactions on Fuzzy Systems*, *13*(4), 517–530. doi:10.1109/TFUZZ.2004.840099

Pant, P. (2022). Blockchain for AI-Enabled Industrial IoT with 5G Network. *2022 14th International Conference on Electronics, Computers and Artificial Intelligence (ECAI),* 1-4. 10.1109/ECAI54874.2022.9847428

Parasuraman, K. (2018). Detection of retinal hemorrhage from fundus images using ANFIS classifier and MRG segmentation. *Biomedical Research, 29*(7).

Parihar, V., & Yadav, S. (2022). *Comparison estimation of effective consumer future preferences with the application of AI.* Academic Press.

Pawar, R., & Kalbande, D. (2020). Use of blockchain technology in wireless body area networks. *Proceedings of the 3rd International Conference on Intelligent Sustainable Systems, ICISS 2020,* 1333–1336. 10.1109/ICISS49785.2020.9316005

Pedrycz, W., & Vulkovich, G. (2004). Fuzzy clustering with supervision. *Pattern Recognition*, *37*(7), 1339–1349. doi:10.1016/j.patcog.2003.11.005

Pêgo, A., & Aguiar, P. (2015). Bioimaging. *4th International Symposium in Applied Bioimaging.* http://www.bioimaging2015.ineb.up.pt/dataset.html

Pham, H. L., Tran, T. H., & Nakashima, Y. (2019). A Secure Remote Healthcare System for Hospital Using Blockchain Smart Contract. *2018 IEEE Globecom Workshops, GC Wkshps 2018 - Proceedings*. doi:10.1109/GLOCOMW.2018.8644164

Pickles, M. D., Gibbs, P., Hubbard, A., Rahman, A., Wieczorek, J., & Turnbull, L. W. (2015). Comparison of 3.0T magnetic resonance imaging and X-ray mammography in the measurement of ductal carcinoma in situ: A comparison with histopathology. *European Journal of Radiology*, *84*(4), 603–610. doi:10.1016/j.ejrad.2014.12.016 PMID:25604907

Prasanna, K., Ramana, K., Dhiman, G., Kautish, S., & Chakravarthy, V. D. (2021). PoC Design: A Methodology for Proof-of-Concept (PoC) Development on Internet of Things Connected Dynamic Environments. *Security and Communication Networks*.

Prensky, M. (2001). *Digital game-based learning*. McGraw-Hill.

Priya, R., & Aruna, P. (2013). Diagnosis of diabetic retinopathy using machine learning techniques. *ICTACT Journal on Soft Computing, 3*(4), 563-575.

Puri, T., Soni, M., Dhiman, G., Ibrahim Khalaf, O., & Raza Khan, I. (2022). Detection of emotion of speech for RAVDESS audio using hybrid convolution neural network. *Journal of Healthcare Engineering*.

Purva Agarwall, P. W. (2016). A Review-Quaternary Signed Digit Number System by reversible Logic Gate. *International Journal on Recent and Innovation Trends in Computing and Communication, 4*(3).

Qadri, Y. A., Nauman, A., Zikria, Y. B., Vasilakos, A. V., & Kim, S. W. (2020). The Future of Healthcare Internet of Things: A Survey of Emerging Technologies. IEEE Communications Surveys & Tutorials, 22(2), 1121-1167. doi:10.1109/COMST.2020.2973314

Rajawat, A.S., Goyal, S.B., Bedi, P., Verma, C., Safirescu, C.O., & Mihaltan, T.C. (2022). Sensors Energy Optimization for Renewable Energy-Based WBANs on Sporadic Elder Movements. *Sensors, 22*(15), 5654. doi:10.3390/s22155654

Rajawat, A. S., Barhanpurkar, K., Shaw, R. N., & Ghosh, A. (2021). Risk Detection in Wireless Body Sensor Networks for Health Monitoring Using Hybrid Deep Learning. In S. Mekhilef, M. Favorskaya, R. K. Pandey, & R. N. Shaw (Eds.), *Innovations in Electrical and Electronic Engineering. Lecture Notes in Electrical Engineering* (Vol. 756). Springer. doi:10.1007/978-981-16-0749-3_54

Rajawat, A. S., Bedi, P., Goyal, S. B., Kautish, S., Xihua, Z., Aljuaid, H., & Mohamed, A. W. (2022). Dark Web Data Classification Using Neural Network. *Computational Intelligence and Neuroscience*.

Rajawat, A. S., Bedi, P., Goyal, S. B., Shaw, R. N., Ghosh, A., & Aggarwal, S. (2022). AI and Blockchain for Healthcare Data Security in Smart Cities. In V. Piuri, R. N. Shaw, A. Ghosh, & R. Islam (Eds.), *AI and IoT for Smart City Applications. Studies in Computational Intelligence* (Vol. 1002). Springer. doi:10.1007/978-981-16-7498-3_12

Rajawat, A. S., Rawat, R., Barhanpurkar, K., Shaw, R. N., & Ghosh, A. (2021). Depression detection for elderly people using AI robotic systems leveraging the Nelder–Mead Method. *Artificial Intelligence for Future Generation Robotics*, *2021*, 55–70. doi:10.1016/B978-0-323-85498-6.00006-X

Ren, S., He, K., Girshick, R., & Sun, J. (2016). Faster R-CNN: Towards real-time object detection with region proposal networks. *IEEE Transactions on Pattern Analysis and Machine Intelligence*, *39*(6), 1137–1149.

Rodríguez Ramos, A., Llanes-Santiago, O., Bernal de Lázaro, J. M., Cruz Corona, C., Silva Neto, A. J., & Verdegay Galdeano, J. L. (2017). A novel fault diagnosis scheme applying fuzzy clustering algorithms. *Applied Soft Computing*, *58*, 605–619. doi:10.1016/j.asoc.2017.04.071

Ronneberger, O., Fischer, P., & Brox, T. (2015). *U-net: Convolutional networks for biomedical image segmentation*. Available: https://arxiv.org/abs/1505.04597

Roth, H. R., Oda, H., Hayashi, Y., Oda, M., Shimizu, N., Fujiwara, M., . . . Mori, K. (2017). *Hierarchical 3D fully convolutional networks for multi-organ segmentation*. arXiv preprint arXiv:1704.06382.

Roychowdhury, S., Koozekanani, D. D., & Parhi, K. K. (2013). DREAM: Diabetic retinopathy analysis using machine learning. *IEEE Journal of Biomedical and Health Informatics*, *18*(5), 1717–1728. doi:10.1109/JBHI.2013.2294635 PMID:25192577

Ruchin, C. M., & Whig, P. (2015). Design and Simulation of Dynamic UART Using Scan Path Technique (USPT). *International Journal of Electrical, Electronics & Computing in Science & Engineering*.

Rupani, A., & Kumar, D. (2020). *Temperature Effect On Behaviour of Photo Catalytic Sensor (PCS)*. Used For Water Quality Monitoring.

Rupani, A., & Sujediya, G. (2016). A Review of FPGA implementation of Internet of Things. *International Journal of Innovative Research in Computer and Communication Engineering*, *4*(9).

Rupani, A., Whig, P., Sujediya, G., & Vyas, P. (2017). A robust technique for image processing based on interfacing of Raspberry-Pi and FPGA using IoT. *2017 International Conference on Computer, Communications and Electronics (Comptelix)*, 350–353. 10.1109/COMPTELIX.2017.8003992

Rupani, A., Whig, P., Sujediya, G., & Vyas, P. (2018). Hardware implementation of IoT-based image processing filters. *Proceedings of the Second International Conference on Computational Intelligence and Informatics*, 681–691. 10.1007/978-981-10-8228-3_63

Safitri, D. W., & Juniati, D. (2017, August). Classification of diabetic retinopathy using fractal dimension analysis of eye fundus image. In AIP conference proceedings (Vol. 1867, No. 1, p. 020011). AIP Publishing LLC.

Saidin, N., Abd Halim, N. D., & Yahaya, N. (2015). A Review of Research on Augmented Reality in Education: Advantages and Applications. *International Education Studies*, *8*(13). Advance online publication. doi:10.5539/ies.v8n13p1

Samaddar, A., Gadepalli, R., Nag, V. L., & Misra, S. (2020). The enigma of low COVID-19 fatality rate in India. *Frontiers in Genetics*, *11*, 854. doi:10.3389/fgene.2020.00854 PMID:32849833

Samsuddin, M. N. M., Raffei, A. F. M., & Rahman, N. S. A. (2021). IoT Based Sport Healthcare Monitoring System. *2021 International Conference on Software Engineering & Computer Systems and 4th International Conference on Computational Science and Information Management (ICSECS-ICOCSIM)*, 316-319. 10.1109/ICSECS52883.2021.00064

Senthilnath, J., Omkar, S. N., & Mani, V. (2011). Clustering using firefly algorithm: Performance study. *Swarm and Evolutionary Computation*, *1*(3), 164–171. doi:10.1016/j.swevo.2011.06.003

Sereno, M., Wang, X., Besançon, L., Mcguffin, M., & Isenberg, T. (2020). Collaborative Work in Augmented Reality: A Survey. *IEEE Transactions on Visualization and Computer Graphics*. doi:10.1109/TVCG.2020.3032761

Shah, S. (2020). Latest Statistics of Breast Cancer in India. *Breast Cancer India*. https://www.breastcancerindia.net/statistics/trends.html

Shah, R., & Chircu, A. (2018). IoT and AI in healthcare: A systematic literature review. *Issues in Information Systems*, *19*(3).

Shapiro, A. F. (2005). Fuzzy regression models. *Article of Penn State University*, *102*(2), 373–383.

Sharma, N. K., Shrivastava, S., & Whig, P. (n.d.). *Optimization of Process Parameters for Developing Stresses in Square Cup by Incremental Sheet Metal (ISM) Technique uses Finite Element Methods*. Academic Press.

Sharma, A., Kaur, S., & Singh, M. (2021). A comprehensive review on blockchain and Internet of Things in healthcare. *Transactions on Emerging Telecommunications Technologies*, *32*(10). Advance online publication. doi:10.1002/ett.4333

Sharma, A., Kumar, A., & Whig, P. (2015). On the performance of CDTA based novel analog inverse low pass filter using 0.35 μm CMOS parameter. *International Journal of Science, Technology & Management*, *4*(1), 594–601.

Sharma, C., Sharma, S., Kautish, S., Alsallami, S. A., Khalil, E. M., & Mohamed, A. W. (2022). A new median-average round Robin scheduling algorithm: An optimal approach for reducing turnaround and waiting time. *Alexandria Engineering Journal*, *61*(12), 10527–10538.

Sharma, O., Sultan, A. A., Ding, H., & Triggle, C. R. (2020). A Review of the Progress and Challenges of Developing a Vaccine for COVID-19. *Frontiers in Immunology*, *11*, 2413. doi:10.3389/fimmu.2020.585354 PMID:33163000

Sharma, S., Gupta, S., Gupta, D., Juneja, S., Gupta, P., Dhiman, G., & Kautish, S. (2022a). Deep Learning Model for the Automatic Classification of White Blood Cells. *Computational Intelligence and Neuroscience*.

Sharma, S., Gupta, S., Gupta, D., Juneja, S., Singal, G., Dhiman, G., & Kautish, S. (2022b). Recognition of Gurmukhi Handwritten City Names Using Deep Learning and Cloud Computing. *Scientific Programming*.

Sharma, T., Nair, R., & Gomathi, S. (2022). Breast cancer image classification using transfer learning and convolutional neural network. *International Journal of Modern Research*, *2*(1), 8–16.

Sharma, T., Nair, R., & Gomathi, S. (2022). Breast Cancer Image Classification using Transfer Learning and Convolutional Neural Network. *International Journal of Modern Research*, *2*(1), 8–16.

Shie, C. K., Chuang, C. H., Chou, C. N., Wu, M. H., & Chang, E. Y. (2015, August). Transfer representation learning for medical image analysis. In *2015 37th annual international conference of the IEEE Engineering in Medicine and Biology Society (EMBC)* (pp. 711-714). IEEE.

Shin, H. C., Roth, H. R., Gao, M., Lu, L., Xu, Z., Nogues, I., ... Summers, R. M. (2016). Deep convolutional neural networks for computer-aided detection: CNN architectures, dataset characteristics and transfer learning. *IEEE Transactions on Medical Imaging*, *35*(5), 1285–1298.

Shi, S., He, D., Li, L., Kumar, N., Khan, M. K., & Choo, K. K. R. (2020). Applications of blockchain in ensuring the security and privacy of electronic health record systems: A survey. *Computers & Security*, *97*, 101966. Advance online publication. doi:10.1016/j.cose.2020.101966 PMID:32834254

Shridhar, J., & Whig, P. (2014). Design and simulation of power-efficient traffic light controller (PTLC). *2014 International Conference on Computing for Sustainable Global Development (INDIACom)*, 348–352. 10.1109/IndiaCom.2014.6828157

Shrivastav, P., Whig, P., & Gupta, K. (n.d.). *Bandwidth Enhancement by Slotted Stacked Arrangement and its Comparative Analysis with Conventional Single and Stacked Patch Antenna*. Academic Press.

Shukla, S. K., Gupta, V. K., Joshi, K., Gupta, A., & Singh, M. K. (2022). Self-aware Execution Environment Model (SAE2) for the Performance Improvement of Multicore Systems. *International Journal of Modern Research*, *2*(1), 17–27.

Simonyan, K., & Zisserman, A. (2015). Very deep convolutional networks for large-scale image recognition. *Proc. Int. Conf. Learn. Represent. (ICLR)*, 1-14.

Singha, A., Bhowmik, M. K., & Bhattacherjee, D. (2020). Akin-based Orthogonal Space (AOS): A subspace learning method for face recognition. *Multimedia Tools and Applications*, *79*(47-48), 35069–35091. doi:10.100711042-020-08892-9

Singhal, S., Bagga, S., Goyal, P., & Saxena, V. (2012). Augmented Chemistry: Interactive Education System. *International Journal of Computers and Applications*, *49*(15), 1–5. Advance online publication. doi:10.5120/7700-1041

Singh, N., Houssein, E. H., Singh, S. B., & Dhiman, G. (2022). HSSAHHO: A novel hybrid Salp swarm-Harris hawks optimization algorithm for complex engineering problems. *Journal of Ambient Intelligence and Humanized Computing*, 1–37.

Singh, S. K., Rathore, S., & Park, J. H. (2020). Blockiotintelligence: A blockchain-enabled intelligent IoT architecture with artificial intelligence. *Future Generation Computer Systems, 110*, 721–743. doi:10.1016/j.future.2019.09.002

Sinha, R., & Ranjan, A. (2015). Effect of Variable Damping Ratio on the design of PID Controller. *2015 4th International Conference on Reliability, Infocom Technologies and Optimization (ICRITO)(Trends and Future Directions)*, 1–4.

Sirinukunwattana, K., Raza, S. E. A., Tsang, Y. W., Snead, D. R., Cree, I. A., & Rajpoot, N. M. (2016). Locality sensitive deep learning for detection and classification of nuclei in routine colon cancer histology images. *IEEE Transactions on Medical Imaging*, *35*(5), 1196–1206.

Spanhol, F. A., Oliveira, L. S., Petitjean, C., & Heutte, L. (2016). Breast cancer histopathological image classification using convolutional neural networks. *Proc. Int. Joint Conf. Neural Netw. (IJCNN)*, 2560-2567. 10.1109/IJCNN.2016.7727519

Srinivasa, N., & Medasani, S. (2004). Active fuzzy clustering for collaborative filtering. *IEEE International Conference on Fuzzy Systems*, *3*, 1697–1702. 10.1109/FUZZY.2004.1375436

Srivastava, N., Mansimov, E., & Salakhudinov, R. (2015, June). Unsupervised learning of video representations using lstms. In *International conference on machine learning* (pp. 843-852). PMLR.

Su. (2021). COVID-19 Vaccine Donations—Vaccine Empathy or Vaccine Diplomacy? A Narrative Literature Review. *Vaccines, 9*(9).

Sumathy, B., Chakrabarty, A., Gupta, S., Hishan, S. S., Raj, B., Gulati, K., & Dhiman, G. (2022). Prediction of Diabetic Retinopathy Using Health Records With Machine Learning Classifiers and Data Science. *International Journal of Reliable and Quality E-Healthcare*, *11*(2), 1–16.

Sun, J., & Binder, A. (2017). Comparison of deep learning architectures for H&E histopathology images. *Proc. IEEE Conf. Big Data Analytics (ICBDA)*, 43-48. 10.1109/ICBDAA.2017.8284105

Sun, T. Q., & Medaglia, R. (2019). Mapping the challenges of Artificial Intelligence in the public sector: Evidence from public healthcare. *Government Information Quarterly*, *36*(2), 368–383.

Swain, S., Bhushan, B., Dhiman, G., & Viriyasitavat, W. (2022). Appositeness of Optimized and Reliable Machine Learning for Healthcare: A Survey. *Archives of Computational Methods in Engineering*, 1–23.

Tajbakhsh, N., Shin, J. Y., Gurudu, S. R., Hurst, R. T., Kendall, C. B., Gotway, M. B., & Liang, J. (2016). Convolutional neural networks for medical image analysis: Full training or fine tuning? *IEEE Transactions on Medical Imaging*, *35*(5), 1299–1312.

Tanaka, H., & Asai, K. (1984). Fuzzy linear programming problems with fuzzy numbers. *Fuzzy Sets and Systems*, *13*(1), 1–10. doi:10.1016/0165-0114(84)90022-8

Tanaka, H., Hayashi, I., & Watada, J. (1989). Possibilistic linear regression analysis for fuzzy data. *European Journal of Operational Research*, *40*(3), 389–396.

Tanaka, H., Uejima, S., & Asai, K. (1980). *Fuzzy linear regression model.* Presented at the *International Congress on Applied Systems Research and Cybernetics*, Acapulco, Mexico.

Tran, D., Bourdev, L., Fergus, R., Torresani, L., & Paluri, M. (2016). Deep end2end voxel2voxel prediction. In *Proceedings of the IEEE conference on computer vision and pattern recognition workshops* (pp. 17-24). IEEE.

Truong, T. D., & Pham, H. T. T. (2020). Breast cancer histopathological image classification utilizing convolutional neural network. *IFMBE Proceedings*, *69*, 531–536. doi:10.1007/978-981-13-5859-3_92

Tymchenko, B., Marchenko, P., & Spodarets, D. (2020). *Deep learning approach to diabetic retinopathy detection.* arXiv preprint arXiv:2003.02261.

Vaghela. (2021). World's largest vaccination drive in India: Challenges and recommendations. *Health Science Reports, 4*(3).

Vaishnav, P. K., Sharma, S., & Sharma, P. (2021). Analytical review analysis for screening COVID-19 disease. *International Journal of Modern Research*, *1*(1), 22–29.

Vashistha, R., Dangi, A. K., Kumar, A., Chhabra, D., & Shukla, P. (2018). Futuristic biosensors for cardiac health care: an artificial intelligence approach. *Biotech, 8*(8), 1-11.

Velu, A., & Whig, P. (2022). Studying the impact of the COVID vaccination on the world using data analytics. *Vivekananda J Res*, *10*(1), 147–160.

Verma, T., Gupta, P., & Whig, P. (2015). Sensor Controlled Sanitizer Door Knob with Scan Technique. *Emerging ICT for Bridging the Future-Proceedings of the 49th Annual Convention of the Computer Society of India CSI, 2*, 261–266.

Viriyasitavat, W., Da Xu, L., Dhiman, G., Sapsomboon, A., Pungpapong, V., & Bi, Z. (2021). Service Workflow: State-of-the-Art and Future Trends. *IEEE Transactions on Services Computing*.

Viriyasitavat, W., Xu, L. D., Sapsomboon, A., Dhiman, G., & Hoonsopon, D. (2022). Building trust of Blockchain-based Internet-of-Thing services using public key infrastructure. *Enterprise Information Systems*, 1–24.

Vu, Q. D., Graham, S., Kurc, T., To, M. N. N., Shaban, M., Qaiser, T., Koohbanani, N. A., Khurram, S. A., Kalpathy-Cramer, J., Zhao, T., Gupta, R., Kwak, J. T., Rajpoot, N., Saltz, J., & Farahani, K. (2019). Methods for segmentation and classification of digital microscopy tissue images. *Frontiers in Bioengineering and Biotechnology*, *7*(53), 1–15. doi:10.3389/fbioe.2019.00053 PMID:31001524

Wang, D., Khosla, A., Gargeya, R., Irshad, H., & Beck, A. H. (2016). *Deep learning for identifying metastatic breast cancer*. Available: https://arxiv.org/abs/1606.05718

Wang, H., Xian, M., & Vakanski, A. (2020). Bending Loss Regularized Network for Nuclei Segmentation in Histopathology Images. *Proc. 2020 IEEE 17th International Symposium on Biomedical Imaging (ISBI)*, 1-5.

Wang, J., MacKenzie, J. D., Ramachandran, R., & Chen, D. Z. (2016, October). A deep learning approach for semantic segmentation in histology tissue images. In *International Conference on Medical Image Computing and Computer-Assisted Intervention* (pp. 176-184). Springer.

Wang, J., Peng, Y., Xu, H., Cui, Z., & Williams, R. O. III. (2020). The COVID-19 vaccine race: Challenges and opportunities in vaccine formulation. *AAPS PharmSciTech*, *21*(6), 1–12. doi:10.120812249-020-01744-7 PMID:32761294

Wang, P., Hu, X., Li, Y., Liu, Q., & Zhu, X. (2016). Automatic cell nuclei segmentation and classification of breast cancer histopathology images. *Signal Processing*, *122*, 1–13. doi:10.1016/j.sigpro.2015.11.011

Wang, R., Liu, H., Wang, H., Yang, Q., & Wu, D. (2019). Distributed Security Architecture Based on Blockchain for Connected Health: Architecture, Challenges, and Approaches. *IEEE Wireless Communications*, *26*(6), 30–36. doi:10.1109/MWC.001.1900108

Wang, Y., Lei, B., Elazab, A., Tan, E.-L., Wang, W., Huang, F., Gong, X., & Wang, T. (2020). Breast Cancer Image Classification via Multi-Network Features and Dual-Network Orthogonal Low-Rank Learning. *IEEE Access: Practical Innovations, Open Solutions*, *8*, 27779–27792. doi:10.1109/ACCESS.2020.2964276

Whig, P., & Ahmad, S. N. (2011). Performance analysis and frequency compensation technique for low power water quality monitoring device using ISFET sensor. *International Journal of Mobile and Adhoc Network*, 80–84.

Whig, P., & Ahmad, S. N. (2013a). A novel pseudo NMOS integrated CC -ISFET device for water quality monitoring. *Journal of Integrated Circuits and Systems*. https://www.scopus.com/inward/record.url?eid=2-s2.0-84885357423&partnerID=MN8TOARS

Whig, P., & Ahmad, S. N. (2014). Simulation of linear dynamic macro model of photo catalytic sensor in SPICE. *COMPEL: The International Journal for Computation and Mathematics in Electrical and Electronic Engineering*.

Whig, P., & Ahmad, S. N. (2016). Ultraviolet Photo Catalytic Oxidation (UVPCO) sensor for air and surface sanitizers using CS amplifier. *Global Journal of Research in Engineering*.

Whig, P., Nadikattu, R. R., & Velu, A. (2022). COVID-19 pandemic analysis using application of AI. *Healthcare Monitoring and Data Analysis Using IoT: Technologies and Applications*, 1.

Whig, P., Nadikattu, R. R., & Velu, A. (2022). COVID-19 pandemic analysis using the application of AI. *Healthcare Monitoring and Data Analysis Using IoT: Technologies and Applications*, 1.

Whig, P., Velu, A., & Sharma, P. (2022). Demystifying Federated Learning for Blockchain: A Case Study. In Demystifying Federated Learning for Blockchain and Industrial Internet of Things (pp. 143–165). IGI Global. doi:10.4018/978-1-6684-3733-9.ch008

Whig, P., & Ahmad, S. N. (2013b). A novel pseudo-PMOS integrated ISFET device for water quality monitoring. *Active and Passive Electronic Components*, *2013*. doi:10.1155/2013/258970

Whig, P., & Ahmad, S. N. (2014a). CMOS integrated VDBA-ISFET device for water quality monitoring. *International Journal of Intelligent Engineering and Systems*, *7*(1), 1–7. doi:10.22266/ijies2014.0331.01

Whig, P., & Ahmad, S. N. (2014b). Development of economical ASIC for PCS for water quality monitoring. *Journal of Circuits, Systems, and Computers*, *23*(06), 1450079. doi:10.1142/S0218126614500790

Whig, P., & Ahmad, S. N. (2014d). *Simulation of a linear dynamic macro model of the photocatalytic sensor in SPICE. COMPEL The International Journal for Computation and Mathematics in Electrical and Electronic Engineering*.

Whig, P., & Ahmad, S. N. (2015). *Impact of Parameters on Characteristics of Novel PCS*. Academic Press.

Whig, P., & Ahmad, S. N. (2016a). Modeling and simulation of economical water quality monitoring device. *Journal of Aquaculture & Marine Biology*, *4*(6), 1–6. doi:10.15406/jamb.2016.04.00103

Whig, P., & Ahmad, S. N. (2016b). *Novel SPICE model for Ultraviolet Photo Catalytic Oxidation (UVPCO)*. Sensor for Air and Surface Sanitizers.

Whig, P., & Ahmad, S. N. (2017a). Controlling the Output Error for Photo Catalytic Sensor (PCS) Using Fuzzy Logic. *Journal of Earth Science & Climatic Change*, *8*(4), 1–6.

Whig, P., & Ahmad, S. N. (2017b). Fuzzy logic implementation of the photocatalytic sensor. *Int. Robot. Autom. J*, *2*(3), 15–19.

Whig, P., & Ahmad, S. N. (2019). Methodology for Calibrating Photocatalytic Sensor Output. *International. Journal of Sustainable Development in Computing Science*, *1*(1), 1–10.

Whig, P., Kouser, S., Velu, A., & Nadikattu, R. R. (2022). Fog-IoT-Assisted-Based Smart Agriculture Application. In *Demystifying Federated Learning for Blockchain and Industrial Internet of Things* (pp. 74–93). IGI Global. doi:10.4018/978-1-6684-3733-9.ch005

Whig, P., Velu, A., & Bhatia, A. B. (2022). Protect Nature and Reduce the Carbon Footprint With an Application of Blockchain for IIoT. In *Demystifying Federated Learning for Blockchain and Industrial Internet of Things* (pp. 123–142). IGI Global. doi:10.4018/978-1-6684-3733-9.ch007

Whig, P., Velu, A., & Naddikatu, R. R. (2022). The Economic Impact of AI-Enabled Blockchain in 6G-Based Industry. In *AI and Blockchain Technology in 6G Wireless Network* (pp. 205–224). Springer. doi:10.1007/978-981-19-2868-0_10

Whig, P., Velu, A., & Nadikattu, R. R. (2022). Blockchain Platform to Resolve Security Issues in IoT and Smart Networks. In *AI-Enabled Agile Internet of Things for Sustainable FinTech Ecosystems* (pp. 46–65). IGI Global. doi:10.4018/978-1-6684-4176-3.ch003

Whig, P., Velu, A., & Ready, R. (2022). Demystifying Federated Learning in Artificial Intelligence With Human-Computer Interaction. In *Demystifying Federated Learning for Blockchain and Industrial Internet of Things* (pp. 94–122). IGI Global. doi:10.4018/978-1-6684-3733-9.ch006

World Health Organization. (2021). *Cohort study to measure COVID-19 vaccine effectiveness among health workers in the WHO European Region: Guidance document*. Author.

Wu, L., Xin, Y., Li, S., Wang, T., Heng, P. A., & Ni, D. (2017, April). Cascaded fully convolutional networks for automatic prenatal ultrasound image segmentation. In *2017 IEEE 14th international symposium on biomedical imaging (ISBI 2017)* (pp. 663-666). IEEE.

Xie, Y., Zhang, Z., Sapkota, M., & Yang, L. (2016, October). Spatial clockwork recurrent neural network for muscle perimysium segmentation. In *International Conference on Medical Image Computing and Computer-Assisted Intervention* (pp. 185-193). Springer.

Xing, F., & Yang, L. (2016). Robust nucleus/cell detection and segmentation in digital pathology and microscopy images: A comprehensive review. *IEEE Reviews in Biomedical Engineering*, *9*, 234–263. doi:10.1109/RBME.2016.2515127 PMID:26742143

Xingjian, S. H. I., Chen, Z., Wang, H., Yeung, D. Y., Wong, W. K., & Woo, W. C. (2015). Convolutional LSTM network: A machine learning approach for precipitation now casting. In Advances in neural information processing systems (pp. 802-810). Academic Press.

Xu, J., Meng, X., Liang, W., Zhou, H., & Li, K. C. (2020). A secure mutual authentication scheme of blockchain-based in WBANs. *China Communications*, *17*(9), 34–49. doi:10.23919/JCC.2020.09.004

Xu, J., Xiang, L., Liu, Q., Gilmore, H., Wu, J., Tang, J., & Madabhushi, A. (2016). Stacked sparse autoencoder (SSAE) for nuclei detection on breast cancer histopathology images. *IEEE Transactions on Medical Imaging*, *35*(1), 119–130. doi:10.1109/TMI.2015.2458702 PMID:26208307

Yadav, K., Alshudukhi, J. S., Dhiman, G., & Viriyasitavat, W. (2022). iTSA: An improved Tunicate Swarm Algorithm for defensive resource assignment problem. *Soft Computing*, *26*(10), 4929–4937.

Yadav, K., Jain, A., Osman Sid Ahmed, N. M., Saad Hamad, S. A., Dhiman, G., & Alotaibi, S. D. (2022). Internet of Thing based Koch Fractal Curve Fractal Antennas for Wireless Applications. *Journal of the Institution of Electronics and Telecommunication Engineers*, 1–10.

Yaeger, K., Martini, M., Rasouli, J., & Costa, A. (2019). Emerging Blockchain Technology Solutions for Modern Healthcare Infrastructure. *Journal of Scientific Innovation in Medicine*, *2*(1), 1. Advance online publication. doi:10.29024/jsim.7

Yang, J., Onik, M. M. H., Lee, N. Y., Ahmed, M., & Kim, C. S. (2019). Proof-of-Familiarity: A Privacy-Preserved Blockchain Scheme for Collaborative Medical Decision-Making. *Applied Sciences, 9*(7), 1370. doi:10.3390/app9071370

Yang, M. S., Hwang, P. Y., & Chen, D. H. (2004). Fuzzy clustering algorithms for mixed feature variables. *Fuzzy Sets and Systems*, *141*(2), 301–317. doi:10.1016/S0165-0114(03)00072-1

Yari, Y., Nguyen, T. V., & Nguyen, H. T. (2020). Deep Learning Applied for Histological Diagnosis of Breast Cancer. *IEEE Access: Practical Innovations, Open Solutions*, *8*, 162432–162448. doi:10.1109/ACCESS.2020.3021557

Yasmin, M., Sharif, M., & Mohsin, S. (2013). Survey paper on diagnosis of breast cancer using image processing techniques. *Research Journal of Recent Sciences*, *2*, 8898.

Yeom, S.-J. (2011). Augmented Reality for Learning Anatomy. Proceedings ASCILITE 2011 Hobart: Concise Paper, 1377-1384.

Yosinski, J., Clune, J., Bengio, Y., & Lipson, H. (2014). *How transferable are features in deep neural networks?* arXiv preprint arXiv:1411.1792.

Zadeh. (1971). Similarity relations and fuzzy orderings. *Information Sciences, 3*, 177–200.

Zadeh, L. A. (1965, June). Fuzzy sets. *Information and Control*, *8*(3), 338–353. doi:10.1016/S0019-9958(65)90241-X

Zeadally, S., & Bello, O. (2021). Harnessing the power of Internet of Things based connectivity to improve healthcare. *Internet of Things*, *14*, 100074.

Zeidabadi, F. A., Dehghani, M., Trojovský, P., Hubálovský, Š., Leiva, V., & Dhiman, G. (2022). Archery algorithm: A novel stochastic optimization algorithm for solving optimization problems. *Computers, Materials and Continua*, *72*(1), 399–416.

Zeidabadi, F. A., Doumari, S. A., Dehghani, M., Montazeri, Z., Trojovsky, P., & Dhiman, G. (2022a). MLA: A new mutated leader algorithm for solving optimization problems. *Computers. Materials & Continua*, *70*(3), 5631–5649.

Zeidabadi, F. A., Doumari, S. A., Dehghani, M., Montazeri, Z., Trojovsky, P., & Dhiman, G. (2022b). AMBO: All members-based optimizer for solving optimization problems. *CMC-Comput. Mater. Contin*, *70*, 2905–2921.

Zeiler, M. D., & Fergus, R. (2014, September). Visualizing and understanding convolutional networks. In *European conference on computer vision* (pp. 818-833). Springer.

Zeng, G., & Zheng, G. (2018, April). Multi-stream 3D FCN with multi-scale deep supervision for multi-modality isointense infant brain MR image segmentation. In *2018 IEEE 15th International Symposium on Biomedical Imaging (ISBI 2018)* (pp. 136-140). IEEE.

Zeng, G., He, Y., Yu, Z., Yang, X., Yang, R., & Zhang, L. (2015). Going deeper with convolutions Christian. *Proc. IEEE Conf. Comput. Vis. Pattern Recognit. (CVPR)*, 1-9.

Zeng, G., Yang, X., Li, J., Yu, L., Heng, P. A., & Zheng, G. (2017, September). 3D U-net with multi-level deep supervision: fully automatic segmentation of proximal femur in 3D MR images. In *International workshop on machine learning in medical imaging* (pp. 274-282). Springer.

Zeng, G., & Zheng, G. (2018). Deep learning-based automatic segmentation of the proximal femur from MR images. In *Intelligent Orthopaedics* (pp. 73–79). Springer.

Zhang, P., White, J., Schmidt, D. C., & Lenz, G. (2017). *Applying Software Patterns to Address Interoperability in Blockchain-based Healthcare Apps*. https://arxiv.org/abs/1706.03700v1

Zhang, P., Schmidt, D. C., White, J., & Lenz, G. (2018). Blockchain Technology Use Cases in Healthcare. *Advances in Computers*, *111*, 1–41. doi:10.1016/bs.adcom.2018.03.006

Zhao, H., Shi, J., Qi, X., Wang, X., & Jia, J. (2017). Pyramid scene parsing network. *Proc. IEEE Conf. Comput. Vis. Pattern Recognit.*, 2881-2890.

Zheng, S., Jayasumana, S., Romera-Paredes, B., Vineet, V., Su, Z., Du, D., ... Torr, P. H. (2015). Conditional random fields as recurrent neural networks. In *Proceedings of the IEEE international conference on computer vision* (pp. 1529-1537). IEEE.

Zhou, J., Wang, Y., Ota, K., & Dong, M. (2019). AAIoT: Accelerating artificial intelligence in IoT systems. *IEEE Wireless Communications Letters*, *8*(3), 825–828. doi:10.1109/LWC.2019.2894703

Zhou, X., Takayama, R., Wang, S., Hara, T., & Fujita, H. (2017). Deep learning of the sectional appearances of 3D CT images for anatomical structure segmentation based on an FCN voting method. *Medical Physics*, *44*(10), 5221–5233.

About the Contributors

Sandeep Kautish is working as Professor & Dean-Academics with LBEF Campus, Kathmandu Nepal running in academic collaboration with Asia Pacific University of Technology & Innovation Malaysia. I am seasoned academician and accomplished professor with over 16 Years of work experience including over 05 years in academic administration in various institutions of India and abroad. I earned my bachelors, masters in Computer Science and a doctorate degree in Computer Science in the area of Intelligent Systems in Social Networks.

Gaurav Dhiman is an Assistant Professor within the Department of Computer Science, Government Bikram College of Commerce, Patiala. The editor's current research interests include bio-inspired and evolutionary-based metaheuristic techniques for solving single-, multi-, and many-objective large-scale complex problems.

* * *

Mayank Anand completed Masters in Computer Applications from Guru Gobind Singh Indraprastha University, Delhi in 2020. Before completing his Post Graduation, he started working on NLP based research on AI Virtual Assistants. He has worked with V-Force (UNV India) in raising awareness towards society for International Youth Day 2021. He has also been certified in Data Science from Edwisor where he went through rigorous training in the year 2020-21. He is currently working as a Data Engineer at BridgeLabz Solutions where he builds pipelines for data-centric processes and mentors Engineering Freshers to get into companies in his field. His research has been published over 5 international journals and his research areas are Machine Learning, Natural Language Processing and Artificial Intelligence.

Pradeep Bedi received the B.Tech. degree in computer science and engineering from Uttar Pradesh Technical University (UPTU), Lucknow, India, in 2005 and M.Tech. in computer science and engineering from Guru Gobind Singh Indraprastha University (GGSIPU), Delhi, India, in 2009. He is GATE, UGC-NET qualified and currently pursuing Ph.D from Indira Gandhi National Tribal University, Amarkantak (Regional Campus Manipur). He started his academic career from Mahatma Gandhi Mission's College of Engineering and Technology in 2005 and served various reputed colleges and universities in India and abroad. Currently, he holds the position of assistant professor in the department of computer science and engineering, Galgotias University, Greater Noida, Uttar Pradesh, India. He has authored or co-authored over 40 technical papers published in national and international journals and conferences and also published 15 patents in India and abroad. He is a member of reputed professional bodies such as CSI, ACM etc. His research interests include applications of artificial intelligence, machine learning, deep learning and IoT in healthcare, automation, etc.

Robin Chouhan is a final year student in Shri Vaishnav Vidyapeeth.

S. B. Goyal completed PhD in the Computer Science & Engineering in 2012 from India and served many institutions in many different academic and administrative positions. He is holding 19+ years experience at national and international level. He has peerless inquisitiveness and enthusiasm to get abreast with the latest development in the IT field. He has good command over Industry Revolution (IR) 4.0 technologies like Big-Data, Data Science, Artificial Intelligence & Blockchain, computer networking, deep learning etc. He is the first one to introduce IR 4.0 including Blockchain technology in the academic curriculum in Malaysian Universities. He had participated in many panel discussions on IR 4.0 technologies at academia as well as industry platforms. He is holding 19+ years' experience in academia at National & International level. He is serving as a reviewer or guest editors in many Journals published by Inderscience, IGI Global, Springer. He is contributing as a Co-Editor in many Scopus books. He had contributed in many Scopus/ SCI Journal/ conferences. Currently, Dr Goyal is associated as a Director, Faculty of Information Technology, City University, Malaysia.

Ketan Gupta is PMP certified with 10 years of experience as a professional in Information technology, Supply Chain, and Healthcare domains. Ketan is currently pursuing a Ph.D. in Information Technology at the University of the Cumberlands focusing on Artificial Intelligence and Machine Learning tools. As a research graduate student, he has various research papers published in renowned journals. Currently, Ketan is working as a Program Manager for the company Meta (formerly Facebook) where he is accountable to enrich CBOM management, ERP system architecture implementation, pricing models, risk opportunities, cost-benefit analysis, supplier plan of record, data analysis using data visualization for AR, VR, and Portal Products.

G. Jayanthi was awarded a doctorate in Computer science and Engineering in the year 2021. She is the recipient of Pondicherry University gold medal in the year 2017 at Pondicherry University, India. She was awarded silver medal for proficiency in the subject Satellite Image Processing for the degree M.Tech Remote Sensing during the Alumni Meet at Anna University, India in the year 2017. She has professional teaching experience of 12 years in computer science and Engineering. Her research interests include Data Science, Geoinformatics, Artificial Intelligence, Machine Learning, Deep Reinforcement Learning etc. She is member of IEEE and published science citation indexed research articles in journals like IET Intelligent Transport Systems, IETE Journal of Research, Internal Journal of Intelligent Information Technologies, and IEEE Xplore. She has been the reviewer in many international conferences held in the year 2021 and 2022. She has authored many book chapters in the domain of Machine learning, Deep learning, and Reinforcement Learning and published in CRC Press, Springer, and IGI Global.

Nasmin Jiwani is a graduate PHD student at University of the Cumberlands currently in her second year. Her area of research is Into Machine learning and Artificial intelligence in healthcare sector. She has various conference paper published in renowned journals and conferences. Nasmin professionally has been working as a project manager at an IT based firm where she manages and drives various technology-based projects. she is PMP, Product Owner and Scrum master certified along with 11 years of IT based project related experience.

Jugnesh Kumar is working as a Director in St. Andrews Institute of Technology and Management, Gurugram, Haryana affiliated to the Maharshi Dayanand University, Rohtak, Haryana. He is an IT specialist in the area of machine learning, big-data. Dr Kumar is received academic cum professional degrees MCA, M.Tech. and PhD (CSE). He is holding 20+ year administrative experience in addition to academic expertise in the area of Database System, Mobile Computing, Software Engineering, Computer Architecture, Java programming, Computer Networking, Deep Learning etc. He had organized many conferences/ events at Indian level. He had published many research papers/ book chapters in the Scopus Journals/ International Conferences/ Edited books. He had got the grant of International Patent for eight years from Australia in data analytics.

Supriya M. S. has a B E. in telecommunications and M Tech. in real-time embedded systems. She's currently pursuing her PhD on employing machine learning techniques for classifying cardiac arrhythmia. She is currently employed as an Assistant Professor in Computer Science and Engineering department at Ramaiah University of Applied Sciences, where she has worked for the past six years. She has two Indian patents filed in the field of Multi-Sensor Data Fusion bearing patent number 201641044563 and Artificial Intelligence bearing patent number 202241004577 and she has published papers in several national and international journals and conferences. She is also the author of various book chapters. Software Engineering, Real-Time Embedded Systems, Multi-Sensor Data Fusion, Healthcare, Machine Learning, and Artificial Intelligence are some of her research interests.

Nikil Kumar P. has earned his Bachelor of Engineering in Information Science. He was a software engineer for Healthfore Technologies and is now a team leader for Torry Harries Business Solutions. He holds an ISTQB certification as a software tester. His areas of interest in research include software engineering, the Internet of Things, Healthcare, Machine Learning, Robotic Process Automation.

Piyush Pant is a scholar at Sandip University currently pursuing a Bachelor of Science in Computer Science specialization in Artificial Intelligence, Machine learning, and Virtual Reality (BSc CS AIML & VR). His Areas of interest are Artificial Intelligence, machine learning, deep learning, and Data science, which he studied the concepts and practically applied to his research works which were - AI and IIoT in Industry 5.0, Blockchain and AI, Environment Conservation using AI, Space and Planet Exploration using AI, providing Security using Machine learning, AGI and its future etc. Along with having good knowledge and working experience in the field of Artificial Intelligence, he is also a full stack web developer proficient in MERN stack. He used his knowledge to help and contribute to NGOs (Non-Governmental organizations) where he was nominated as one of the Co-founders of a start-up that was focused on developing and empowering women and children. He is a "Rashtrapati Puruskar" and "Rajya Puruskar" holder in Bharat Scouts and guides, the highest honor given to a scout. He was also chosen as the School Captain of Kendriya Vidyalaya in his Intermediate for the session 2018-2020. Along with academic excellence, he also participated in Cricket and Boxing and represented his school in the regional level. He participated in various extra-curricular activities like Debate, story-telling, elocution, essay writing, painting, etc. and represented his school in the regional level. He is focused and aims to pursue a master's and Ph.D. in the field of machine learning and deep learning to help society in progressive ways and do research.

Anand Singh Rajawat is an Associate Professor in Computer science and Engineering department, the School of Computer Science and Engineering, Sandip University Nashik, India. He has published 90+ research publications in various reputed peer-reviewed international journals, book chapters, and conferences. His area of interest are mainly in developing health care data security, privacy and Industry 4.0/5.0 processing algorithms for the multidisciplinary field of computer science. Patient data (image, video, text) has become the most potent tool in bio informatics.

Kalpana Ramanujam is currently working as Professor in Dept. of CSE at Puducherry Technological University. She completed Bachelor of Technology in Computer Science from Pondicherry Engineering College, during 1992-96. She completed Master of Technology in Computer Science from Pondicherry University in 1998. She obtained her Ph.D from Pondicherry University. Her area of interest includes Parallel and Distributed Systems Algorithm design and Optimization.

Anu Singha received his Master's Degrees in Computer Applications (MCA) from South Asian University, New Delhi, and in Computer Science & Engineering (M.Tech CSE) from Tripura University (A Central University), India in 2013 and 2015, respectively. In 2021, he received his PhD in CSE from Tripura University (A Central University), India. Currently, he is working as an Assistant Professor in Faculty of Engineering and Technology, Sri Ramachandra Institute of Higher Education and Research, Chennai. He has an experience of three years as Research Fellow in a Defense Research and Development Organization (DRDO) funded project. His research interests include computer vision, image processing, deep learning, and medical imaging.

Sowmiya is a PhD scholar in Dept. of CSE at Puducherry Technological University. She completed Bachelor of Technology in Information Technology from Adhiparasakthi Engineering College, during 2008-12. She completed Master of Technology in Information Technology from Pondicherry Engineering College in 2017. Her area of research is Artificial intelligence in healthcare sector.

Pawan Whig did B.Tech in Electronics and Communication Engineering in 2005. After successfully completing his graduation he completed M.Tech in VLSI in 2008. His educational Journey is not stop here, he was awarded "Doctorate" from Jamia Millia Islamia. He has been working in the field of Electronics and Communication for the last 21 years. He is an editor and reviewer of several internationally refereed journals. He is designing and mentoring several projects in universities across India. He is member of international association of engineers Hong Kong, ISTE, IEEE, SCI, IEI and state student coordinator of Rajasthan of Computer Society of India(CSI).

He published technical articles in more than 80 national and international journals. He has a wide area of research like Analog Signal Processing, Sensor Modeling, Water Quality Monitoring Applications and Simulation & design. He has invented a Low Power Water Quality Monitoring Device which is under Patent Process. He has proposed a SPICE Model for Novel Photo catalytic Sensor (PCS) which can be the area of interest for new researchers in the same field.

Index

H

I

M

N

O

P

R

S

T

U

V

W

Printed in the United States
by Baker & Taylor Publisher Services